ALLERGY AND ALLERGEN IMMUNOTHERAPY

New Mechanisms and Strategies

ALLERGY AND ALLERGEN IMMUNOTHERAPY

New Mechanisms and Strategies

Edited by

A. B. Singh

Former Scientist Emeritus
CSIR Institute of Genomics and Integrative Biology
Delhi University Campus
Delhi–110007, India

AAP APPLE ACADEMIC PRESS

Apple Academic Press Inc.
3333 Mistwell Crescent
Oakville, ON L6L 0A2 Canada

Apple Academic Press Inc.
9 Spinnaker Way
Waretown, NJ 08758 USA

Exclusive worldwide distribution by CRC Press, a member of Taylor & Francis Group
No claim to original U.S. Government works
Printed in the United States of America on acid-free paper
International Standard Book Number-13: 978-1-77188-542-3 (Hardcover)
International Standard Book Number-13: 978-1-315-20752-0 (CRC Press/Taylor & Francis eBook)
International Standard Book Number-13: 978-1-77188-543-0 (AAP eBook)

Library and Archives Canada Cataloguing in Publication

Allergy and allergen immunotherapy : new mechanisms and strategies / edited by A.B. Singh, Former Scientist Emeritus, CSIR Institute of Genomics and Integrative Biology Delhi University Campus, Delhi–110007, India.

Includes bibliographical references and index.
Issued in print and electronic formats.
ISBN 978-1-77188-542-3 (hardcover).--ISBN 978-1-315-20752-0 (PDF)
1. Allergy--Immunotherapy. 2. Allergens--Therapeutic use. I. Singh, A. B., author, editor

RC588.I45A45 2016 616.97'071 C2016-907482-X C2016-907483-8

Library of Congress Cataloging-in-Publication Data

Names: Singh, A. B., editor.
Title: Allergy and allergen immunotherapy : new mechanisms and strategies / editor, A.B. Singh.
Description: Toronto ; New Jersey : Apple Academic Press, 2017. | Includes bibliographical references and index.
Identifiers: LCCN 2016051241 (print) | LCCN 2016051497 (ebook) | ISBN 9781771885423 (hardcover : alk. paper) | ISBN 9781771885430 (eBook) | ISBN 9781315207520 ()
Subjects: | MESH: Allergens--immunology | Hypersensitivity--immunology | Hypersensitivity--therapy | Immunotherapy--methods Classification: LCC RC582.17 (print) | LCC RC582.17 (ebook) | NLM QW 900 | DDC 616.97/071--dc23
LC record available at https://lccn.loc.gov/2016051241

Apple Academic Press also publishes its books in a variety of electronic formats. Some content that appears in print may not be available in electronic format. For information about Apple Academic Press products, visit our website at **www.appleacademicpress.com** and the CRC Press website at **www.crcpress.com**

ABOUT THE EDITOR

Dr. A. B. Singh has more than 40 years of research experience in pollen and fungal allergy and was the coordinator of multi-centered project on "Aeroallergen and Human Health," sponsored by the Ministry of Environment and Forest, New Delhi, India. He has completed many projects from United States Environmental Protection Agency (EPA), the Indian Council of Medical Research, and the Ministry of Environment and Forest of India, surveying pollen and fungal allergens and identifying the important allergens that trigger allergic symptoms, such as asthma, rhinitis, and dermatitis etc. He worked at the Nebraska University (USA) as the Borlaug Fellow on genetically modified food safety assessments and has been involved in a EPA-funded project on Legume Food Allergies in India. He has also compiled a National Pollen Calendar of India for allergy diagnosis and treatment. He was formerly Vice President of the Asia Pacific Association of Allergy, Asthma and Clinical Immunology (2010–2013) and served on several committees of World Allergy Organization (WAO). Other roles included Secretary General of South Asia Association of Allergy, Asthma, and Clinical Immunology (SAAACI), Secretary of the Indian College of Asthma and Applied Immunology (ICAAI), and Member Executive Council of the Indian Aerobiological Society (IAS). He has reviewed many projects from different funding organizations and is a regular reviewer of several international journals of allergy and immunology.

He has been the founding Editor-in-Chief of the *Indian Journal of Aerobiology* since its inception in 1982 and is also Associate Editor of the *Indian Journal of Allergy and Immunology*. He has delivered more than 250 guest lectures and invited talks at international and national conferences on allergy, asthma, and aerobiology in different countries and in India. He has extensively traveled abroad to USA, Canada, Europe, Australia, and South East Asia, etc., as a visiting faculty and guest speaker. The awards and honors he has received include the Charles Richet Prize for Fundamental Work in Allergy and Scientist of the Year by the National Environmental Science Academy (India). In addition, Dr. Singh has received a life-time achievement award from International Asthma Services (USA). He has delivered many oration lectures at various scientific forums, supervised more than 20 PhD and MPhil students, and has published more than 200 research papers in international and national journals of repute and chapters in different books.

CONTENTS

LIST OF CONTRIBUTORS

S. Narmada Ashok
Consultant Pediatrician and Director, Nalam Medical Centre and Hospital, Tamilnadu, India

Mohammad-Ali Assarehzadegan
Immunology Department, School of Medicine, Iran University of Medical Sciences (IUMS), Tehran, Iran, Tel: +98-(21) 86703285, Fax: +98-21-44357329, E-mail: assarehma@gmail.com, assareh.ma@iums.ac.ir

Jeff Bennert
Air Oasis, Research and Development, Amarillo, Texas 79118, USA, E-mail: drj@airoasis.com

Jon Bennert
Air Oasis, Research and Development, Amarillo, Texas 79118, USA, E-mail: jon@airoasis.com

Danius Bouyi
Life, Earth and Environmental Sciences, West Texas A&M University, Canyon, Texas 79015, USA, E-mail: emersonbouyi@hotmail.com

Gennaro D'Amato
Division of Respiratory and Allergic Diseases, Department of Chest Diseases, High Speciality A. Cardarelli Hospital, Napoli Italy; University "Federico II," Medical School, Naples, Italy, E-mail: gdamatomail@gmail.com

Maria D'Amato
First Division of Pneumology, High Speciality Hospital "V. Monaldi" and University "Federico II" Medical School Naples, Italy

A. Dahl
Department of Biological Environmental Science, University of Gothenburg, Gothenburg, Sweden

Griselda Estrada
Life, Earth and Environmental Sciences, West Texas A&M University, Canyon, Texas 79015, USA, E-mail: gestrada1@buffs.wtamu.edu

G. Frenguelli
Department of Agriculture, Food and Environmental Sciences, University of Perugia, Italy

C. Galán
Department of Botany, Ecology and Plant Physiology, University of Córdoba, Spain

R. Gehrig
Federal Office of Meteorology and Climatology MeteoSwiss, Zurich, Switzerland

Nabarun Ghosh
Life, Earth and Environmental Sciences, West Texas A&M University, Canyon, Texas 79015, USA, E-mail: nghosh@wtamu.edu

R. E. Goodman
Food Allergy Research and Resource Program, Dept. of Food Science and Technology, University of Nebraska-Lincoln, 1901 North 21st Street, P.O. Box 886207, Lincoln, NE, 68588-6207, USA

G. Hassan
Postgraduate, Department of Medicine, Government Medical College, University of Kashmir, Srinagar, Jammu and Kashmir – 190010, India, Mobile: +91-9419007335

Amrutha D. Holla
Director, Allergy Asthma Associates, Mysore, India

M. Ismail
Postgraduate, Department of Medicine, Government Medical College, University of Kashmir, Srinagar, Jammu and Kashmir – 190010, India, Mobile: +91-9419007335

Paranjothy Kanni
Allergy Center, Bengaluru, India

Nagendra Prasad Komarla
Allergy Center, Bengaluru, India

P. A. Mahesh
Professor, Department of Pulmonary Medicine, JSS Medical College, JSS University, Mysore, India

T. Masood
Postgraduate, Department of Medicine, Government Medical College, University of Kashmir, Srinagar, Jammu and Kashmir – 190010, India, Mobile: +91-9419007335; E-mail: lungkashmir@rediffmail.com

Chandni Mathur
CSIR-Institute of Genomics and Integrative Biology, Delhi University Campus, Delhi – 110007, India

Antonio Molino
First Division of Pneumology, High Speciality Hospital "V. Monaldi" and University "Federico II" Medical School Naples, Italy

P. A. Mridula
Research Associate, Allergy Asthma Associates, Mysore, India

Major K. Nagaraju
Consultant Allergist, Apollo Children's Hospital, Director, VN, Paediatric Allergist Saveetha Medical College and Hospital, Allergy and Asthma Research Centre, Chennai, India

Jae-Won Oh
Department of Pediatrics, Division of Allergy and Despiratory Diseases, Hanyang University College of Medicine, Seoul, Korea

H. Paramesh
Pediatric Pulmonologist and Environmentalist and Chairman, Sirona Center for Health Promotion, Bangalore, India

Chandini Revanna
Department of Environmental Health and Safety, Texas Tech University, Lubbock, TX 79409, E-mail: c.revanna@ttu.edu

Constantine Saadeh
Allergy A.R.T.S., Amarillo, Texas 79124, USA, E-mail: csaadeh@allergyarts.com

Rajiv R. Sahay
Environmental Diagnostics Laboratory at Pure Air Control Services, Inc.4911-C Creekside Drive Clearwater, FL, 33760, USA

S. Saheer
Specialist Pulmonologist, International Modern Hospital, Bur Dubai, Dubai

Alessandro Sanduzzi
University "Federico II," Medical School, Naples, Italy; Second Division of Pneumology, High Speciality Hospital "V. Monaldi" and University "Federico II" Medical School Naples, Italy, E-mail: gdamatomail@gmail.com

Shifa Wiqar Shaikh
Allergy and Asthma Clinic, Shakti Sadan Co-op Housing Society Ground Floor, B-Block, Opp. Navjeevan Society Lamington Road, Mumbai–400007, India

Wiqar Shaikh
Professor of Medicine, Grant Medical College and Sir J.J. Group of Hospitals, Mumbai, India, E-mail: drwiqar@gmail.com

A. B. Singh
CSIR-Institute of Genomics and Integrative Biology, Delhi University Campus, Delhi – 110007, India; Allergy Center, Bengaluru, India

Alessandro Vatrella
Department of Medicine and Surgery, University of Salerno, Via Giovanni Paolo II, 132, 84084 Fisciano SA, Italy

P. K. Vedanthan
University of Colorado, Denver, Colorado, USA; Christian Medical College, Vellore, Tamilnadu, India

Mitsy Veloz
Life, Earth and Environmental Sciences, West Texas A&M University, Canyon, Texas 79015, USA, E-mail: velozfam6401@yahoo.com

Carolina Vitale
First Division of Pneumology, High Speciality Hospital "V. Monaldi" and University "Federico II" Medical School Naples, Italy

Agam Vora
Assistant Hon. & In Charge - Department of Chest & TB, Dr. R. N. Cooper Muni. Gen. Hospital, Mumbai.

Anura Weerasinghe
Fellowship of the Ceylon College of Physicians, Member of the Indian Association for Allergy Asthma and Applied Immunology, Professor of Medicine and Immunology Dr. Neville Fernando Teaching Hospital of South Asian Institute of Technology and Medicine, Sri Lanka, Professor on Assignment, Rajarata University of Sri Lanka, Sri Lanka

Alan L. Wozniak
Environmental Diagnostics Laboratory at Pure Air Control Services, Inc. 4911-C Creekside Drive Clearwater, FL, 33760, USA

LIST OF ABBREVIATIONS

AAAAI	American Academy of Allergy Asthma and Immunology
ABCD	asthma, rhinitis and air-borne contact dermatitis
AHR	airway hyper reactivity
AHU	air handler unit
AICP	All India Coordinated Project
AIT	allergen immunotherapy
APCs	antigen presenting cells
API	Annual Pollen Index
AR	allergic rhinitis
ARIA	allergic rhinitis and its impact on asthma
AU	allergy units
BAU	bioequivalent allergy unit
BBG	Beijing Botanical Garden
BCA	bicinchoninic acid
BHR	basophil activation or basophil histamine release
BRI	building related illness
BRS	building related symptoms
Bt	*Bacillus thuringiensis*
BU	biological units
CAAMP	Computer Assisted Air Management Program
CAgM	Commission for AgroMeteorology
CCD	cross-reactive carbohydrate binding
CCD	cross-reactive carbohydrate determinants
CD	celiac disease
CDC	Centers for Disease Control
CFU	colony-forming unit
COPD	chronic obstructive pulmonary disease
CP	coat protein
CPM	critical path management
DBAS	dysfunctional beliefs and attitudes about sleep
DBPCFC	double blind placebo controlled food challenge

DCs	dendritic cells
DDS	dirty duct syndromes
DECC	diethylcarbamazine citrate
DFH	dematiaceous fungal hyphal elements
DFS	dematiaceous fungal spore elements
DMDs	disease modifying drugs
DSS	dirty sock syndrome
DT	drum trap
EAACI	European Academy of Allergy and Clinical Immunology
EACA	epsilon-amino caproic acid
EAN	European Aeroallergen Network
EAS	European Aerobiology Society
EEA	European Environment Agency
EMA	European Medical Agency
EPIT	epicutaneous route
EPR	early phase reaction
ESD	electrostatic sampling device
ET	electrostatic trap
FACE	free air CO_2 experiments
FAO	Food and Agricultural Organization
FT	filter trap
Gal	galanin
GDD	growing degree day
GDH	growing degree hour
GE	genetically engineered
GFD	gluten-free diet
GINA	global initiative for asthma
GM	genetically modified
GP	gravity or settle plates
GPM	Global Phenological Programme
HAVC	heating, ventilation and air conditioning system
HD MITE	house dust MITE
HIST	histamine
HRT	histamine release test
HVAC	heating ventilation and air conditioning systems
IAQ	indoor air quality

ICMR	Indian Council of Medical Research
ICS	inhaled corticosteroids
IgE	immunoglobulin-E
IHR	in-house reference
IHRP	in-house reference preparation
IL	interleukin
IP	impinger trap
IPG	International Phenological Gardens
ISAAC	International Study of Asthma and Allergies in Childhood
ISAC	immuno-solid-phase allergen chip
ISU	ISAC Standard Units
JSAP	job specific action plan
LABA	long-acting β2-agonists
LBIT	local bronchial immunotherapy
LC	locus coeruleus
LDT	laterodorsal tegmental
LNIT	local nasal immunotherapy
LPR	late phase reaction
LSI	laser induced fluorescence
MAC	mold associated conditions
MCS	multiple chemical sensitivity
MED	middle eastern dust
MLI	mold linked illness
MRSA	methicillin-resistant *Staphylococcus aureus*
MVOC	microbiological volatile compounds
NA	noradrenaline
NO_x	nitrous oxides
NSAID's	non-steroidal anti-inflammatory drugs
ODTS	organic dust toxic syndrome
OIT	oral immunotherapy
PACS	pure air control services
PAH	polynuclear aromatic hydrocarbons
PAMP's	pathogen associated molecular patterns
PAT	preventive allergy treatment
PBT	persistent, bio-accumulative, and toxic
PCB	Polychlorinated biphenyls

PEF	peak expiratory flow
PEG	polyethylene glycol
PNIFR	peak nasal inspiratory flow rate
PNU	protein nitrogen units
PPT	pedunculopontine tegmental nuclei
PRR	pattern recognition receptors
PRSV	pathogenic ringspot virus
PT	pore trap
RAST	radioimmunosorbent test
RCEES	Research Center for Eco-Environmental Sciences
RIA	radioimmunoassay
RT	rotorod trap
SBS	sick building syndrome
SCF	skin cell fragments
SCFA	short chain fatty acids
SCIT	subcutaneous immunotherapy
SIT	specific immunotherapy
SLIT	sublingual immunotherapy
SO_x	sulfur oxides
SPT	skin prick test
ST	spore trap
TCR	T-cell receptor
TGF-α	transforming growth factor
TJ	tight junction
TLR	toll-like receptors
TMN	tuberomammillary nucleus
TP	thermal trap
VIT	venom immunotherapy
VLPO	ventrolateral preoptic nucleus
VOC	volatile organic compounds
WHO	World Health Organization
WMO	World Meteorological Organization

ACKNOWLEDGMENTS

This book, *Allergy and Allergen Immunotherapy: New Mechanisms and Strategies*, is the product of more than two years of work, and we could not have completed it without the support and contributions of our many talented international experts from the field of allergy, aerobiology and immunology. I wish to extend my greatest appreciation to Prof. Carmen Galan and Prof. D'Amato, who have been the greatest source of inspiration and guidance to me and have always stood to make suggestions at various stages of the book. I extend my sincere thanks to all the contributors of the different chapters in the book without whose cooperation and help it would not have been possible to complete this task.

Most importantly, I am very grateful for the crucial guidance, mentorship, and inspiration given to me by my teachers, late Prof. D. N. Shivpuri, and Prof. C. R. Babu. Prof. Richard Goodman, Prof. N. Ghosh, and Dr. P. K. Vedanthan have been very cooperative and have always encouraged and inquired at every stage of this book. Many of my colleagues and mentors, such as Dr. S. V. Gangal, Prof. S. K. Brahmchari, Dr. Rajesh Gokhale, and Prof. S. N. Gaur cooperated in the formation of this book and have inspired me to make it physician/allergologist/aerobiologist friendly. Dr. Rajesh Gokhale, a man of exceptional vision, provided me with the necessary administrative support and guidance for the benefit of allergy patients and physicians. Prof. Connie Katelaris from Australia, who has not been only my well-wisher but also the mentor for clinical aerobiology, deserves special thanks.

I acknowledge with a deep sense of reverence and affection my wife Pushpa Singh, who stood with me during my deep involvement during this period and long absence from household responsibilities. It will be unfair on my part if I do not acknowledge the assistance and computational help provided my sons and their spouses.

Finally, I thank Sandy Jones Sickels and Ashish Kumar, Publisher, as well as Rakesh Kumar of Apple Academic Press for their professionalism and quality concerns in shaping the book.

—A. B. Singh

FOREWORD

Although pollen grains constitute only a small part of the viable particulates in the atmosphere, they can be causative agents of allergic responses in susceptible humans. A characteristic feature of pollen sensitivity is its seasonal pattern of occurrence at the time when pollen is most frequent in the atmosphere. The vast numbers of species involved together with the differences in climate and vegetation make studies of allergenic pollen and pollinosis of great complexity.

During the last years, aeropalynological studies in several parts of the world developed rapidly. Knowledge about the various pollen seasons in the different countries is necessary in order to understand the appearance of symptoms in the allergic population. Moreover, as a result of greater mobility people who travel for work or leisure need to have reliable information about the likelihood of seasonal allergy when they visit another country. For this reason, knowledge of the atmospheric pollen concentration encountered in different regions of the World is of great interest to clinicians and allergic patients, in order to achieve better management of their hay fever symptoms.

In this book, prevention, diagnosis and management of allergic disorders are treated in the light of the more recent literature.

The development and phenotypic expression of atopic diseases depends on a complex interaction between genetic factors, environmental exposure to allergens,and non-specific adjuvant factors, such as tobacco smoke, air pollution and infections. Preventive measures may include both exposure to allergens and adjuvant risk/protective factors and pharmacological treatment. These measures may address the general population, children at risk for development of atopic disease, children with early symptoms of allergic disease or children with chronic disease. Furthermore, potential risks of food allergy from genetically engineered crops are also discussed.

In regard to therapy, the Authors review exhaustively the clinical efficacy and safety of allergen immunotherapy and of Anti IgE Therapy in patients with allergic asthma and rhinitis.

In this very interesting book Prof Singh has brought together authorities from several different countries and together they have produced a detailed account of the regional differences in allergenic pollen, providing a wealth of information for allergists, aerobiologists, botanists and others interested in this fascinating branch of medical science.

— **Prof. Gennaro D'Amato, MD, FAAAAI.**
University Professor of Respiratory Medicine, Naples, Italy;
Chairman Committee World Allergy Organization on "Climate change, biodiversity and Allergy";
Director, Division of Respiratory and Allergic Diseases Department of Chest Diseases High Speciality A. Cardarelli Hospital, Napoli Italy

PREFACE

Humans are known to suffer from various allergic disorders such as allergic rhinitis, allergic asthma, atopic dermatitis, urticaria, etc., since times immemorial. Allergic diseases affect 20–30% of the global population and are considered epidemic of 21st century. The latter part of 20th century has seen an increase in prevalence of allergy and asthma implicating changing environment and lifestyle as significant causes. Pollen grains, fungal spores, dust mites, insect debris and epithelia, etc., are known to trigger allergic symptoms beside other factors. Among these agents pollen are the most predominant allergens in different geographical regions, including tropics. For efficient and effective diagnosis and therapeutic management of these ailments, a detailed knowledge of their prevalence and season is a prerequisite.

In this book, *Allergy and Allergen Immunotherapy: New Mechanisms and Strategies*, an effort has been made to provide information on allergy, asthma and Immunology not only from tropical countries such as India, Sri Lanka, Iran, South Korea, but also from temperate regions of the globe. The chapters have been contributed by experts from these countries in areas of allergy, and immunology, including genetically modified plant allergens. The concept of this book originated about two years back but took shape in 2016 with authors who are internationally recognized experts in their fields; the have contributed their chapters to make the book globally interesting.

There is a total of 43 authors contributing 19 chapters on different aspects of allergy and allergen immunotherapy from different continents. The book deals not only on the basics of allergy and allergen immunotherapy but also on indoor environments and safety considerations of genetically modified food allergens. The book is first of its kind from the Indian subcontinent to cater to the needs of clinicians, aerobiologists, environmentalists, and regulatory agencies.

I am glad that all the authors have been extremely cooperative in submitting their respective chapters as per our guidelines provided by the publisher. I am highly grateful to Prof. D'Amato and Prof. Carmen Galan for their constant encouragement and support during the course of finalizing the book. Thus the book will be of immense interest for clinicians and patients of allergy as diagnostic and therapeutic management of allergy in tropics.

I also profusely thank the publisher, Apple Academic Press (AAP), and the authors who contributed, helped, and cooperated to bring out this book after two years of long efforts.

—*A. B. Singh*

INTRODUCTION

There are bodies of evidence that suggest that allergic diseases are increasing world over including developing countries. The latter part of 20th century has seen an abnormal, increase in prevalence of allergic diseases covering as high as 30% of population world over. However, development of civilization often at the expense of the natural environment by pollution or biopollution stimulates the appearance of new health problems beside increase in allergic diseases. The most common allergic diseases are allergic rhinitis, allergic asthma, atopic dermatitis, urticaria, etc. Since air borne induced respiratory allergy cannot be limited to National boundaries, exposure to allergens is key factor among environmental determinants of allergic rhinitis and asthma.

There has been an increasing interest in allergens and their impact on allergy in recent decades. Among all bioparticulates, pollen grains and fungal spores are most predominant allergens in air. However, for effective diagnosis and therapeutic management of allergies, a detailed information on seasonal and annual variations in concentration of allergens from different countries is of paramount importance. Today there are emerging studies on pollen aeroallergens as phenological indicator of both flowering time and intensity in airborne pollen producing species. These studies also provide evidence of increasing temperature on pollen season advancement in spring. As pollen allergens represent one of the main causes of allergic diseases it has a high social and economic relevance at different levels.

On one hand the information on aeroallergens is an important tool not only for environmental management but also for therapeutic management of allergies. Tropical countries, including India with teaming population of more than 1.2 billion and with divergent geographical backdrop ranging from Deccan Plateau in south, flat to rolling plain along the Ganges river, Thar desert in the west, Himalayas in North has very rich pollen diversity and hence variable pollen season and symptomatology in Indian subcontinent. Like variation in pollen concentration and season, pollen causing allergy are also quite variable in different geographical regions which makes it very important to identify pollinosis-causing species in tropics and temperate regions of the world.

There are broadly four ways by which symptoms of allergy patients are relieved:

1. Environmental management
2. Pharmacological Management
3. Immunomodulation or Allergen Specific Immunotherapy
4. Patient Education

Allergen Immunotherapy (AIT) is now widely used in clinical practice of patients with moderate to severe allergic rhinitis and moderate allergic asthma to inhalant allergens. AIT may be delivered via subcutaneous (SCIT) or sublingual (SLIT) routes. However, the quality of evidence for individual AIT products are heterogeneous. There is scientific consensus on evidence based AIT which ultimately may lead to a more efficacious treatment of allergic patients and appropriate recognition of AIT. During the last decades, substantial progress has been made in development AIT products based on current state of the art and high quality clinical trials. It has been possible to evaluate therapeutic efficacy of specific allergen products by clinicoimmunologic tools.

In this book "Allergy and Allergen Immunotherapy: New Mechanisms and Strategies" an effort has been made by the editor to provide a balanced approach to enumerating pollen allergens for allergy diagnosis and therapeutic management and safety assessment of genetically engineered food allergens.

I hope book will be of immense use to allergologists, clinicians, aerobiologists, and environmentalists and will aid in appropriate allergen selection for diagnosis and immunotherapy of respiratory allergy patients.

PART I

EPIDEMIOLOGY, PATHOPHYSIOLOGY, AND DIAGNOSIS OF ALLERGY

CHAPTER 1

SENSITIZATION TO ALLERGENS: EPIDEMIOLOGY AND PATHOPHYSIOLOGY

P. A. MAHESH[1] and AMRUTHA D. HOLLA[2]

[1]*Professor, Department of Pulmonary Medicine, JSS Medical College, JSS University, Mysore, India*

[2]*Director, Allergy Asthma Associates, Mysore, India*

CONTENTS

1.1 BACKGROUND

Sensitization to different allergens is a prelude to the development of clinical allergies in different age groups (Nwaru et al., 2010; Viswanathan and Mathur, 2011). Early sensitization to inhalant allegens predicts development of wheezing and asthma till adolescence (Piippo-Savolainen et al., 2007). The development of sensitization needs a multifactorial interplay of various host factors such as a genetic predisposition, immunological pathways skewed towards the Th2 phenotype, and a gut microbiome with predominant Fermicutes and less of Xylanibacter and Prevotella of the Bacteroides species and environmental factors including diet, early life exposures related to the hygiene hypothesis, allergen characteristics and load, and parasitic infestations (Glick-Bauer and Yeh, 2014; Janse et al., 2014; Kalliomaki et al., 2010; Mahesh et al., 2010; Maslowski and Mackay, 2011; Palm et al., 2012; Rosenkranz et al., 2012; van Ree et al., 2014). Vegetarian Diet and diet rich in 3-Omega Fatty acids are likely strong factors influencing expression of clinical allergies and both of these modifies the gut microbiome (Maslowski and Mackay, 2011). Strachan generated the Hygiene hypothesis (Strachan, 1989) to explain that early life exposures that could increase microbial exposure in childhood affects sensitization and is relevant in both children and adults (Matricardi et al., 1998; Matheson et al., 2011; Rhodes et al., 2001; Svanes et al., 1999).

1.2 EPIDEMIOLOGY

1.2.1 PREVALENCE OF SENSITIZATION

The prevalence of sensitization varies in different geographies and different populations (Sunyer et al., 2004). The prevalence also varies depending on the allergen being evaluated and whether the studies are being done in the community or in diseased subjects in the hospital. Few studies have shown an increase in the prevalence of sensitization over time, though the exact reasons for such an increase is not clear (Warm et al., 2013). India has among the highest sensitization rates in the world (Mahesh PA et al., 2016). Table 1.1 lists the prevalence of sensitization in different countries. The summary of the key factors involved in the epidemiology of sensitization is listed in Figure 1.1.

TABLE 1.1 Prevalence of Aeroallergen Sensitization in Different Countries—Key Studies

Year	Country	Prevalence	Antigens
2004 **Adults**	**ECRHS, Multicenter study, Europe, USA and Australia, N = 13,558**	USA (43%), Australia (45%), New Zealand (46%), UK (44%), Netherlands (41%), Germany (40%), France (43%), Sweden (32%), Italy (30%), Spain (42%), Iceland (23%), Estonia (18%)	**Any allergen** House dust mite, cat, timothy grass, *C. herbarum*, and birch, *P. judaica*, ragweed
2008 **Children**	**ISAAC, Multicenter study, N = 54,178**	Albania (12.4%), Brazil (12.1%), China (22.9%), Hong Kong (45.2%), Ecuador (18.1%), Estonia (12.6%), Georgia (27.4%), Ghana (1.6%), Greece (9.2%), India (5.8%), Spain (41.5%), Palestine (10.3%), Norway (20.1%), Turkey (15.8%), UK (10.6%)	Any Allergen Tree pollen, grass pollen, House dust mite, Cat hair, Alternaria

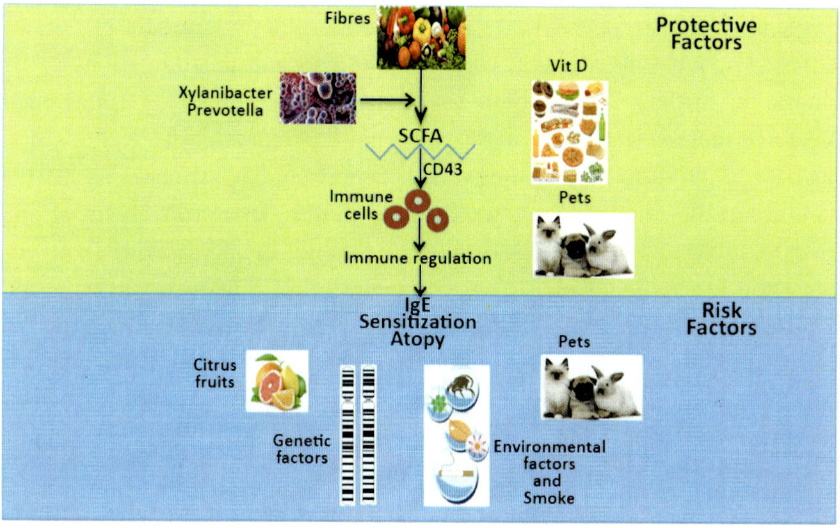

FIGURE 1.1 The summary of various epidemiological factors involved in increasing the risk of sensitization and those offering protection against sensitization. (Data from the ECRHS and the ISAAC Studies, listed above.)

1.2.2 GENETICS OF SENSITIZATION

It was discovered in the early 20th century that allergies and asthma were heritable. Hopp estimated that around 50% of the risk of developing atopy and allergy was genetic and the other half due to environmental exposures. Atopy is a complex trait and is influenced by several genes with each gene carrying a small weight and different genes being important at different levels in each individual. Most of the genes that are associated with atopy are present in the region of Chromosome 5q including regions encoding IL-3, IL-4, IL-5, IL-9, IL-13 and GM-CSF (Steinke et al., 2003). The other important chromosome that is involved in regulating the total IgE is Chromosome 12 (Nickel et al., 1997). MHC II complex is also involved in regulating specific IgE to different allergens such as grasses, ragweed and mite antigens (Marsh et al., 1982; Steinke et al., 2003).

1.2.3 DIET AND SENSITIZATION

Evidence is accumulating that diet is an important determinant of sensitization. The key pathway that connects diet and immune deviations is the alterations in the gut microbiome with alterations in the diet. It has been observed that even changes in the maternal diet can alter the sensitization profiles in children. In a Finnish birth cohort study (Nwaru et al., 2010) examining the effects of maternal diet and allergies until 5 years of age observed that increased consumption of Vitamin D decreased risk of sensitization to foods and increased consumption of Citrus foods increased the risk of sensitization to inhalant allergens. Similar observations of increased maternal consumption of Citrus fruits and increase in sensitization to both inhalant and food allergens in children until 2 years of age have been reported from Germany (Sausenthaler et al., 2007). Nutrients including allergens are transported to the fetus via the placenta and influence immune development in the offspring and the effect of diet starts in utero itself. The reasons for the relation between increased maternal citrus fruit consumption and increased risk of sensitization in the children could be due to the transfer of pan allergens such as Profilin and Germin-like proteins which are known to be important allergens in oranges and have strong pro-inflammatory properties (Nwaru et al., 2010). Other birth cohort studies from the US (Camargo et al., 2007) has shown beneficial benefits in decreased sensitization in children with increased maternal consumption of Vitamin D and the study from UK (Devereux et al., 2007) showed benefit on asthma but not on sensitization. The effect of supplementation of *n*–3 PUFA mainly from fish oils during pregnancy and sensitization in children is controversial. Observational and Randomized controlled studies have shown both benefits (Almqvist et al., 2007; Dunstan et al., 2003) and no benefits (Fitzsimon et al., 2007; Marks et al., 2006).

There is some evidence regarding the role of Vitamin E, Selenium and flavonoids such as Quercetin in the diet, which along with their anti-oxidant effects also have specific effects on the Th differentiation (Devereux and Seaton, 2005). They promote Th1 differentiation and suppress Th2 differentiation and thus have an effect on decreasing sensitization. Human T cells exposed to physiologic amounts of Vitamin E show a reduced gene expression of IL-4 by inhibiting the transcription (Devereux and Seaton, 2005). The key age for their beneficial effects is likely to be during pregnancy and early childhood until 5 years of age (Devereux and Seaton, 2005). Therefore supplementation studies in adults have not yielded any positive results. There is also a possible protective role for regular fruits and vegetable consumption and decreasing consumption in a more westernized life-style could be associated with increasing sensitization and clinical allergies. However, further studies are needed to confirm these associations as true associations.

1.2.4 GUT MICROBIOME AND SENSITIZATION

There is a close relation also to the diet and the gut microbiome of the individual and is one of the most exciting areas of research today. About 90% of the cells in the human body are not human but part of the microbiome, that is bacterial cells in the skin, oral cavity and the largest numbers are present in the gut. There is very strong evidence that diet influences the gut microbiome, which can change quickly with changes in the diet. Higher fibers in the diet lead to higher proportion of the gut microbiome of the Bacteroides group, with predominance of the Xylanibacter and Prevotella species (Maslowski and Mackay, 2011). These are highly beneficial gut microbes that help in the digestion of the insoluble fiber and help release Short Chain Fatty Acids (SCFA), one of the most important metabolites having very potent anti-inflammatory effects not only in the gut but also systemically that helps to reduce sensitization to allergens and clinical allergy (Maslowski and Mackay, 2011). On the other hand, consumption of a more western diet with more of meat and refined wheat (Burgers and Pizza) and less of fiber would lead to the predominance of Fermicutes in the gut microbiome which increases the risk of systemic inflammatory disorders. Studies in mice have shown that introduction of a western diet would change the gut microbiome in a matter of few weeks (Maslowski and Mackay, 2011). Studies in children from Burkina Faso (Africa) and Europe with their vastly different diets have shown similar changes in their gut microbiome (Maslowski and Mackay, 2011) with the children from Africa having predominantly Bacteroides species and the European Children having the Fermicutes species. It is necessary to study the effect of the typical Indian diet and the gut microbiome and sensitization as it would help in the primary and secondary prevention of sensitization. The high consumption of fermented products in the Indian diet could contribute to a better and more beneficial microbiome.

1.2.5 BACTERIAL INFECTION, PARASITIC INFESTATION AND SENSITIZATION

Field studies investigating whether foodborne and orofecal infections affect sensitization have shown inconsistent results. Few studies in adults have supported the concept of hygiene hypothesis and observed that prior infection with hepatitis A, *Toxoplasma gondii* and *Helicobacter pylori* lowers the risk of allergic sensitization and allergic diseases (Janse et al., 2014). While other studies did not find significant association for *T. gondii* or hepatitis A. Studies in young children observed protection against sensitization with prior infection with *T. gondii* and *H. pylori*, and not with hepatitis A (Janse et al., 2014). Another study on hospitalized children, found a protective effect of salmonella on respiratory allergies (Janse et al., 2014). In the Europrevall study evaluating the risk of sensitization and prior infection with Hepatitis A, *Salmonella* and *Toxoplasma gondii*, a significant positive association was found between prior exposure to hepatitis A and lower sensitization to food allergens, but not with Salmonella and Toxoplasma (Janse et al., 2014).

The hygiene hypothesis proposed that a reduced stimulation of the immune system by microbial infections and parasitic infestations due to better sanitation, use of antibiotics and various lifestyle factors including a change in the diet, use of antiseptics, decreasing number of siblings has contributed to increased risk of sensitization. A bacterial or a viral infection would shift the balance towards Th2, which would increase the risk of sensitization and allergic diseases. Even though helminthic infestation exerts a strong Th2 stimulus there is a protective effect against sensitization. This dichotomy is due to the simultaneous strong stimulation of regulatory T cells, which increases IL-10 and TGF-beta that prevents development of sensitization and clinical allergies. Studies have observed that worm infestation can reduce the prevalence of sensitization by more than 25% (Schafer et al., 2005).

1.2.6 PET OWNERSHIP AND SENSITIZATION TO PETS

There are conflicting evidences relating to the pet ownership and sensitization to the same pets (Park et al., 2013). In some studies, owning a dog is shown to be protective, whereas in other studies, it is a risk factor for sensitization to the dog. Similar conflicting studies exist for cats as well. Presence of sensitization to other allergens such as House dust mites increases the risk of sensitization to pets such as dogs and rabbits (Park et al., 2013).

There are also conflicting evidence related to exposure to animals in the farms including pets and overall sensitization to any allergen (Mandhane et al., 2009). Some reports show that it is protective while others show an increased risk or no effect. There is also the possibility on evaluation of exposure to pets in children that parents of sick children with allergies avoid pets at home and so cross-sectional studies may show a beneficial effect that children with pets have fewer allergies (Mandhane et al., 2009). Even among adults, only healthy workers continue to work on the farms as compared to people who suffer from allergies and so studies may erroneously observe that fewer people working in farms have allergies (healthy worker effect) (Mandhane et al., 2009). One study demonstrated that the protective effect in children living in farms against allergies is not due to exposure to animals but due to drinking unpasteurized milk (Mandhane et al., 2009).

1.2.7 EARLY LIFE FACTORS AND SENSITIZATION

Key early life factors that are associated with risk of sensitization are the family size (sib-ship effect) and the number of older siblings (birth order effect) (Matricardi et al., 1998). The hypothesis is part of the hygiene hypothesis that states that larger families have higher rates of cross-infection among family members and infections early in life help immune maturation (Matricardi et al., 1998). Many studies (UK, Italy, Germany) have shown that having a higher number of siblings reduce the risk of sensitization to common aeroallergens (Matricardi et al., 1998). There is also evidence that having a higher number of older siblings reduces the risk of Atopy in the child. The hypothesis again is related to the increased frequency of infections in the younger child from their older siblings. Some of the infections shown to have protective effect against sensitization include respiratory, Hepatitis A, measles and tuberculin reactivity or BCG vaccination. A possibility of a better maternal-fetal interaction in subsequent births towards immune priming in the fetus has been considered, but is yet to be proven (Matricardi et al., 1998). This effect of sib-ship size and birth order effect is relevant not only in children but also in adults (Matricardi et al., 1998).

1.2.8 CIGARETTE SMOKING AND SENSITIZATION

Cigarette smoking reduces the number of T helper cells and is known to enhance suppressor T cell function (Hancox et al., 2008). There are conflicting evidence regarding exposure to tobacco smoke and risk for sensitization (Strachan and Cook, 1998). Different situations may lead to different outcomes contributing to the confusion. What are the effects of maternal smoking versus paternal smoking on the atopic sensitization in children, prenatal smoking by the mothers and the effect on the fetus and active smoking by children in adolescence and risk of sensitization? There is still need of studies to answer these questions effectively. The prevailing data from three longitudinal studies suggest that cigarette smoking probably reduces the risk of atopic sensitization both in children and adults although there are other studies that point to an increased risk (Barbee et al., 1987; Hancox et al., 2008; Linneberg et al., 2001). The type of allergen also may matter. Smoking may increase sensitization to House dust mites while reducing sensitization to pets such as cats and dogs. There are many confounders that usually affect interpretation of these studies and it is difficult to design a study to answer this question. There is also the possibility that healthy subjects continue to smoke, whereas subjects who have developed allergic symptoms avoid smoking and therefore, subjects who smoke may show lesser degree of sensitization (healthy bias effect) (Hancox et al., 2008).

1.3 PATHOPHYSIOLOGY

In a genetically susceptible individual, the process of sensitization starts at a certain age, the cause for which remains unknown to date. Why does the process not start earlier or later? What are the sequences of events or exposure that culminates in the initiation of the sensitization? How many critical processes need to happen during the initiation of sensitization that primes the individual to develop IgE antibodies? Is the load of allergen important? Why do some subjects develop sensitization to indoor allergens such as house dust mites and others outdoor-allergens such as pollens? A lot remains to be understood. The key mechanisms involved in the pathophysiology of sensitization are depicted in Figure 1.2.

1.3.1 ANTIGEN PRESENTING CELLS

However, once the subject is primed to develop sensitization, the further mechanisms of development of IgE have been understood to some extent. One of the most important cells is the antigen-presenting cell (APC) called the dendritic cells (von Bubnoff et al., 2001). The dendritic cells process the allergens and some of the peptides are presented to the Naive T lym-

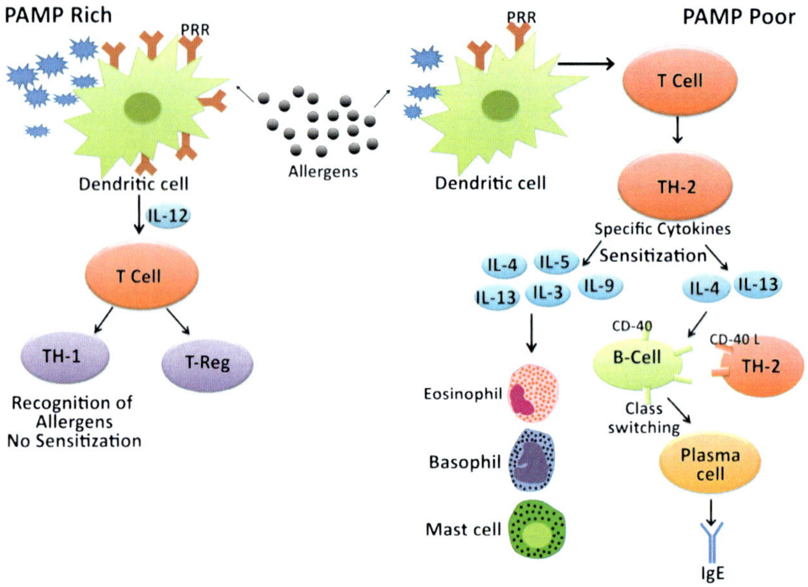

FIGURE 1.2 Key mechanisms involved in the pathogenesis of sensitization. Exposure to allergens in the presence of a PAMP rich environment with increase in PRR's on the Dendritic cells skews the immune system towards the Th1 pathway with absence of sensitization, though there is recognition of the allergens via development of IgM and IgG antibodies. On the other hand, in a PAMP poor environment, with low number of PRR's on the dendritic cells, there is a skew towards the Th2 pathway with resultant cytokine profile leading to the B cell switch to IgE producing cells and activation of other cells relevant to sensitization and clinical allergy. (Adapted from Andrew H Liu; J Allergy Clin Immunol 2008;122:846-58)

phocytes in association with the Major Histocompatibility complex II. Exposure to the allergen for sensitization can occur via the inhaled route (most common), ingestion (important for food allergens) or cutaneous. The cross talk between the dendritic cells and the T lymphocytes occur via the allergen and MHC II complex on the dendritic cell and the T-cell receptor (TCR) on the T-lymphocyte (Min, 2010). The response may be different when this cross talk happens in the presence of plenty of Pathogen associated molecular patterns (PAMP's) such as endotoxins versus PAMP poor environments (Liu, 2008). The PAMP's influence the cross talk between the APC's and T-lymphocytes via the Toll-like receptors such as TLR-4. In a PAMP poor environment, the APC's can divert the differentiation of the naive T lymphocyte to an allergen specific Th2 lymphocyte. This can further lead to secretion of specific cytokines that can lead to class switching of the B lymphocyte. The cross talk between the Th2 lymphocyte and the B-lymphocyte occurs via the binding of CD40 on the B lymphocyte to the CD40 ligand on the Th2 lymphocyte. Normally on exposure to various allergens, an individual produces IgM and IgG antibodies. But once there is class switching of the B-lymphocyte, they produce IgE antibodies. These IgE antibodies bind to high affinity receptors on mast cells and basophils. The other cells that can present the allergen to the Th lymphocytes are macrophages and B-lymphocytes (Johansson-Lindbom and Borrebaeck, 2002).

1.3.2 CD4 LYMPHOCYTES

CD4 T cells are of different types (van Ree et al., 2014). There are the effector T lymphocytes, which are further divided depending on the types of cytokines they release as Th1, Th2 and Th17 cells. Th1 cells release gamma interferon and IL-2 inducing a cell mediated response. Th2 cells are critical for the development of allergy and the naive T cells under influences above can differentiate into a Th2 lymphocyte, which produces IL-4 and IL-13 that leads to the class switching of the B lymphocyte, IL-5 leads to activation and recruitment of eosinophils, while IL-9 plays a role in mast cell activation. Th17 cells are important in combating extracellular pathogens and promote neutrophilic inflammation. Other than the effector T lymphocytes, there are memory T cells and T reg cells. Memory T cells can quickly change to effector T cells when required. T reg cells are important regulatory cells maintaing appropriate immune regulation and homeostasis. CD4+ CD25+ FOXP3+ T reg cells are key in maintaining tolerance to allergens via secretion of IL-10 and TGF-beta. Abnormalities in this cell population of T reg cells lead to the development of sensitization to allergens.

1.3.3 AIRWAY EPITHELIUM

The first barrier for the allergen in the airways is the airway epithelium, which forms a physical, chemical and an immunological barrier. Some of the allergens such as house dust mite antigens are proteases and can alter the physical barrier by affecting the tight junction (TJ) proteins. The airway epithelium expresses innate immune system receptors such as the pattern recognition receptors (PRR's). These can interact with various bacteria, viruses and fungi and activate immune cells underlying the epithelium such as dendritic cells, T cells, eosinophils and mast cells. The airway epithelium is damaged on exposure to cigarette smoke and possibly other pollutants as also with certain viral infections. Damage to the airway epithelium allows easy access to the other immune cells in the airways.

1.3.4 TOLL-LIKE RECEPTORS

Toll-like receptors (TLR) are widely expressed in various cells including the airway epithelial cells, dendritic cells, macrophages and regulatory T cells. Each of the TLR's can be activated via various microbial products. For example, TLR-4 can be activated by the lipopolysaccharide from the gram-negative bacteria such as endotoxin, as well as products from the gram-positive bacteria and viruses such as respiratory syncitial virus. Stimulation of TLR's lead to activation of the T regulatory cell and skewing of the Th1/Th2 balance towards Th1.

Sensitization, an intermediate phenotype of clinical allergies such as allergic rhinitis and asthma, is a complex interaction of gene-gene and gene-environment interaction, with significant impact of various epigenetic and metagenetic factors. The diagnosis of sensitization is by identifying specific IgE in the blood via RAST or Immunocap or by skin prick tests, which will be discussed in a subsequent chapter. Further research is necessary to understand sensitization further and discover mechanisms to delay or prevent the onset of sensitization, which can help to delay or prevent clinical allergic diseases.

ACKNOWLEDGEMENTS

I am thankful to Sangeetha Vishweswaraiah, Research Scholar, Genetics and Genomics Lab, Department of Studies in Zoology, University of Mysore, Karnataka for help in designing both the figures in this chapter.

KEYWORDS

- **allergy**
- **antigen presenting cells**
- **asthma**
- **intermediate phenotype**
- **microbiome**
- **pets**
- **sensitization**
- **T-helper 2 cells**
- **toll-like receptors**

REFERENCES

Almqvist, C., Garden, F., Xuan, W., Mihrshahi, S., Leeder, S. R., Oddy, W., et al. Omega-3 and omega-6 fatty acid exposure from early life does not affect atopy and asthma at age 5 years. *J Allergy Clin Immunol,* 2007, 119(6), 1438–1444. doi: 10.1016/j.jaci.2007.01.046.

Barbee, R. A., Kaltenborn, W., Lebowitz, M. D., Burrows, B. Longitudinal changes in allergen skin test reactivity in a community population sample. *J Allergy Clin Immunol,* 1987, 79(1), 16–24.

Camargo, C. A., Jr., Rifas-Shiman, S. L., Litonjua, A. A., Rich-Edwards, J. W., Weiss, S. T., Gold, D. R., Gillman, M. W. Maternal intake of vitamin D during pregnancy and risk of recurrent wheeze in children at 3 years of age. *Am J Clin Nutr,* 2007, 85(3), 788–795.

Devereux, G., Seaton, A. Diet as a risk factor for atopy and asthma. *J Allergy Clin Immunol,* 2005, 115(6), 1109–1117; quiz 1118. doi: 10.1016/j.jaci.2004.12.1139.

Devereux, G., Litonjua, A. A., Turner, S. W., Craig, L. C., McNeill, G., Martindale, S., Weiss, S. T. Maternal vitamin D intake during pregnancy and early childhood wheezing. *Am J Clin Nutr,* 2007, 85(3), 853–859.

Dunstan, J. A., Mori, T. A., Barden, A., Beilin, L. J., Taylor, A. L., Holt, P. G., Prescott, S. L. Maternal fish oil supplementation in pregnancy reduces interleukin-13 levels in cord blood of infants at high risk of atopy. *Clin Exp Allergy,* 2003, 33(4), 442–448.

Fitzsimon, N., Fallon, U., O'Mahony, D., Loftus, B. G., Bury, G., Murphy, A. W., Lifeways Cross Generation Cohort Study Steering, Group. Mothers' dietary patterns during pregnancy and risk of asthma symptoms in children at 3 years. *Ir Med J,* 2007, 100(8), Suppl. 27–32.

Glick-Bauer, M., Yeh, M. C. The health advantage of a vegan diet: exploring the gut microbiota connection. *Nutrients,* 2014, 6(11), 4822–4838. doi: 10.3390/nu6114822.

Hancox, R. J., Welch, D., Poulton, R., Taylor, D. R., McLachlan, C. R., Greene, J. M., Sears, M. R. Cigarette smoking and allergic sensitization: a 32-year population-based cohort study. *J Allergy Clin Immunol,* 2008, 121(1), 38–42, e33. doi: 10.1016/j.jaci.2007.09.052.

Janse, J. J., Wong, G. W., Potts, J., Ogorodova, L. M., Fedorova, O. S., Mahesh, P. A., Yazdanbakhsh, M et al. The association between foodborne and orofecal pathogens and allergic sensitization—EuroPrevall study. *Pediatr Allergy Immunol,* 2014, 25(3), 250–256. doi: 10.1111/pai.12175

Johansson-Lindbom, B., Borrebaeck, C. A. Germinal center B cells constitute a predominant physiological source of IL-4: implication for Th2 development in vivo. *J Immunol,* 2002, 168(7), 3165–3172.

Kalliomaki, M., Antoine, J. M., Herz, U., Rijkers, G. T., Wells, J. M., Mercenier, A. Guidance for substantiating the evidence for beneficial effects of probiotics: prevention and management of allergic diseases by probiotics. *J Nutr,* 2010, 140(3), 713S–721S. doi: 10.3945/jn.109.113761

Linneberg, A., Nielsen, N. H., Madsen, F., Frolund, L., Dirksen, A., Jorgensen, T. Smoking and the development of allergic sensitization to aeroallergens in adults: a prospective population-based study. The Copenhagen Allergy Study. *Allergy,* 2001, 56(4), 328–332.

Liu, A. H. Innate microbial sensors and their relevance to allergy. *J Allergy Clin Immunol,* 2008, 122(5), 846–858; quiz 858–860. doi: 10.1016/j.jaci.2008.10.002.

Mahesh, P. A., Kummeling, I., Amrutha, D. H., Vedanthan, P. K. Effect of area of residence on patterns of aeroallergen sensitization in atopic patients. *Am J Rhinol Allergy,* 2010, 24(5), e98–103. doi: 10.2500/ajra.2010.24.3529.

Mahesh, P. A., Gary W. K. Wong , L. Ogorodova , J. Potts , T. F. Leung , O. Fedorova, Amrutha D. Holla, M. Fernandez-Rivas, E. N. Clare Mills, I. Kummeling, S. A. Versteeg, R. van Ree, M. Yazdanbakhsh & P. Burney. Prevalence of food sensitization and probable food allergy among adults in India: the EuroPrevall INCO study. Allergy 2016, 71 (7);1010–19.

Mandhane, P. J., Sears, M. R., Poulton, R., Greene, J. M., Lou, W. Y., Taylor, D. R., Hancox, R. J. Cats and dogs and the risk of atopy in childhood and adulthood. *J Allergy Clin Immunol,* 2009, 124(4), 745–750 e744. doi: 10.1016/j.jaci.2009.06.038.

Marks, G. B., Mihrshahi, S., Kemp, A. S., Tovey, E. R., Webb, K., Almqvist, C., Leeder, S. R. Prevention of asthma during the first 5 years of life: a randomized controlled trial. *J Allergy Clin Immunol,* 2006, 118(1), 53–61. doi: 10.1016/j.jaci.2006.04.004.

Marsh, D. G., Hsu, S. H., Roebber, M., Ehrlich-Kautzky, E., Freidhoff, L. R., Meyers, D. A., Bias, W. B. HLA-Dw2: a genetic marker for human immune response to short ragweed pollen allergen Ra5. I. Response resulting primarily from natural antigenic exposure. *J Exp Med,* 1982, 155(5), 1439–1451.

Maslowski, K. M., Mackay, C. R. Diet, gut microbiota and immune responses. *Nat Immunol,* 2011, 12(1), 5–9. doi: 10.1038/ni0111-5.

Matheson, M. C., Dharmage, S. C., Abramson, M. J., Walters, E. H., Sunyer, J., de Marco, R., Svanes, C. Early-life risk factors and incidence of rhinitis: results from the European Community Respiratory Health Study—an international population-based cohort study. *J Allergy Clin Immunol,* 2011, 128(4), 816–823 e815. doi: 10.1016/j.jaci.2011.05.039.

Matricardi, P. M., Franzinelli, F., Franco, A., Caprio, G., Murru, F., Cioffi, D., Rosmini, F. Sibship size, birth order, and atopy in 11,371 Italian young men. *J Allergy Clin Immunol,* 1998, 101(4 Pt 1), 439–444.

Min, Y. G. The pathophysiology, diagnosis and treatment of allergic rhinitis. *Allergy Asthma Immunol Res,* 2010, 2(2), 65–76. doi: 10.4168/aair.2010.2.2.65.

Nickel, R., Wahn, U., Hizawa, N., Maestri, N., Duffy, D. L., Barnes, K. C., Marsh, D. G. Evidence for linkage of chromosome 12q15–q24.1 markers to high total serum IgE concentrations in children of the German Multicenter Allergy Study. *Genomics,* 1997, 46(1), 159–162. doi: 10.1006/geno.1997.5013.

Nwaru, B. I., Ahonen, S., Kaila, M., Erkkola, M., Haapala, A. M., Kronberg-Kippila, C., Virtanen, S. M. Maternal diet during pregnancy and allergic sensitization in the offspring by 5 yrs of age: a prospective cohort study. *Pediatr Allergy Immunol,* 2010, 21(1 Pt 1), 29–37. doi: 10.1111/j.1399-3038.2009.00949.x.

Palm, N. W., Rosenstein, R. K., Medzhitov, R. Allergic host defences. *Nature,* 2012, 484(7395), 465–472. doi: 10.1038/nature11047.

Park, Y. B., Mo, E. K., Lee, J. Y., Kim, J. H., Kim, C. H., Hyun, I. G., Choi, J. H. Association between pet ownership and the sensitization to pet allergens in adults with various allergic diseases. *Allergy Asthma Immunol Res,* 2013, 5(5), 295–300. doi: 10.4168/aair.2013.5.5.295

Piippo-Savolainen, E., Remes, S., Korppi, M. Does early exposure or sensitization to inhalant allergens predict asthma in wheezing infants? A 20-year follow-up. *Allergy Asthma Proc,* 2007, 28(4), 454–461. doi: 10.2500/aap.2007.28.3022

Rhodes, H. L., Sporik, R., Thomas, P., Holgate, S. T., Cogswell, J. J. Early life risk factors for adult asthma: a birth cohort study of subjects at risk. *J Allergy Clin Immunol,* 2001, 108(5), 720–725. doi: 10.1067/mai.2001.119151

Rosenkranz, R. R., Rosenkranz, S. K., Neessen, K. J. Dietary factors associated with lifetime asthma or hayfever diagnosis in Australian middle-aged and older adults: a cross-sectional study. *Nutr J,* 2012, 11, 84. doi: 10.1186/1475-2891-11-84.

Sausenthaler, S., Koletzko, S., Schaaf, B., Lehmann, I., Borte, M., Herbarth, O., et al. Maternal diet during pregnancy in relation to eczema and allergic sensitization in the offspring at 2 yrs of age. *Am J Clin Nutr,* 2007, 85(2), 530–537.

Schafer, T., Meyer, T., Ring, J., Wichmann, H. E., Heinrich, J. Worm infestation and the negative association with eczema (atopic/nonatopic) and allergic sensitization. *Allergy,* 2005, 60(8), 1014–1020. doi: 10.1111/j.1398-9995.2005.00801.x.

Steinke, J. W., Borish, L., Rosenwasser, L. J. Genetics of hypersensitivity. *J Allergy Clin Immunol,* 2003, 111(2 Suppl), S495–501.

Strachan, D. P. Hay fever, hygiene, and household size. *BMJ,* 1989, 299(6710), 1259–1260.

Strachan, D. P., Cook, D. G. Health effects of passive smoking. Parental smoking and allergic sensitization in children. *Thorax,* 1998, 53(2), 117–123.

Sunyer, J., Jarvis, D., Pekkanen, J., Chinn, S., Janson, C., Leynaert, B., et al. European Community Respiratory Health Survey Study, Group. Geographic variations in the effect of atopy on asthma in the European Community Respiratory Health Study. *J Allergy Clin Immunol,* 2004, 114(5), 1033–1039. doi: 10.1016/j.jaci.2004.05.072

Svanes, C., Jarvis, D., Chinn, S., Burney, P. Childhood environment and adult atopy: results from the European Community Respiratory Health Survey. *J Allergy Clin Immunol,* 1999, 103(3 Pt 1), 415–420.

van Ree, R., Hummelshoj, L., Plantinga, M., Poulsen, L. K., Swindle, E. Allergic sensitization: host-immune factors. *Clin Transl Allergy,* 2014, 4(1), 12. doi: 10.1186/2045-7022-4-12.

Viswanathan, R. K., Mathur, S. K. Role of allergen sensitization in older adults. *Curr Allergy Asthma Rep,* 2011, 11(5), 427–433. doi: 10.1007/s11882-011-0204-9.

von Bubnoff, D., Geiger, E., Bieber, T. Antigen-presenting cells in allergy. *J Allergy Clin Immunol,* 2001, 108(3), 329–339. doi: 10.1067/mai.2001.117457.

Warm, K., Lindberg, A., Lundback, B., Ronmark, E. Increase in sensitization to common airborne allergens among adults—two population-based studies 15 years apart. *Allergy Asthma Clin Immunol,* 2013, 9(1), 20. doi: 10.1186/1710-1492-9-20.

CHAPTER 2

IN-VIVO AND *IN-VITRO* DIAGNOSIS OF ALLERGY

P. A. MRIDULA,[1] AMRUTHA D. HOLLA,[2] and P. A. MAHESH[3]

[1]*Research Associate, Allergy Asthma Associates, Mysore, India*

[2]*Director, Allergy Asthma Associates, Mysore, India*

[3]*Professor, Department of Pulmonary, Medicine, JSS Medical College, Mysore, India*

CONTENTS

2.1 INTRODUCTION

The clinical diagnosis of atopy in an individual depends on the demonstration of sensitization to specific allergens. Sensitization can usually be demonstrated either by skin prick testing (SPT) or by the measurement of allergen specific IgE in the serum. Out of the above two techniques, skin prick testing is the preferred method of demonstration of clinically relevant sensitization since it is two tests in one. It demonstrates, on one hand, the presence of allergen specific IgE and on the other, it confirms that these allergen specific IgE are appropriately positioned on the mast cells and basophils to elicit an allergic reaction on exposure to the allergen, since that is the mechanism of a positive test on skin prick testing. To have the same information, one needs to measure the allergen specific IgE in the serum as well as demonstrate release of mediators by a basophil histamine release assay which is a very difficult assay to standardize and perform on a regular basis. The measurement of allergen specific IgE in the serum only measures the free IgE in the blood, but does not confirm how these would be located on the mast cells or basophils and therefore may have less clinical relevance than a skin prick test.

2.2 SKIN PRICK TESTING

2.2.1 INDICATIONS

SPT is indicated on clinical suspicion based on a detailed history of a Type I hypersensitivity reaction to any of the following allergens; inhalants or aeroallergens, foods, drugs or occupational allergens (Heinzerling et al., 2013). It is important to realize for the clinician that not all positive tests are clinically important and a detailed history of clinical symptoms and the temporal relationships between the onset of symptoms on exposure to the allergen, its reproducibility are critical to identify the clinically relevant allergen in each individual patient.

2.2.2 KEY PERFORMANCE PARAMETERS FOR SPT'S

The following are important performance parameters for SPT's (Bousquet et al., 2012). Always use standardized extracts. Manufacturer would give details of their standardization in the form of Allergen units (AU), Bioequivalent Allergen Units (BAU), Biological units (BU), micrograms of the major allergens, Protein Nitrogen Units (PNU). When it is not standardized, the manufacturer will simply give a weight by volume. Always use both negative and positive controls. Always test on a normal skin. Read the reactions and wheal sizes after 15–20 minutes. Rule out dermographism before performing SPT's. Ask for medications taken and which of those can affect the SPT and its last dose. The extracts should be stored between +2 to +8 degree centigrade to maintain their potency. Histamine dihydrochloride at a concentration of 10 mg/mL is used as a positive control and glycerinated buffer saline is used as a negative control. Make sure you have checked the expiration date of the extracts and have always maintained the cold chain.

2.2.3 MEDICATIONS INTERFERING WITH SPT'S

It is always important to elicit medication history before performing SPT's. Some medications can significantly interfere with the results of the SPT's and can be falsely negative if they are not avoided and avoided for a sufficient period of time. For most medications avoidance for a period of 4–7 days would be sufficient. The list of medications and the possible duration of their interference with the SPT results are given in Table 2.1. The wheal size would also be reduced in subjects with immunosuppressive disorders such as cirrhosis, renal failure, cancer or chemotherapy.

2.2.4 PRECAUTIONS TO BE TAKEN DURING SPT

In majority of the cases, SPT is very safe and has no adverse events. Extremely rarely, severe reactions have been noted (Lockey et al., 1987). Therefore, it is always advisable to have a health care professional experienced in handling allergic reactions at hand while testing, along with emergency medications and resuscitation facilities. This is especially true, when patients with history of anaphylaxis to foods and drugs are tested (Lockey et al., 1987). Asthma has to be under good control before performing the allergy testing. Uncontrolled asthma is a risk factor for adverse events during a SPT (Lockey et al., 1987). In patients with severe pollen allergy, testing to these pollens during the pollen season is associated with

TABLE 2.1 Medications That Can Interfere With the SPT Results

Medication	Interference	Duration
Oral anti-histamine	Yes	2–7 days
Intranasal anti-histamine	No	–
H2 blockers	No	–
Oral steroids (short term)	No	–
Oral steroids (long term)	Possible	–
Inhaled steroids	No	–
Topical steroids (area of SPT)	Yes	Up to 7 days
Immunotherapy	No	–
Montelukast	No	–
Imipramine	Yes	21 days
UV treatment (PUVA)	Yes	28 days
Omazulimab	Yes	>4 weeks
Cyclosporin	No	–
Theophylline	No	–
Salmeterol, Formoterol	No	–

increased respiratory symptoms after SPT. Similarly, adverse reactions to SPT is increased in patients with an elevated basal levels of tryptase (Rueff et al., 2009). Care is to be taken when SPT is performed in patients taking beta-blockers or ACE inhibitors due to reduced response to epinephrine. Another relative contraindication is SPT in pregnancy due to the very rare possibility of a systemic reaction that would mandate the use of adrenaline that may cause uterine contractions or spasm of the umbilical artery (Bernstein and Storms, 1995). It is better to test with high dilutions rather than the standard concentration and then titrate to reach the regular concentration while SPT is performed in patients with severe systemic reactions to food or drugs.

2.2.5 SPT PROCEDURE

The recommended technique is the modified prick testing introduced by Pepys and involves a prick with a skin-testing lancet through a drop of the antigen placed on the skin.

Confirm that the patient is not on any drug that can inhibit skin sensitivity or accentuate systemic reaction before beginning to test. The ideal test site is the volar surface of the forearm. Leave a gap of at least 2–3 cm from the wrist and the ante-cubital fossa. A gap of at least 2 cm is necessary between two allergens to avoid a false positive test due to direct contamination of the adjacent site of skin prick test or due to secondary axonal reflex (Heinzerling et al., 2013). There are special lancets for SPT from reputed companies that have a tip of 1 mm. One should not use blood lancets, which usually have a tip size of 3–4 mm. The lancet is held pressed after the prick for at least for 1 second (Heinzerling et al., 2013). The antigen solution should enter the epidermis and there should be no bleeding at the site of the prick. If there is bleeding, the test should be repeated. It is important for the technician performing the SPT to apply equal pressure at every site. Each technician should first train and confirm their proficiency by performing the histamine standardization test. Each of the 4–6 histamine sites should give similar wheal size and this helps to reduce intra-observer variability. This histamine standardization is also used to compare different technicians in an epidemiological study to assess inter-observer variation. The SPT is measured after 15–20 minutes after the test procedure. The longest diameter of the wheal size is preferred to using the mean of the longest diameter and its perpendicular diameter (Heinzerling et al., 2013).

2.2.6 COMMON ERRORS DURING SPT

It is important to ensure that the minimum space between two skin prick test sites is >2 cms to prevent overlap between 2 large reactions when present. Also, give sufficient space away from the wrist and the cubital fossa. If sufficient pressure is not applied, antigen will not enter the epidermis and will lead to false negative results. This is especially important when using plastic needles. Too much pressure on the other hand can lead to bleeding and a false positive result, which is due to trauma. Care must be taken as in some patients the allergen tends to spread quickly over the skin especially when a small drop is used and may lead to a false negative result and when wiping the antigens after testing care to be taken to avoid mixing of allergens. It is important to test only on healthy skin. If the skin on the forearms is diseased, the test can be done on the back. Skin diseases can interfere with the test and some diseases like leprosy also can give a false negative test.

2.2.7 CHOOSING AN ALLERGEN PANEL FOR SPT

This depends on the local aerobiology. Some of the allergens need to be tested in most countries such as House dust mites, cockroach, molds such as Aspergillus and Alternaria. If patient has pets in the house, dog, cats and birds can be tested. The pollens such as weeds, grasses, shrubs and trees need to be decided based on the local aerobiological survey if available. Generally carefully chosen 30–35 allergen panel should be good enough to identify most important allergens in the community.

2.2.8 REASONS FOR A FALSE NEGATIVE SPT

If a subject is using any drug that interfere with the SPT, patient has an immunosuppressive disease, allergens tested are of low potency or have lost potency, poor technique such as a weak or no puncture, diseased skin, atrophic skin in the elderly or in some subjects who have only limited local production of IgE in the nose, eyes or lungs only (Bousquet et al., 2012).

2.2.9 INTERPRETATION OF A SPT

It is extremely important to be able to correlate SPT results with clinical history to have a meaningful interpretation that can help your patients. Though it is possible that the larger the SPT wheal size, higher the clinical relevance, it is not true in many cases. There has to be a strong clinical history of having symptoms with temporal correlation with the antigen exposure. It is important to repeat the history after the SPT and confirm the clinical relevance for each of the positive test. For example, if a patient is found to be highly sensitized to pollens and is a farmer and he says that he is regularly involved in deweeding his farm and he has no symptoms during this exposure, then he is sensitized to pollens but those are not causing his symptoms. He is found to be moderately sensitized to house dust mite, but has severe symptoms on waking up in the early morning and on handling his blankets, then it is likely that the mites are responsible for his clinical symptoms, though he has much greater sensitization to the pollens. One can ask whether the symptoms are predominantly indoors or outdoors and what happens on exposure to each of the antigens that the patient is sensitized to and tease out those that are clinically relevant for that patient.

2.2.10 FOOD ALLERGY AND RELATION TO RESPIRATORY ALLERGIES (RHINITIS AND ASTHMA)

Many subjects with allergic rhinitis and asthma do complain of symptoms on exposure to foods even satisfying the requirement of suffering from symptoms within two hours after consumption of a food, but they may not be having food allergy. The most common of these foods people complain are banana, cold juices, cold water, ice-creams, Brinjal (egg plant), some fishes, crab and shrimp, oily and fried foods and sour fruits such as orange. A skin prick test can be done for many of these and are found to be mostly negative. These foods can elicit symptoms even on a challenge. How does one explain this dichotomy?

Most of these foods act as irritants, which can elicit symptoms of sneezing, throat itching and are not allergens. Some foods such as banana contain chlorogenic acid, which can irritate an already inflamed mucosa. Some foods such as Brinjal, certain fish (scromboids), crab and shrimp actually contain histamine, bradykinin or serotonin, which can elicit symptoms. Certain other foods such as ice-creams elicit symptoms due to their physical nature, simply being cold irritate the exposed nerves with the inflamed mucosa in an allergic subject.

2.2.11 FUTURE DIRECTIONS FOR SPT

Recombinant allergens can be used in the future for allergy testing. Nearly 1800 different allergens have been identified and using recombinant allergens can lead to better standardization and eliminate irritant and nonspecific reactions, especially related to food extracts (Heinzerling et al., 2013). These should also lead to better sensitivity and specificity.

2.3 CHALLENGE TESTS

2.3.1 ORAL CHALLENGE TESTING

Oral Challenge testing can be performed in both adults and children for the confirmation of food allergies. Skin prick testing as well as serum specific IgE's can only confirm that the patient is sensitized but does not demonstrate clinical allergy, which means that the patient reacts with a particular symptom complex on exposure to the offending allergen. The benefits of an oral challenge would include a confirmation whether a patient who is sensitized to the food does indeed have clinical allergy and if negative helps the patient to avoid unnecessary food restrictions, which may be detrimental to the subject.

2.3.2 TYPES OF CHALLENGE

Oral Challenge testing can be open, single blind or double blind and placebo controlled. Open challenge is done with the food that is usually consumed by the patient. Here both the patient as well as the physician is aware of the food being tested. The key disadvantage is that when the patient complains of only subjective symptoms such as skin itching, but there are no visible rashes on the skin, throat and oral mucosa itching, but no visible changes or has nausea it becomes difficult to ascertain its clinical relevance. In a single blind oral food challenge, the patient is unaware of the food being tested but the physician is and in a double blind placebo controlled food challenge (DBPCFC), both the physician and the patient are unaware of the food being tested and this is considered as the gold standard test for the diagnosis of food allergy. Blinding helps to remove patient bias. The key disadvantages to conduct the DBPCFC for most foods is the lack of data on the dose that is to be initiated, the dose increments and the final threshold dose beyond which the patient can be safely categorized as not to have food allergy. Many of the foods such as Brinjal (egg plant) are very difficult to mask when conducting the DBPCFC and further research is needed to identify good masking matrixes for these foods.

2.3.3 TECHNIQUE OF ORAL CHALLENGE

The total food protein that is generally recommended is 4 g for children less than 4 years of age and 8 g for those above 4 years of age (Perry et al., 2004). For example, for children aged 10 years, the dose can be started at 5% of the recommended dose that is 0.4 g and increased every 15 minutes as follows; 0.8 g, 1.2 g, 1.6 g, 2 g, 2 g, thus a total of 8 g are completed in a period of 90 minutes.

2.3.4 PRECAUTIONS

Make sure a physician is present in the premises at all times. There is a possibility of severe reaction including anaphylaxis. The following drugs and instruments should be available at hand; Adrenaline, oral and parenteral Chlorpheniramine maleate, oral and parenteral steroids, Nebuliser with beta-agonist nebulizing solution, Glucagon, IV fluids and IV canula, oxygen source, Pulse oxymeter, equipments for securing the airways and a Defibrillator. Symptoms that may warrant immediate treatment are cough, breathing difficulty, tongue or throat swelling that may precede anaphylaxis.

2.3.5 ORGAN SPECIFIC CHALLENGES

These are performed to confirm the clinical relevance of inhalant allergens. The organ specific challenges that can be performed are conjunctival, nasal and bronchial challenges. These need special expertise and are not routinely performed.

2.3.5.1 Conjunctival Challenges

Conjunctival challenges are usually used to diagnose local eye allergies. Evaluation is by both subjective and objective symptoms such as tear volume, mucus quantity and erythema in palpebral and bulbar conjunctiva. The allergens can be applied both in the dry and wet forms. The concentrations used for the challenge are usually 3–4 log fold less than the concentration that is used for skin testing solution and if there is no reaction, dose can be increased to reach a maximum concentration of 1:1000 (Bernstein and Storms, 1995). A placebo of an inert solution (saline) is tested in the opposite eye before the actual challenge. After the introduction of the antigen, both subjective symptoms and objective signs are documented at baseline, 5, 10 and 15 minutes. Itching is usually the first symptom to occur followed by erythema, which can be objectively measured by spectroradiometry. Edema can be measured using the SLIT-lamp microscope. Tears and mucus can be collected for estimation of cytokines, mediators, inflammatory cells and specific IgE (Bernstein and Storms, 1995).

2.3.5.2 Nasal Challenges

These are used to confirm clinical sensitivity in patients who have a positive in-vivo or in-vitro test to the allergen, to confirm a condition called Local Allergic Rhinitis when skin prick testing or serum specific IgE are negative and to evaluate the efficacy of medications. Evaluation of the challenge is by both subjective responses such as number of sneezes and by objective measures such as nasal resistance by rhinomanometry and by measuring inflammatory mediators (Bernstein and Storms, 1995). Using the allergen in either the dry or the wet forms via a pipette, atomizer, paper disc or direct introduction can perform the allergen challenge. It is important to ensure that the particle size is large to prevent the allergen from reaching the lower airways, which can lead to severe bronchospasm. Paper disc soaked in allergen containing fluid is the ideal form to ensure only local exposure to the allergen and prevent spread of allergen to other areas (Bernstein and Storms, 1995). A large number of subjects can be tested in rooms with controlled allergen exposure simulating a natural exposure to pollens.

Nasal challenges takes a longer time than conjunctival challenges. The room should be temperature and humidity controlled. Objective measures are conducted at the beginning of the study with inspiratory and expiratory nasal flow rates and by rhinomanometry. After nasal challenge, the measurements are taken every minute for 5 minutes, every 2 minutes for the next 15 minutes and every 5 minutes beyond 15 minutes. Nasal secretions can be collected for further evaluation such as cytokines, mediators, inflammatory cells and specific IgE. In addition, nasal brushings or biopsy can be done (Bernstein and Storms, 1995).

2.3.5.3 Bronchial Challenges

These are the most difficult to perform and should be done only in specialized centers with experience in conducting bronchial challenges. Both early and late phase responses are to be evaluated. A histamine or a methacholine challenge test is performed a day before the specific allergen bronchial challenge and is also performed again after the bronchial challenge to assess increased bronchial hyper-responsiveness. Short acting beta agonists are to be stopped 8 hours before the test and long acting beta agonists, leukotriene receptor antagonists and theophyllines are avoided 48 hours before the test. Systemic steroids and antihistamines are withheld 72 hours before and inhaled steroids need to be avoided for one month before testing. Patient's FEV1 should be more than 70% predicted to avoid any false positives as well as to avoid dangers to the patient during testing. If the allergen is soluble, the best method of exposure is by inhalation via a nebulizer. The initial concentration to be used may depend on the degree of sensitivity of the patient and a serial titration skin prick testing can be done to identify the initial dose of the challenge (Bernstein and Storms, 1995). The dose can be increased every 15 minutes until there is a drop in FEV1 of 20%. Patient must be further observed for late-phase reactions and medical team should be available throughout the period in case resuscitation is required. The other method of exposure is via challenge chambers, which simulate natural exposures to the allergen.

2.4 IN-VITRO TESTING

2.4.1 INTRODUCTION

Allergic diseases are on the rise worldwide. Diagnosis of allergy for a particular individual involves a detailed clinical history and clinical examination. When these tests do not provide confirmatory evidence of allergy, specific IgE antibody, histamine release and B-tryptase analyses by serological methods is essential. Nowadays these serve as an integral part of the diagnostic evaluation for a patient, since they clarify and provide a better picture about the patient's state of sensitization. This section provides information on the past and present analytical methods for IgE antibody detection and quantitation in the serum.

2.4.2 HISTORY

Allergy, IgE antibodies and detection and quantitation of IgE (SPT, provocation tests, RAST) are all phenomenal discoveries of the 20th Century (Bergmann, 2014). RAST-short for Radioallergosorbent test is an immunological method to detect sensitization to allergens in an individual/subject. Upon exposure to allergens, in a predisposed individual, the subject's immune system produces IgE antibodies specific to that allergen (Type I hypersensitivity), the quantitation of which is an indication that the subject is sensitized to that particular allergen. Quantification helps in assessing the severity of sensitization to that allergen and the higher the levels of specific IgE, it is more likely to be clinically relevant (Sicherer, Wood, 2012). Similarly, measurement of mediators like histamine and B-tryptase in whole blood, isolated basophils and mast cells also serve as valuable research tools for *in vitro* investigations of allergy.

2.4.3 RAST TECHNIQUE

RAST as an allergy detection technique was first described in the year 1967 by Wide, Bennich and Johansson as an *in vitro* diagnostic test for allergen antibodies (Wide, Bennich, & Johansson, 1967). It had been widely used for detection of various allergic manifestations caused by food, common environmental allergens such as dust mite, pollen, animal dander, mould and parasitic infections, to name a few (Asser and Hamburger, 1984; Chodirker, 1985; Dreborg et al., 1986; Sampson and Ho, 1997; Wahyuni et al., 2003). The basic principle behind the test is the antigen-antibody reaction. The allergens are covalently bound to solid-phase polysaccha-

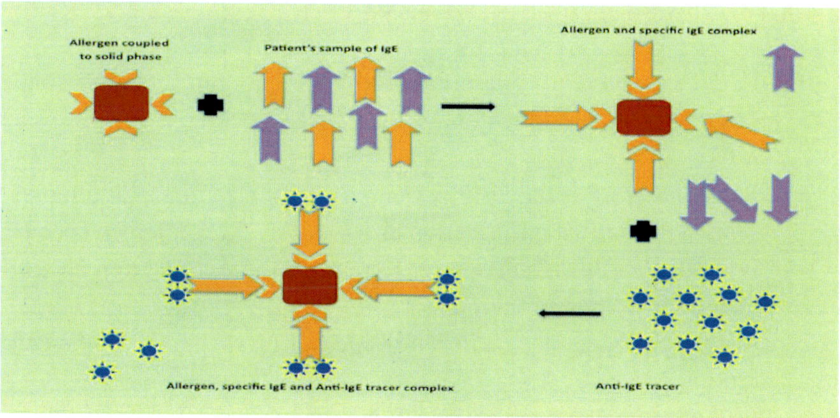

FIGURE 2.1 Diagramatic representation of Radioallergosorbent test.

rides (cellulose disk) activated by reaction with cyanogen bromide. The test (Figure 2.1) as outlined in Gleich and Yunginger (1981) involves the following steps:

1. Sera is collected from allergic patients and allowed to react to this solid phase allergen complex by overnight incubation. Antibodies produced against the allergen will bind to this complex.
2. Unbound antibodies are washed and the solid-phase allergen-antibody complex is allowed to react with radioiodinated affinity chromatography purified antibody to IgE. After overnight incubation, unbound antibodies are washed and the amount of radioactivity is measured by a scintillation counter.
3. The quantity of radioactive antibodies bound to the solid-phase allergen-antibody complex is proportional to the amount of IgE antibodies produced by the subject against the allergen.

2.4.4 *COMPARISON OF SPT AND RAST*

Skin prick test and RAST are the two widely used tests to detect allergen sensitization. Adults and children both can undergo these tests. Advantages and disadvantages of the two techniques (Chodirker, 1985; Sicherer et al., 2012) can be summarized as follows:

2.4.4.1 Advantages of RAST Over Skin Prick Test

- RAST is an *in vitro* test, more suitable for children because a single prick to draw blood is gentler than several pricks as in skin prick tests.
- RAST is more reliable in patients on antihistamines, antidepressants with antihistamine action as it measures free allergen specific IgE. It is not always necessary to remove the patient from an antihistamine treatment regimen.
- Measuring range is excellent-full measuring range across the calibration curve.
- Preferred method in patients who have skin diseases such as eczema, psoriasis, dermographism, etc., where it is difficult to perform SPT.
- Can be performed with patients who exhibit very high sensitivity to certain antigens since a skin prick test may have a risk for serious side effects. This is especially true in patients who have anaphylaxis on exposure to very low levels of the allergen.

2.4.4.2 Drawbacks of the RAST Method

- Cross-reactivity by homologous proteins may occur which lead to false positive results. Cross-reactivity among homologous proteins of aeroallergens and food allergens may result in false positive results without clinical allergy, for example, birch pollen with hazelnut or peanut and dust mite with shrimp, etc. (Sicherer et al., 2012).
- The test takes longer to perform and is less cost-effective.
- May fail to detect clinically relevant allergies that can be detected by skin prick tests.

2.4.5 MEASUREMENT AND SCALE

The RAST is scored on a scale from 0 to 6 (Almogren et al., 2013). RAST test results are expressed as Total Radioactive counts bound (cpm), Arbitrary units (RAST class, PRU/mL) or Units of IgE (IU/mL, kU/L). To express IgE levels in microgram per liter (μg/L), multiply kU/L value with 2.4 (Hamilton and Adkinson, 2003).

2.5 HISTAMINE RELEASE TEST (HRT)

Histamine is an inflammatory mediator released from both mast cells and basophils in response to an allergen challenge or natural exposure to the allergen. The interaction of specific allergen with IgE antibodies fixed to Fc receptors on basophils triggers the release of preformed histamine and other pharmacologic mediators, which are indicators of immediate hypersensitivity, into the blood and other biological fluids. In recent days, sensitive immunoassays have been developed to measure the histamine released by basophils into whole blood, serum and peripheral blood. This is considered to be a valuable research tool for investigating allergies *in vitro*.

Usually the HRT is performed by incubating allergen/antigen with isolated leukocytes from venous blood. Another simplistic method is to skip the leukocyte isolation and add the allergen to heparinized whole blood and incubate. The released histamine in the supernatant can then be determined by using antibodies to histamine. Assay kits are commercially available and mostly follow the competitive inhibition method.

Results of the HRT are expressed as a percentage of total cellular histamine. Histamine released into the supernatant without addition of allergen is taken as control measurement and is subtracted to calculate the release of histamine specific to an allergen. A positive control is usually the addition of different dilutions of anti-IgE antiserum to the cells.

There are two parameters for expressing histamine release results. (a) Cell sensitivity: concentration of allergen/antigen required to release 30–50% of total cellular histamine. (b) Cell reactivity: maximum amount of histamine release obtained with any amount of antigen. False-positive reactions may happen wherein the subjects have a negative skin test result and a positive histamine release test with an allergen. False-negative reactions may occur and is a more critical factor in interpreting HRTs. In such patients, there is a little histamine release at any concentration of allergen, but they are sensitive to skin tests.

There are several advantages of HRT over other serological tests:

(a) Smaller amounts of allergen are sufficient.
(b) No injection of allergen into the patient.
(c) Coupling of allergen to immobilized support systems is not required.

Disadvantages are that large amount of blood is required and the test needs to be carried out within a short time after the sample is obtained. This is because histamine levels peak quickly within 5 to 10 minutes of an allergic event and may return to baseline levels in less than an hour.

Commercial assay kits are available from various manufacturers. Measurement technique could be ELISA or ImmunoCAP. Normal range of histamine is usually obtained from the manufacturer. Unit of expression of histamine levels is nm/mL.

2.6 DETERMINATION OF B-TRYPTASE LEVELS IN SERUM

Tryptase is a neutral serine esterase (MW 134,000 kDa) with trypsin-like substrate specificity found in large quantities in mast cells. It is stored in secretory granules as an active enzyme complexed to and stabilized by heparin. Many forms of tryptase have been described, i.e., I, IIB, IIIa, T, but the B form is the one that is clinically relevant, since a considerable amount of this is found in basophils.

During an anaphylactic episode, when mast cell degranulation happens, stored histamine, proteases, B-tryptase and other vasoactive mediators are released to the surrounding tissue. This can be measured in serum and is a strong clinical marker of mast cell activation. Elevated levels of plasma histamine (>10 nmol/L), serum total tryptase (>15 ng/mL) and B-tryptase (>1 ng/mL) have been detected by competitive ELISA in patients with acute allergic reactions.

2.7 CURRENT AND NEWER METHODS OF IN-VITRO DIAGNOSTIC TESTING FOR ALLERGEN SENSITIZATION

In the advent of fluorescence enzyme-based assays gaining popularity by being more sensitive and more specific, needing no radioactive compounds, health organizations have recommended that RAST be abandoned. Moreover, handling radioactivity is also very risky and cumbersome. As per NIH guidelines, it is abandoned since 2010. Modern day assays are automated procedures with minimum intervention by the technician. The assay procedures have retained the same basic steps as RAST. Allergen-specific IgE is bound to solid-phase allergen and the bound IgE is detected with labeled antihuman IgE. So, it can be said that these procedures are improved or advanced versions of RAST. The evolution of *in vitro* serological tests from manually handled radioimmunoassays to the modern day, third generation automated and quantitative allergen-specific IgE assays is discussed extensively in a review by Hamilton et al. (2004).

Component resolved diagnostics are the newer methods of testing specific allergenic molecules or components instead of the whole allergenic extracts. More than 130 such components are available for commercial testing at present and more are likely to be available in the future (Canonica et al., 2013). Such molecular diagnostics offer increased accuracy and help to resolve few key issues that are not taken care of by regular in-vitro specific IgE testing. They help to identify genuine sensitization to the primary allergen as compared to a positive test due to cross-reactivity or sensitization to a pan-allergen. Some of the components such as profillin are present in a wide variety of plant foods and pollens and can explain multiple sensitizations across seemingly unrelated pollens and foods. Similarly sensitizations to cross-reactive carbohydrate determinants (CCD's), which are the carbohydrate moieties of glycoproteins, which are present in a wide spectrum of plant foods. CCD sensitization actually explains a lot of positive in-vitro (specific IgE) positive tests for multiple foods in patients and even in normal subjects. On component resolved diagnostics it is observed that these multiple food sensitization in a patient is due to sensitization to a common component in all these foods, the CCD's. But CCD sensitization does not cause any clinical symptoms. Therefore, patients usually confirm that on consumption of these foods they do not have any clinical symptoms within two hours. They also help in a group of patients whether their sensitization can lead to severe systemic reactions or are they likely to cause only mild symptoms on exposure to the allergen, especially in patients with food allergy. For example, patients who show a positive serology for storage proteins, which are heat stable such as Ara h2 from peanut of Cor a9 from nuts are likely to have severe systemic reactions on exposure to the food, whereas some of the other components in the same food (Ara h8 from peanut) elicit only mild reactions. It can help in identifying the allergenic components for specific immunotherapy.

The component resolved diagnostics can be evaluated by singleplex (one assay per sample) or multiplex (multiple assays per sample) measurement platforms. Example for singleplex platform is ImmunoCAP and in the multiplex platform the classical one is the Immuno Solid-Phase Allergen Chip (ISAC) biochip technology measuring more than 100 components from 50 allergen sources in one sitting. In a singleplex platform the doctor can select the allergenic components to be tested based on the clinical history whereas in the multiplex platform the broad sensitization pattern of the patient to a predetermined set of allergenic components will be assessed. Multiplex platforms may be useful in the clinical setting of polysensitized patients with complex clinical history and symptoms. The interpretation of these systems must take into account the patient environment, exposure, temporal relation of exposure versus development of clinical symptoms and without clinical correlation these tests are not meaningful.

2.7.1 IMMUNOCAP TEST PRINCIPLE

The RAST methodology was brought into the market by Pharmacia Diagnostics AB, Uppsala, Sweden, under the brand name RAST in the year 1974 (Makhija and O'Gorman, 2012). In 1989, a superior version of RAST namely ImmunoCAP specific IgE blood test was introduced by the same company. The literature may describe this method as CAP RAST, CAP FEIA (Flurenzyme immunoassay) or Pharmacia CAP. Hence in the recent years, ImmunoCAP has taken over RAST as a technology that provides fast and accurate measurement of a patient's IgE levels, thus confirming the atopic condition of the subject (Lee et al., 2015).

ImmunoCAP uses cellulose as its solid phase with the following qualities:

- high binding capacity per mg of cellulose;
- hydrophilic and highly branched;
- binds the allergen covalently/irreversibly with their native structure intact.

This solid phase is similar to that of cellulose paper disk used in RAST, but has a three dimensional structure, thus increasing the surface area and binds three times more protein than the paper disk solid phase used in RAST (Bousquet et al., 1990).

The assay is designed as a sandwich immunoassay. Performance of the ImmunoCAP procedure (Figure 2.2) can be outlined as follows:

- Sera from the patients are allowed to react with the allergen/allergen component bound to the solid phase CNBr-activated cellulose enclosed in a capsule (CAP).

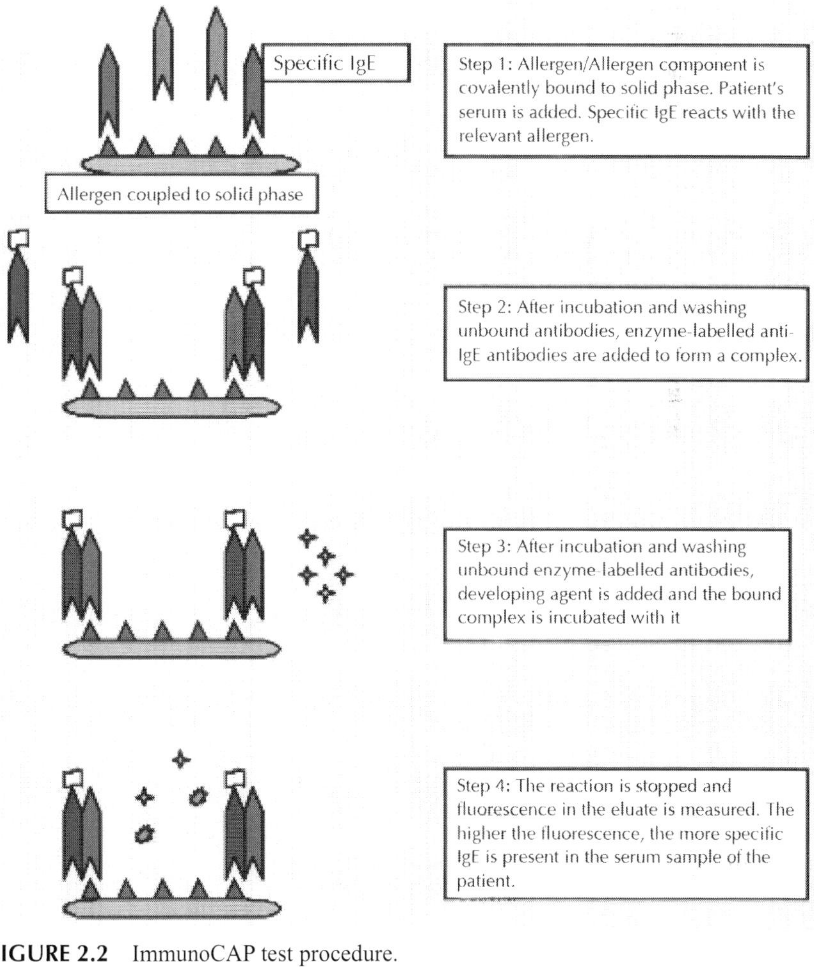

FIGURE 2.2 ImmunoCAP test procedure.

TABLE 2.2 ImmunoCAP Measurement and Score

Score	IgE level (kU/L)	Comment
0	<0.35	Absent or undetectable allergen specific IgE
1	0.35–0.69	Low level of allergen specific IgE
2	0.70–3.49	Moderate level of allergen specific IgE
3	3.50–17.49	High level of allergen specific IgE
4	17.50–49.99	Very high level of allergen specific IgE
5	50.00–100.00	Ultra high level of allergen specific IgE
6	>100.00	Extremely high level of allergen specific IgE

- Specific IgE antibodies in the patient's sera react with the allergen.
- Enzyme-linked anti-IgE antibodies are added after washing away unbound/non-specific IgE antibodies.
- The bound complex is then incubated with a developing agent and fluorescence is measured. Higher the fluorescence, higher the IgE production and higher the sensitivity of the patient towards that particular allergen.

The assay can be performed as a Radioimmunoassay (RIA) or a fluorimetric assay. The assay is calibrated against the WHO standard for IgE. Results are quantitatively expressed in kilounits per liter KU/L for both total and serum specific IgE. Range of measurement and score is the same as for RAST (Table 2.2) (Bousquet et al., 1990).

2.7.2 IMMUNOCAP ISAC TECHNIQUE

ImmnunoCAP immuno-solid-phase allergen chip (ISAC) (Figure 2.3) is a fluorescence-based immunossay, which allows measurement of IgE sensitivity to multiple allergens in a single test using only 20–30 μL of serum/plasma. Capillary blood sample may be used, making the procedure less invasive for infants and children. ImmunoCAP ISAC 112 platform is the only commercially available multiplexing diagnostic assay so far. It is based on the principle of microarray, a biochip based technology where purified and/or biotechnologically produced recombinant allergen/allergen components are immobilized on a solid support-microarray chip. It is a

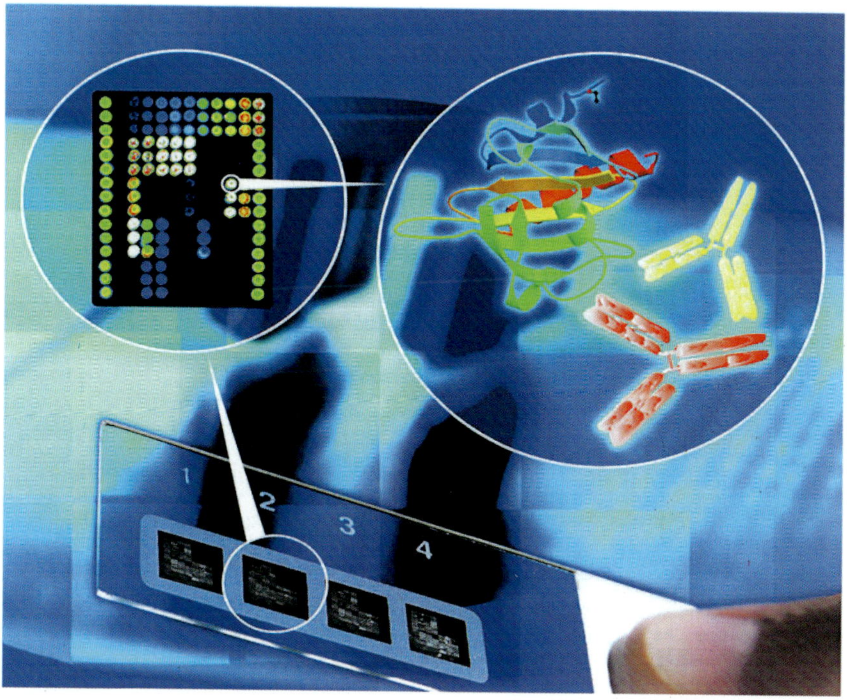

FIGURE 2.3 Immuno-solid-phase allergen chip (ISAC) (*Image courtesy:* Google images: http://leistungsverzeichnis.labor-gaertner.de/Entry/1866).

two-step procedure. In the first incubation step, IgE antibodies from the patient's serum bind to immobilized allergen components on the chip. In the second incubation step, the bound IgE antibodies are detected by fluorescence labeled anti-IgE antibody. Fluorescence is measured with a laser scanner. The total duration of the assay including incubation and washing is 4 hours.

With a broad spectrum of antigens (as many as 112 from 51 sources), one can easily generate the patient's IgE antibody profile. This cutting edge technology is particularly useful when the patient is multi-sensitized or the symptoms and case history are inconsistent or when response to an allergy treatment regimen is unsatisfactory. Test results are measured with biochip scanner and evaluated using appropriate software. This is a semi quantitative test and results are expressed as ISAC Standard Units (ISU). Categorization was done as per the manufacturer's instructions (Table 2.3) (Hamilton and Oppenheimer, 2015; Santosa et al., 2015).

TABLE 2.3 ISU and Categorization As Per Manufacturer's Instructions

Manufacturer's cutoff value (ISU)	Category
<0.3	Undetectable or very low
0.3–0.9	Low
1–14.9	Moderate/High
>=15	Very high

TABLE 2.4 Comparison of Common Modalities of Testing for Sensitization

Skin Prick test	ImmunoCAP	ISAC
Advantage: • High sensitivity • Good specificity • Immediate results	Advantage: • Automatic • Component resolved diagnostics possible • High sensitivity Low variation • Useful for monitoring sensitization	Advantage: • >100 components assessed in one assay • Even low levels of allergens can be detected
Disadvantage: • Lack of availability of standardized extracts • Only crude extracts are available • Not useful for monitoring	Disadvantage: • One allergen per assay • Expensive • Assays may not be suitable for local pollens and foods	Disadvantage: • Lower sensitivity than ImmunoCAP • More variation than ImmunoCAP • Not suitable for sensitization • Semiquantitative assay

The allergen components are spotted in triplicates and immobilized on a polymer-coated slide. Each slide contains four microarrays and can take four different samples (sera). The comparison between different diagnostic tests for sensitization are enumerated in Table 2.4.

2.8 SUMMARY

Skin prick tests and *in vitro* serological tests have their own importance in diagnosing and determining sensitization in patients. The traditional wheal and flare reaction elicited by SPTs is still considered the "gold standard" amongst diagnostic techniques for IgE due to extreme sensitivity. But the results are not quantitative. A detailed clinical history may give a picture of a patient's allergenicity, but may be sometimes unreliable. Similarly, the presence of IgE antibodies alone does not confirm an allergic disease state. The results have to be correlated with clinical symptoms that can be derived from a thorough clinical history. In case of food allergy cases, oral provocation tests are a must alongside serological tests. When there is a positive serological test and no clinical symptoms, it may be considered that the patient is tolerant or has high total serum IgE levels that cause non-specific interactions with the allergosorbent. Not to forget cross-reactivity by CCDs. On the other side, when there is a negative serological test and clinical symptoms exist with a strong positive clinical history, it may be considered that the specific IgE/total IgE ratio is high enough to elicit a mediator response or the result is due to missing allergen component in the crude allergen extract. IgE antibodies may not bind due to low specificity and high interference by competing IgG antibodies. It is at this point that we turn towards Molecular allergology, which involves component-based allergen testing, which takes care of cross-reactivity and IgG interference. *In vitro* serological tests have evolved and come a long way from the first ever diagnostic measurement assay called RAST in the late 1960s to an advanced automated version called ImmunoCAP in the 1990s and the latest version, the third generation multiplexing platform called the ISAC. As seen and understood, each method has its own advantages and disadvantages. We could conclude that a thorough clinical history, a record of recurring clinical symptoms, Provocation tests and confirmatory serological tests all go hand-in-hand in determining sensitization and subsequently, allergic disease condition. An allergy specialist is the best person to evaluate the test results and proceed to patient management and therapy.

Although MA diagnostics are gaining popularity, they have not reached out to most of the population in developing countries. Hence, both singleplex and multiplex assays have to be made cost-effective and reach out to as many allergy centers as possible. Data output from multiplex assays may seem complicated and hard to interpret. Allergists need to be trained to handle and comprehend the large amount of data generated by these assays so as to suggest a suitable treatment plan for the patient. Advantages like a small volume of blood sample and a broad-spectrum analysis of the patient's IgE antibody profile have made multiplex assays the method of choice for polysensitized individuals and children in whom food allergies are common. Despite all the hitches, multiplex assays are all set to become a standard tool of diagnosis in every allergist's clinic.

KEYWORDS

- **allergy**
- **asthma**
- **bronchial challenge**
- **histamine release test**
- **immunoCAP**
- **ISAC**
- **multiplex**
- **nasal challenge**
- **organ challenge**
- **sensitization**
- **singleplex**
- **skin prick test**

REFERENCES

Allergy testing in childhood: using allergen-specific IgE tests. *Pediatrics,* 129(1), 193–197. doi: 10.1542/peds.2011-2382.

Almogren, A., Shakoor, Z., Adam, M. H. Garlic and onion sensitization among Saudi patients screened for food allergy: a hospital based study. *Afr Health Sci,* 2013, 13(3), 689–693. doi: 10.4314/ahs.v13i3.24.

Asser, S., Hamburger, R. N. Allergy-important advances in clinical medicine: the radioallergosorbent test. *West J Med,* 1984, 141(4), 511.

Bergmann, K. C. Milestones in the 20th century. *Chem Immunol Allergy,* 2014, 100, 27–45. doi: 10.1159/000358478.

Bernstein, I. L., Storms, W. W. Practice parameters for allergy diagnostic testing. Joint Task Force on Practice Parameters for the Diagnosis and Treatment of Asthma. The American Academy of Allergy, Asthma and Immunology and the American College of Allergy, Asthma and Immunology. *Ann Allergy Asthma Immunol,* 1995, 75(6 Pt 2), 543–625.

Bousquet, J., Chanez, P., Chanal, I., Michel, F. B. Comparison between RAST and Pharmacia CAP system: a new automated specific IgE assay. *J Allergy Clin Immunol,* 1990,85(6), 1039–1043.

Bousquet, J., Heinzerling, L., Bachert, C., Papadopoulos, N. G., Bousquet, P. J., Burney, P. G., Practical guide to skin prick tests in allergy to aeroallergens. *Allergy,* 2012, 67(1), 18–24. doi: 10.1111/j.1398-9995.2011.02728.x.

Canonica, G. W., Ansotegui, I. J., Pawankar, R., Schmid-Grendelmeier, P., van Hage, M., Baena-Cagnani, C. E., Wao-Aria-Ga2Len Task Force: Katrina Allen, Riccardo Asero Barbara Bohle Linda Cox Frederic de Blay Motohiro Ebisawa Rene Maximiliano-Gomez Sandra Gonzalez-Diaz Tari Haahtela Stephen Holgate Thilo Jakob Mark Larche Paolo Maria Matricardi John Oppenheimer Lars K. Poulsen Harald E. Renz Nelson Rosario Marc Rothenberg Mario Sanchez-Borges Enrico Scala Rudolf Valenta. A WAO-ARIA-GA(2)LEN consensus document on molecular-based allergy diagnostics. *World Allergy Organ J,* 2013, 6(1), 17. doi: 10.1186/1939-4551-6-17.

Chodirker, W. B. The diagnosis of allergy: assays for specific IgE antibodies. *Can Med Assoc J,* 1985, 132(12), 1355–1357.

Dreborg, S., Agrell, B., Foucard, T., Kjellman, N. I., Koivikko, A., Nilsson, S. A double-blind, multicenter immunotherapy trial in children, using a purified and standardized Cladosporium herbarum preparation. I. Clinical results. *Allergy,* 1986, 41(2), 131–140.

Gleich, G. J., Yunginger, J. W. The radioallergosorbent test: a method to measure IgE antibodies, IgG blocking antibodies, and the potency of allergy extracts. *Bull N Y Acad Med,* 1981,57(7), 559–567.

Hamilton, R. G., Adkinson, N. F., Jr. Clinical laboratory assessment of IgE-dependent hypersensitivity. *J Allergy Clin Immunol,* 2003, 111(2 Suppl), S687–701.

Hamilton, R. G., Franklin Adkinson, N., Jr. In vitro assays for the diagnosis of IgE-mediated disorders. *J Allergy Clin Immunol,* 2004, 114(2), 213–225; quiz 226.

Hamilton, R. G., Oppenheimer, J. Serological IgE Analyses in the Diagnostic Algorithm for Allergic Disease. *J Allergy Clin Immunol Pract,* 2015, 3(6), 833–840. doi: 10.1016/j.jaip.2015.08.016.

Heinzerling, L., Mari, A., Bergmann, K. C., Bresciani, M., Burbach, G., Darsow, U., Lockey, R. The skin prick test—European standards. *Clin Transl Allergy,* 2013, 3(1), 3. doi: 10.1186/2045-7022-3-3.

Lee, J. H., Park, H. J., Park, K. H., Jeong, K. Y., Park, J. W. Performance of the PROTIA Allergy-Q(R) System in the Detection of Allergen-Specific IgE: A Comparison With the ImmunoCAP(R) System. *Allergy Asthma Immunol Res,* 2015, 7(6), 565–572. doi: 10.4168/aair.2015.7.6.565.

Lockey, R. F., Benedict, L. M., Turkeltaub, P. C., Bukantz, S. C. Fatalities from immunotherapy (IT) and skin testing (ST). *J Allergy Clin Immunol,* 1987, 79(4), 660–677.

Makhija, M., O'Gorman, M. R. Chapter 31: Common *in vitro* tests for allergy and immunology. *Allergy Asthma Proc,* 2012, 33 *Suppl* 1, S108–111. doi: 10.2500/aap.2012.33.3564.

Perry, T. T., Matsui, E. C., Kay Conover-Walker, M., Wood, R. A. The relationship of allergen-specific IgE levels and oral food challenge outcome. *J Allergy Clin Immunol,* 2004, 114(1), 144–149. doi: 10.1016/j.jaci.2004.04.009.

Rueff, F., Przybilla, B., Bilo, M. B., Muller, U., Scheipl, F., Aberer, W., Wuthrich, B. Predictors of severe systemic anaphylactic reactions in patients with Hymenoptera venom allergy: importance of baseline serum tryptase—a study of the European Academy of Allergology and Clinical Immunology Interest Group on Insect Venom Hypersensitivity. *J Allergy Clin Immunol,* 2009, 124(5), 1047–1054. doi: 10.1016/j.jaci.2009.08.027.

Sampson, H. A., Ho, D. G. Relationship between food-specific IgE concentrations and the risk of positive food challenges in children and adolescents. *J Allergy Clin Immunol,* 1997, 100(4), 444–451.

Santosa, A., Andiappan, A. K., Rotzschke, O., Wong, H. C., Chang, A., Bigliardi-Qi, M., Bigliardi, P. L. Evaluation of the applicability of the Immuno-solid-phase allergen chip (ISAC) assay in atopic patients in Singapore. *Clin Transl Allergy,* 2015, 5, 9. doi: 10.1186/s13601-015-0053-z.

Sicherer, S. H., Wood, R. A., American Academy of Pediatrics Section on Allergy and Immunology, 2012.

Wahyuni, S., Van Ree, R., Mangali, A., Supali, T., Yazdanbakhsh, M., Sartono, E. Comparison of an enzyme linked immunosorbent assay (ELISA) and a radioallergosorbent test (RAST) for detection of IgE antibodies to Brugia malayi. *Parasite Immunol,* 2003, 25(11–12), 609–614. doi: 10.1111/j.0141-9838.2004.00673.x.

Wide, L., Bennich, H., Johansson, S. G. Diagnosis of allergy by an in-vitro test for allergen antibodies. *Lancet,* 1967, 2(7526), 1105–1107.

PART II

AEROBIOLOGY AND ALLERGIC DISEASES

CHAPTER 3

AEROBIOLOGY ASSOCIATED WITH ALLERGY

A. B. SINGH and CHANDNI MATHUR

CSIR-Institute of Genomics and Integrative Biology, Delhi University Campus, Delhi –110007, India

CONTENTS

3.1 INTRODUCTION

Pollen grains are amongst the earliest known aeroallergens and are found to be the major cause of bronchial asthma and allergic rhinitis. Seasonal Allergic Rhino conjunctivitis is an important condition afflicting increasing number of individuals. Pollen from trees, weeds and grasses are generally the most common aeroallergens. The information on pollen count can be an important tool in the management of seasonal allergic disease as it alerts the patient to the need to commence effective and preventive treatment.

Respiratory allergy is prevalent among all populations with increasing trend all over the world. However, development of civilization often at the expense of the natural environment by pollution or biopollution stimulates the appearance of new health problems, besides increase in allergic diseases. India, with the teaming population of more than one and half billion and with the divergent geographical backdrop ranging from upland plain (Deccan Plateau) in south, flat to rolling plain along the Ganges, deserts in west, Himalayas in north, has a rich aerobiological diversity. This diversity is further enhanced with the climate, which varies from tropical monsoon in south to temperate in north. The latter part of the 20th century has seen an increase in the prevalence of allergic diseases, implicating changing environment and lifestyle as significant causes. With the alarming increase in allergic disorders, such as allergic rhinitis, bronchial asthma and atopic dermatitis covering as high as 30% of the population world over, there is an increasing interest in the presence and movement of bioparticulate matters in the earth's atmosphere and their impact on human health. This interdisciplinary approach is known as aerobiology. The bioparticulates implicated to cause allergic symptoms are pollen grains, fungal spores, insect debris, house dust mites, animal dander, chemicals and foods, etc. (Kino and Oshima, 1978; Gravesen, 1979; Kang et al., 1979; Shivpuri, 1980; Salvaggio and Aukrust, 1981; Peterson et al., 1983; Lacey and Crook, 1988; Loureiro et al., 2005; Singh and Chandni, 2012). Among all these agents, pollen grains and fungal spores are the most predominant allergens in the air. However, for the effective diagnosis and therapeutic management of these ailments, a detailed information on the daily, seasonal and annual variations of various bioparticles is essential (Singh and Singh, 1994).

3.2 HISTORICAL PERSPECTIVE

Pollen grains as aeroallergen are well studied from across the world and are important cause of allergy. Respiratory system is the direct target organ of airborne pollen taken in by inhalation. This result in immediate hypersensitivity disorders, in genetically predisposed individuals and late hypersensitivity in others causing clinical manifestations of allergic rhinitis, allergic alveolitis, asthma, atopic dermatitis etc. John Bostock (1819) was the first to suspect pollen as the cause of hayfever (allergic rhinitis). Later Blackley (1873) established that grasses are important cause of hay fever in U.K. After more than 40 years, Scheppegrell (1916) from U.S.A., felt the need for field exploration and aerial surveys to record aeroallergens from the atmosphere. Subsequent studies from all over the world-established pollen grains as the major causative agent for respiratory allergic disorders (Feinber, 1946; Naranjo, 1958; Shivpuri et al., 1960; Leuschner, 1974; Lewis, 1984; Singh and Singh, 1994; Groenewoud et al., 2002; Rawat et al., 2004; Masuda et al., 2006; Singh and Chandni, 2012).

Although pollen have been widely studied as aeroallergens throughout the world, far less is known about the fungal aerosols, which are present in much higher concentration than the pollen grains in air. The fungi that produce spores and get airborne are called 'aerospores.' These are implicated in the causation of allergic diseases and infections in immunocompromised patients. They are established to cause Type I hypersensitive diseases with IgE mediated response. The common symptoms of hypersensitivity are bronchial asthma, allergic rhinitis and atopic dermatitis. The first case of fungal sensitivity was reported as early as 1726 (Floyer, 1726). More than a century later, Blackley also suggested the association of species of *Chaetomium* and *Penicillium* with attacks of bronchial catarrh (Blackley, 1873). Feinberg reported respiratory allergic reactions to fungi in his patients and attributed outdoor environment as a source of fungi (Feinberg, 1935). With the studies establishing the role of fungal spores as a major causative agent for the respiratory allergic disorders (Shivpuri et al., 1960; Nilsson et al., 1977; Lewis, 1984; Lugauskas et al., 2004), the seasonal and annual variations in the bioaerosols have been extensively studied in different parts of the world including India (Al-Doory et al., 1982; Ren et al., 1999; Burch and Levetin, 2002; Singh and Deval, 2005; Sharma and Singh,

2005, Sharma et al., 2011). Their knowledge is of paramount importance for diagnosis and therapeutic management of allergic diseases.

3.3 SOURCE OF BIOALLERGENS

3.3.1 POLLEN ALLERGENS

The transport of pollen grains by wind or by the insects, from floral anther to recipient stigma is the critical reproductive event among higher plants. The dispersion of replicate units in massive abundance assures the success of wind pollination as well as its human health effects including asthma, rhinitis, atopic dermatitis, etc. Pollen prevalence (grains per cubic meter) at any point reflects (plant) source strength and location as well as the dynamics of the intervening environment conditions such as climatic factors, pollution and degree of exposure. The presence of pollen, profile of species, concentration, etc. depends on various climatic factors such as temperature, humidity, wind direction, sunshine, substrate precipitation and other seasonal factors. Because of change in the climatic conditions, the study of variations in the diurnal and seasonal prevalence becomes very important (D'Amato et al., 2002).

3.3.2 FUNGAL ALLERGENS

Fungi possess highly evolved mechanism of spore liberation due to which the spores remain suspended in the air for a varying duration, i.e., few hours to several days. Fungi and fungal particles can clearly induce an allergic response in susceptible individuals. Typical symptoms include wheezing, cough, rhinorrhea, itchy nose, sore throat, sinus congestion, etc. (Beaumont et al., 1984; Palmas et al., 1989). The development of allergies to fungi follows the same biological phenomenon as allergies to other environmental allergens. Dead fungi are able to produce symptoms just as well as live fungi (Rose, 1999). Hayward and coworkers reported a separation and characterization of antibodies to moulds in human sera and the role of human precipitins to common fungal antigens in allergic reaction, which was later proved by Pepys (Hayward et al., 1960; Pepys, 1960).

3.3.3 MONITORING AIRBORNE ALLERGENS

Knowledge about diurnal, seasonal and annual variations in airborne pollen and fungal spores in any geographical area are essential for effective diagnosis and treatment of allergic disorders. Aerobiological sampling is therefore carried out to achieve this aim through various sampling devices currently used for monitoring bioparticulates in the air.

The recognition of aeroallergens is divided into two phases: (1) collection of material, and (2) sample analysis (Solomon, 1984).

Different methods employed to achieve the objectives generally exploit the following basic regimes of collection:

1. fall out on a fixed surface through gravitational force;
2. impaction on a rapidly moving surface;
3. impaction through suction of air;
4. filtration;
5. immunochemical assays.

For analysis of data three procedures are followed:

1. microscopic enumeration of individual particles;
2. counting and identification of colonies produced in culture or semisolid media;
3. immunochemical assays for bulk aeroallergens.

3.4 SAMPLING DEVICES

Monitoring of airborne biological particles is carried out by various gravimetric, impaction, and filtration sampling devices (Durham, 1946; Hirst, 1952; Perkins, 1957). In addition, new immunochemical techniques are also used for detecting allergenic pollen and measuring of the size of allergen-carrying particles (Sen et al., 2003).

3.4.1 GRAVIMETRIC SAMPLER

This is based on the principle that bioparticulates settle down on a surface due to gravitational force. The Durham gravity-sampling device (Durham, 1946) consists of two horizontal disks with a diameter of 22.1 cm and 8.1

cm. The upper disc protects the slide from rain and sun. The slides are exposed daily, at a fixed hour, coated with adhesive glycerin jelly. After exposure, the slides are mounted in a drop of molten glycerin jelly, for various allergen types trapped.

It does not give diurnal variation and is dependent on wind velocity. Even in still air the number of large particles collected on the surface are overestimated and smaller particles that have a slower settling velocity are under estimated.

However, this sampler is no more choice of aerobiologists in developed world, but developing countries still report the use of gravity settlement method for pollen and fungal spores/colonies.

3.4.2 IMPACTION SAMPLER

3.4.2.1 Rotorod Sampler

Rotorod sampler developed by Perkins (1951) has leucite rods of 1–3 mm coated with adhesive silicon grease are used to collect air borne particles. It is a lightweight portable sampler operated by DC power. The exposure time can be adjusted according to requirement. There are three models available in the Rotorod Aeroallergen Models (40 s, 85 s and 95 s) and the pollen/spore catch obtained by these three models is almost similar. These three samplers are used to study both pollen and fungal spore types on continuous basis (Figure 3.1).

3.4.3 SUCTION SAMPLERS

The method requires suction of certain volume of air according to a known velocity and for a chosen duration on trapping.

3.4.3.1 Hirst Trap

The Hirst spore trap was most commonly used in UK. In this trap bioparticulates adhere to slides coated with glycerin jelly and slides are replaced

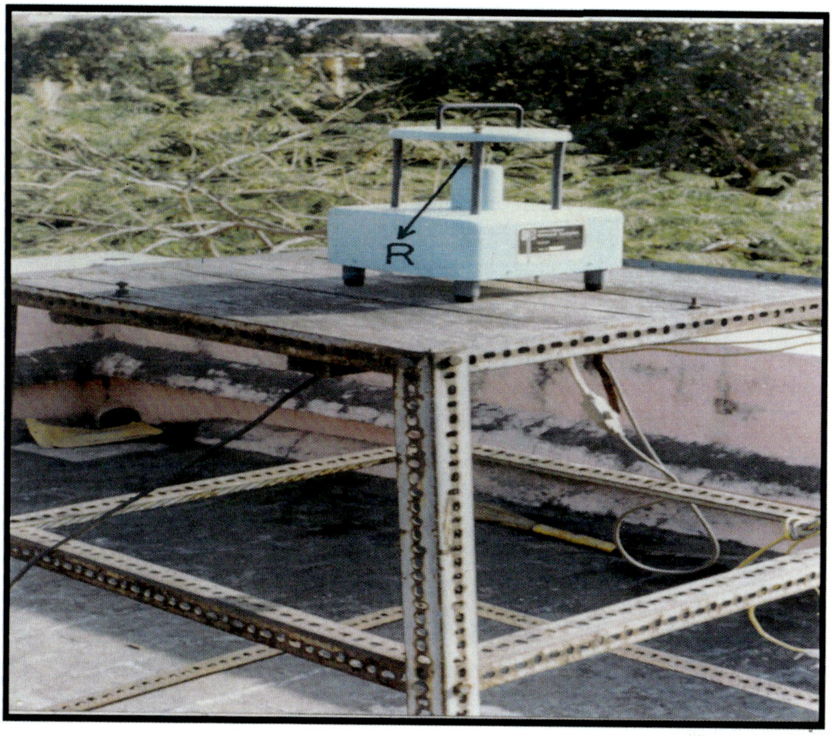

FIGURE 3.1 Rotorod Sampler (Aeroallergen Model 40s) placed at the terrace of Institute of Genomics and Integrative Biology for continuous monitoring of aeroallergens.

each day with fresh slides and provides quantitative data. The method requires suction of certain volume of air according to a known velocity and for a chosen duration on trapping. It records the atmospheric concentration of pollen grains, fungal spores, and other biological particles as a function of time through morphological identification.

3.4.3.2 Burkard Seven Day Volumetric Sampler

The Hirst trap was later modified to Burkard trap in which slides were replaced with a drum, which can rotate and run continuously for seven days with a definite speed with suction rate of 10 L of air per minute (Figure 3.2). Adhesive coated tape mounted is used in on a rotating

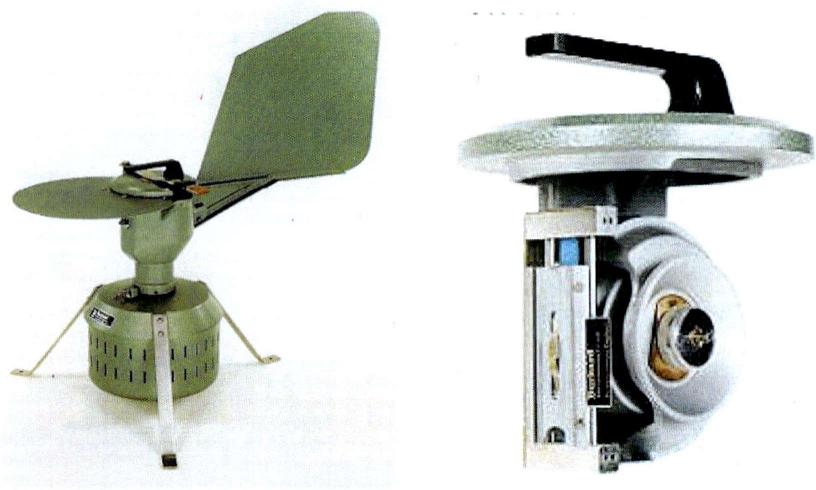

FIGURE 3.2 Burkard Seven Day Volumetric Sampler for studying diurnal, seasonal and annual trends for fungal spores as well as pollen grains.

drum Burkard continuous seven days sampler. The drum is connected to a timer and rotated at constant speed. The tape is changed every seven days. Exposed tape is cut in seven strips corresponding to seven days and mounted on a micro slide. This is one of the most widely used samplers to study diurnal or seasonal trends for pollen grains as well as fungal spores all over the world.

3.4.3.3 Burkard Portable (Slide) Sampler

Burkard slide sampler is a compact battery operated sampler. It has a rectangular orifice at the top end and a slit on the slide to insert microslide (Figure 3.3). The microslide is coated with glycerin jelly. The sampler sucks in 10 L of air per minute. The particles get impacted on the slide in the form of a streak. The slide is then mounted in glycerin jelly and scanned for pollen grains/fungal spores count under research microscope with high resolution.

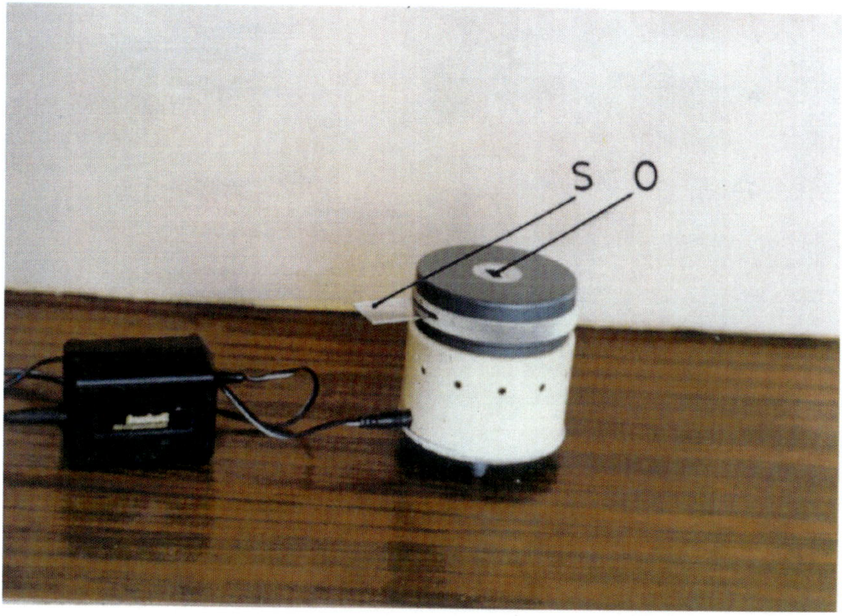

FIGURE 3.3 Burkard Slide Sampler with inserted slide (S) coated with glycerine jelly on which the pollen and fungal spores get impacted through the orifice (O) for spot sampling.

3.4.3.4 Burkard Portable (Petriplate) Sampler

The Burkard Petriplate Sampler is similar to slide sampler except that it has a stage to hold the Petriplate and a sieve to cover the petriplate and on top a lid to cover the sieve. On the cover is a circular opening from where the air is sucked in at the rate of 10 liters per minute (Figure 3.4). These samplers are most convenient for outdoor and spot sampling and places where power connection is not available.

3.4.3.5 Andersen Volumetric Sampler

The best device to obtain culturable fungal spore count is the Andersen Volumetric Sampler. It has 2 stage to 8 stage sampler (Figure 3.5). It uses petriplates in which media is kept under different sieve size present in decreasing order of pore size. Each sieve has 400 pores. The sampler

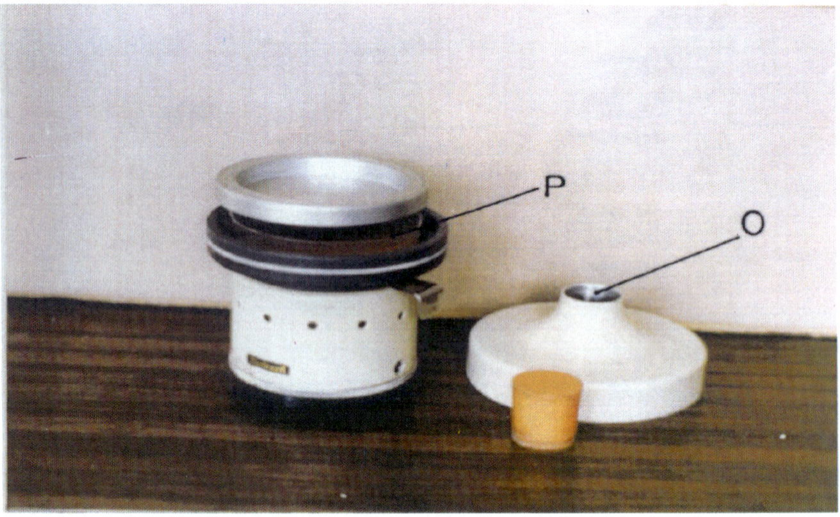

FIGURE 3.4 Burkard Petriplate Sampler shown with a stage to hold the petriplate (P) containing nutrient media along with a sieve and a lid with an orifice (O) for fungal sampling (colony forming units).

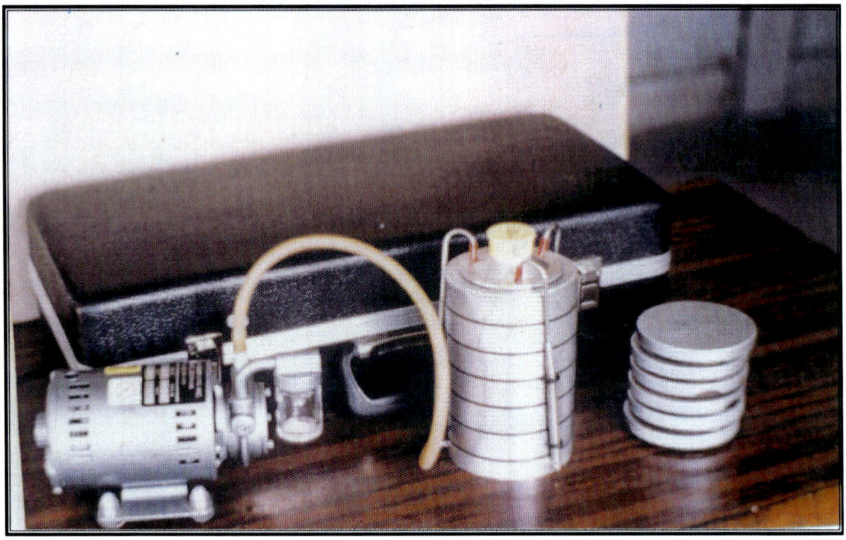

FIGURE 3.5 Andersen Six Stage Volumetric Sampler with six petriplates kept under decreasing pore size of sieves for quantitative assessment of culturable fungi.

sucks in 28.3 L of air per minute. The air passes from the orifice to all the six petriplates before passing out. The particles of similar aerodynamic dimensions are impinged on the same plate. The two stage Andersen Sampler is quiet efficient and less time consuming in number of plates to be examined after exposure.

3.4.3.6 Air-O-Cell Cassette

Air sampling cassette is a device for rapid collection and identification of wide range of airborne aerosols. The principle of the sampler is similar to that of Burkard Portable Sampler. The device is made up of plastic with two cells, namely upper cell and lower cell. The sampler can be run for 5–10 minutes indoor at the suction rate of 5-L air per minute. After the sampling, the seal can be broken and the glass strip (trace) with the sample deposited is mounted in a clean glass slide with a suitable mountant. The slide can be scanned directly under the microscope. With this sampler the total spore in the aerosol can be counted. The quality and quantity of airspores within indoors can be determined. In this species level identification is not feasible.

3.5 LIQUID IMPINGER SAMPLER

In this, the airborne spores are sucked in and suspended in a liquid in the sampler. The suction of the sampler enhances the airborne particles to get in to the flask, which contains sterile water. The suspended particles get dispersed into the liquid and further the liquid can be diluted and studied for the culturable molds using suitable medium. The multistage liquid impinger was devised to separate the collected particles into three fractions corresponding to the size in the upper respiratory tract, bronchi and bronchioles. In this sampler fungal spores can be identified upto species levels. Every principle for separating particle from air, from sedimentation, filtration, internal impaction, impingement in liquids, to thermal and electrical precipitation, has been applied to the collection of microorganisms. Changes in aerosol concentration with time can be followed with the rotation slit or slit-to-agar sampler in which a large petridish of medium is placed on a turntable beneath a stationary slit inlet.

3.6 IMMUNOCHEMICAL ASSAYS

The immunochemical assays for airborne allergens relied on large (e.g., 20 x 25 cm^2) fiber glass filters exposed for 24-hr period in high volume sampler. They are rated for continuous operation and adapted to receive filter support. Hivolume devices are developed to study total suspended particles and devices are operated traditionally with filters surface directed upwards. In a study carried out in Arizona, variability of allergen shedding of airborne cat allergen was carried out by Immunochemical assay. Cats were placed in a lucite chamber with an air sampler attached. Radioallergosorbent (RAST)/Enzyme Linked Immuno Sorbent Assay (ELISA) inhibition type and monoclonal two-site radioimmunosurveys (RIAs) are used to express air concentrations in allergy units (AU) (Chris et al., 1990).

3.7 ANALYSIS OF BIOAEROSOLS

Regardless of their method of collection, samples of mixed biologic aerosols are analyzed by one of the following techniques

3.7.1 DIRECT MICROSCOPY (SLIDES)

The microscopic identification of distinctive particles (pollen/fungi)is an approach validated by years of practical applications of both gravimetric and volumetric samplers. The exposed slides are examined directly by microscope because a variety of particles, including pollen grains, certain basidiospores, ascospores and spores of rust, smuts and downy mildew are recognizable but fails to grow on most laboratory media. The particles/spores are identified based on their characteristics such as shape, size and other morphological features of spores. Therefore, it is a most dependable way to identify most of the pollen/fungal spores.

3.7.2 *CULTURE ANALYSIS (PETRIPLATES)*

This includes the tally of colonies produced in culture or semisolid media. In this the petriplates exposed for sampling are incubated at appropriate temperature (28–30°C) and impacted spores are allowed to grow for a couple of days till colonies start forming. The colonies are identified based on their colony characteristics such as color, shape and other morphological features of the mycelia and spores to the lowest taxonomic rank possible. Each colony represents one spore and considered colony-forming unit (CFU). In addition, different atlases and literature can also be used for authentic identification.

3.7.2.1 Analysis of Data

After suspended particles have been collected on the slide or in a suitable medium, these particles can then be counted and identified. Scientists looking for non-viable particles also used the techniques to extract viable cells and particles carrying them from the air. The most efficient methods of removing suspended particles from the air, example, filtration through fine pore matrices, might be adequate for resistant forms of microorganisms, such as spores, but can be less damaged environmentally resistant vegetative cells. The absence of these sensitive cells from a sample could cause one to mistakenly conclude, thus, they were not present in the environment sampled. The total number of cells present can be estimated by microscopic examination, sometimes with the help of stains or fluorescent tags.

The concentration of pollen/fungal bioparticles are calculated as per the formula given below:

$$\frac{\textbf{Total number of pollen grains/fungal spores}}{\textbf{Total volume of air sampled}} \times \mathbf{1000}$$

The counts are expressed as number of pollen grains/m^3 or colony-forming units (CFU/m^3) as the case may be.

3.7.3 *IMMUNOASSAY*

Immunochemical analysis following descending elution, exposed from filters offers an analytic approach to dust without potential or defined form (e.g., fungi, pollen, dander, seed pomace, arthropod effluvia, etc.). If micronic aerosols do carry pollen allergens, these fractions are also accessible to immunoassay in bulk samples obtained by high vacuum filtration. ELISA base procedures are followed. One advantage in immunoassay for airborne microorganisms is that the amount of materials needed to measure the concentration of viable air contaminants is much lower than that needed to gravimetrically quantitate nonviable particles where only one or a cluster of cell lands on an appropriate solid nutrient medium, or lawn of host cells, a microscopic fungal or bacterial colony, or viral plaque, will develop. These isolates can then be identified specifically using tests of biochemical and immunological reactions conducted on sub cultures of the original material. The researcher, therefore, is not limited to the original amount of the sample but can culture as much material as is needed for the various tests used for identification. The limitations are that a considerable experience is needed to identify particles by their morphology and to distinguish them from debris, and labeled antibodies for only a few clinically important microorganisms are readily available.

3.8 AEROBIOLOGICAL SURVEYS

3.8.1 POLLEN SURVEYS

Airborne pollen and their concentration vary in the different seasons depending upon the flowering seasons and climatic factors, which are quite variable in different geographical regions of the world.

Durham initiated pollen survey in the U.S.A. in 1925. Later, the sampler devised by him (1926) was adopted by the American Academy of Allergy, as a tool to identify airborne particles. In Colarado, pollen patterns were compared between Vail, (8,200 feet elevation), Aspen, (7,900 feet) and Denver, (5,280 feet) from 1984 through 1988. While counts were generally lower in the mountain sites than Denver, certain pollen, especially trees, were quite high. Ragweed was essentially absent from Aspen and Vail, and chenopod-amaranth counts were very low. Cedar, pine, at Aspen frequently pollinated despite active snowfall (Silvers et al., 1992). In U.S.A., most of the investigators have recorded Poaceae,

Ambrosia, *Quercus*, Chenopodiaceae, Amaranthaceae, Pinaceae, Plantaginaceae, *Artemisia*, *Xanthium* as important consistuents of the atmosphere (Anderson et al., 1978; Al-Doory et al., 1982; Ellis and Gallup, 1989). The frequently encounterd pollen at Canada are *Acer*, *Abies*, *Artemisia*, *Populus*, *Betula*, *Quercus*, *Rumex* and *Salix* (Bassett, 1964; Collins – Williams et al., 1973; Bassett et al., 1978). A study at New Jersey-New York City area established that pollen levels have declined from 1993 to the present. The most pronounced drop has been in weed pollen levels. Grass pollen demonstrates a biphasic pattern. Tree pollen composes most annual pollen measured. (Port et al., 2006).

Aerobiological survey was initiated at Cardiff by Hyde and Williams (1944), which was later extended to several other stations in Great Britain. Based on the data, Hyde published an atlas of airborne pollen grains of the U.K. (Hyde and Adams, 1958; Hyde, 1969). The dominant pollen types recorded from the UK are *Alnus*, *Artemisia*, *Betula*, *Corylus*, *Quercus*, *Fagus*, *Pinus*, graminae and others (Davies and Smith, 1973; Mullins et al., 1977; Emberlin et al., 1990). Emberlin (1990) analyzed the annual variation in grass pollen in London during 1961–1990. In Montreal (Quebec, Canada), the influence of meteorological factors on *Ambrosia* pollen concentrations was evaluated between 1994 and 2002 and its adequate monitoring was considered critical (Breton et al., 2006).

In France, studies carried out at Montpellier, Marseilles and Paris, Lyon have shown Chenopodiaceae, Compositae, Cupressaceae, *Pinus*, *Plantain*, Poaceae, *Alnus*, *Betula*, *Quercus* as the pollen species encountered in large numbers (Charpin et al., 1966; Michel et al., 1976). Another important center was Switzerland, where Leuschner (1974) had carried out survey using individual pollen collectors attached to human body, found *Aesculus*, *Artemisia* and *Salix* as important pollen contributors in the atmosphere of Basel.

Survey carried out at Darmstadt, Germany revealed that 70% of the total pollen catch consisted of birch, grasses, nettle, oak and pine (Stix, 1977). As a result of the five-year survey in the Netherlands, Spieksma (1986) demonstrated that in summer 95% of the pollen catch were of weeds namely *Artemisia*, Chenopodiaceae, *Plantago*, *Rumex* and *Urtica*.

Sweden is an important centre for aeropalynological studies. The most abundantly encountered pollen types are *Pinus*, *Betula*, *Urtica*, *Ulmus*, *Quercus*, Poaceae, *Alnus* and some others (Kotzmanidou and Nilsson, 1977; Hjelmroos, 1992; El-Ghazaly et al., 1993). Extensive studies on the airborn pollen and the mode of sampling has been carried out by Kapyla (1984) in Finland, with *Artemisia*, *Betula*, Pinus, Poaceae and *Urtica* being the dominant species. In the air of Denmark, the important pollen contributing species are *Alnus*, *Artemisia*, *Betula*, *Corylus*, Poaceae and *Ulmus* (Goldberg et al., 1988). In Norway, Faegri did pioneering work concerning pollen deposition in the 1940's. The dominant species were *Oxyria digna*, *Salix*, *Betula*, Poaceae, Pinus, *Castanea*, *Corylus*, *Alnus* and *Artemisia* (Johansen, 1991; Ramfjord, 1991). In western Ligurian coast of Italy, a 10-year survey of pollen counts was performed. Over the period a significant increase in the pollen counts was seen for birch and Compositae ($p = 0.001$) (Panzani et al., 1999).

Reports from other European countries like Israel, Portugal, Yugoslavis and Spain revealed that the significant pollen contributors to the atmosphere are *Alnus*, Cheno/Amaranth, *Corylus*, Cupressus, *Morus*, *Olea*, *Pinus*, poaceae, *Populus*, *Quercus* and *Taxus* (Kantoor et al., 1966; Galan et al., 1989; Belmonte and Roure, 1991). In a continuous two year aeropalynological survey of the atmosphere of Bitlis, (Turkey) Gramineae, Urticaceae, *Juglans* spp., *Quercus* spp., Umbellifereae, Cupressaceae/Taxaceae, *Fraxinus* spp., *Salix* spp., *Plantago* spp., *Pinus* spp., *Rumex* spp., *Moraceae* and Chenopodiaceae/Amaranthaceae were responsible for the high amounts of pollen in the investigated region. 58.38 % of total pollen grains were appeared during May and June (Celenk et al., 2005). A 10-year volumetric aerobiologic study was conducted in the city of Heraklion, located in the center of the north-shore of the island of Crete, Greece, main allergenic families and genera encountered in descending order of frequency were, Oleaceae, *Quercus*, Platanaceae, Cupressaceae, Pinaceae, *Populus*, Moraceae, and Corylaceae (Gonianakis et al., 2006). Airborne allergenic pollen spectrum analyzed over a 20-year survey at Trento, Italy recorded taxa like Urticaceae, Graminaceae, Ostyra species and Cupressaceae as highest contributors (Cristofori et al., 2010).

In South Africa, the important pollen types identified in air are *Acacia*, Compositae, *Cupressus, Eucalyptus,* Graminae, *Ligustrum* and *Prosopis* (Ordman, 1970). Latter studies revealed that the airspora mainly comprises *Morus*, *Cannabis*, Poaceae, *Celtis*, *Cynodon*, Compositae, *Pinus*, Asteraceae and Fabaceae (Hawke and Meadows, 1989; Cadman, 1990; Cadman and Dames, 1993).

In Australia, Mercer (1941) had carried out pollen count in Adelaide. The major pollen contributors to the environment were *Casuarina*, grasses, Myrtaceae, *Pinus*, *Plantago*, *Populus*, *Quercus* and few other (Derrick, 1965; Moss 1965). Smart and Knox (1979) had shown that *Lolium* and *Phalaris* are the major sources of atmospheric pollen in Australia. In a recent study at Sydney, of the total airborne pollen, tree pollen comprised 65% of total pollen concentrations, weeds and herbs 11%, grasses 18%, and unidentified pollen (termed other) 6% (Hart et al., 2007).

In Japan, pollen survey started in the 1960's. The most important being Japanese cedar followed by pine (Higuchi et al., 1977; Ishizaka et al., 1987). Chen and Huang (1980) observed that in Taiwan the tree species contribute 56 percent of the total pollen count. *Artemisia*, Casuarinaceae, Euphorbiaceae, Graminae, Moraceae and Pinaceae are the major contributors to the atmosphere of China (Chen and Zhang, 1985; Chen et al., 1988). The important pollen types from West Asia are Gramineae, Chenopodiaceae/Amaranthaceae, Cyperaceae, Pinaceae, Plantaginaceae, *Acer*, *Cupressus*, *Morus*, Poaceae, *Populus*, *Pinus* and others (Saad 1959; Ozkargoz, 1967; Shafiee 1976; Ritchie 1986; Ghazaly and Fawzy, 1988).A revised pollen calendar of South Korea has reported Pine,Oak,Birch.ragweed, Japanese Cedar, Alder,Japanese hop and Mugwort to be densely distributed in different parts of the country (Oh et al., 2012).

Date-Palm trees (*Phoenix dactylifera* L.) are the most abundant crops in the United Arab Emirates (UAE). Pollen counts were about 800 counts/m^3 within the Date-Palm farms and decreased by about 80% just 100 meters away from the farm area and almost diminished beyond 200 meters (Almehdi et al., 2005). Thus the locals handling the tree products are at greater risk of exposure.

3.8.1.1 Pollen Survey in India

In India, first atmospheric survey was initiated in Calcutta by Cunningham (1873). Since then, researchers, all over India have conducted exhaustive studies on airborne pollen types and their concentration. In an All India Coordinated Project on Aeroallergens and Human Health sponsored by the Ministry of Environment and Forests, Govt. of India, was successfully completed by Singh and his colleagues (Anonymous, 2000). Important pollen and fungal allergens from 18 different places have been identified, quantified and characterized for their allergenic properties. This provides the most scientific and up-to-date information on aeroallergens in India. Altogether, 43 types of pollen have been recorded from Northern India. The dominant types are: *Artemesia*, Asteraceae, *Cassia, Casuarina, Cedrus, Eucalyptus, Holoptelea*, *Morus, Pinus,* Poaceae, *Putranjiva*, *Quercus* and *Xanthium* are other important contributors in the air (Anonymous, 2000; Singh and Kumar, 2202; Singh and Chandni 2012).

In an aerobiological survey from Delhi, ninety-four pollen types were recorded and the major contributors included *Morus*, *Cannabis*, Cheno-pod/Amaranth, *Prosopis*, *Artemisia*, and *Eucalyptus* (Singh et al., 2003). A significant reduction in pollen concentration was observed in subsequent years (Figure 3.6). The concentration of *Morus*, *Cannabis*, *Prosopis*, and *Artemisia* pollen decreased considerably (Figures 3.7–3.8). It is suggested that the reduction in pollen numbers from 1990 to 1997 in Delhi is due to massive clearing of vegetation for developmental activities of the city.

From Central India, surveys carried out at Bombay, Gwalior, Nagpur, Bhopal and Kolhapur revealed that the dominant pollen types are from the Poaceae, Asteraceae, Apocynaceae, *Rosa*, *Ricinus*, *Ailanthus*, *Holoptelea*, *Cyperus*, *Cicer*, *Argemone*, *Cocos nucifera* and *Hibiscus* (Anonymous, 2000; Singh and Kumar, 2002). Pollen survey (Anonymous, 1998) at Pune revealed *Parthenium* to be the highest contributor to the pollen load with two peak seasons, i.e., from September to November and January to April. *Cocos* and *Cassia* were observed throughout the year. *Cocos* pollen were recorded in high concentration in April–May and November–December.

In West Bengal, 59 types pollen were revealed from air - their maxi-mum concentration was recorded in May. Important dominant types are *Areca catechu*, Asteraceae, Chenopodiaceae, *Cocos, Pongamia, Trema*

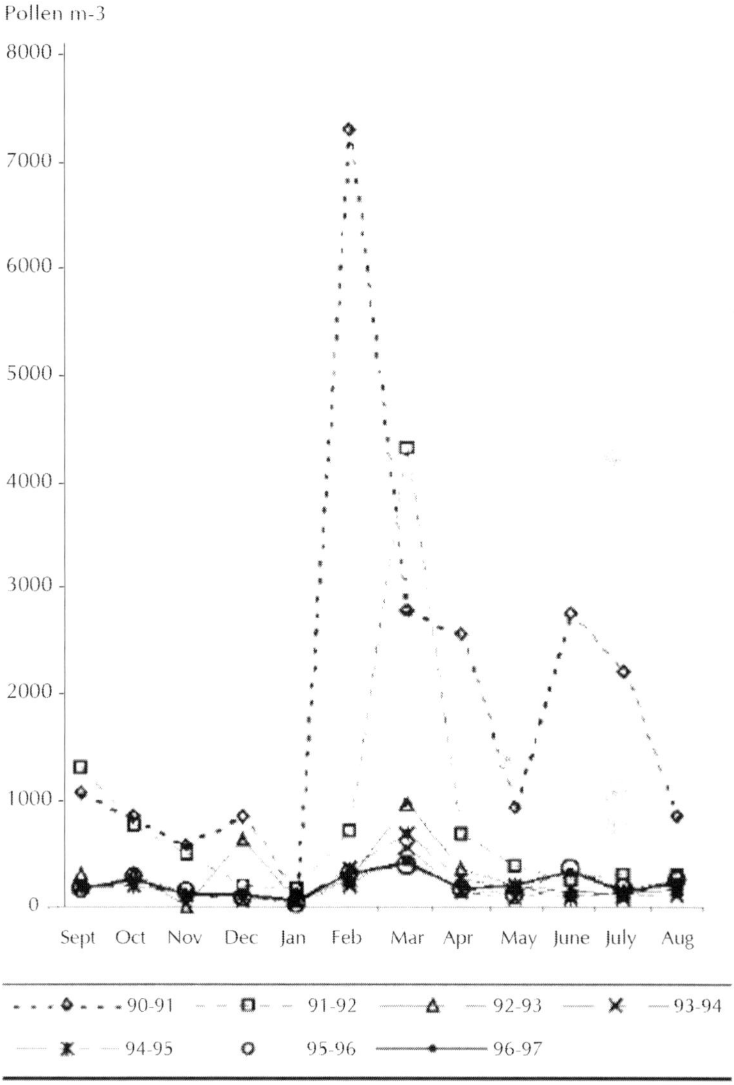

FIGURE 3.6 Seasonal variations in the total atmospheric pollen concentration (pollen m^{-3} air) in Delhi (1990–1997).

orientalis and *Xanthium*. At Gauhati, Asteraceae, *Chenopod/Amaranth*, *Eucalyptus*, Poaceae, *Putranjiva* and *Magnifera* are the dominant types of pollen (Anonymous, 2000; Singh and Kumar, 2002). In the air of Santinik-

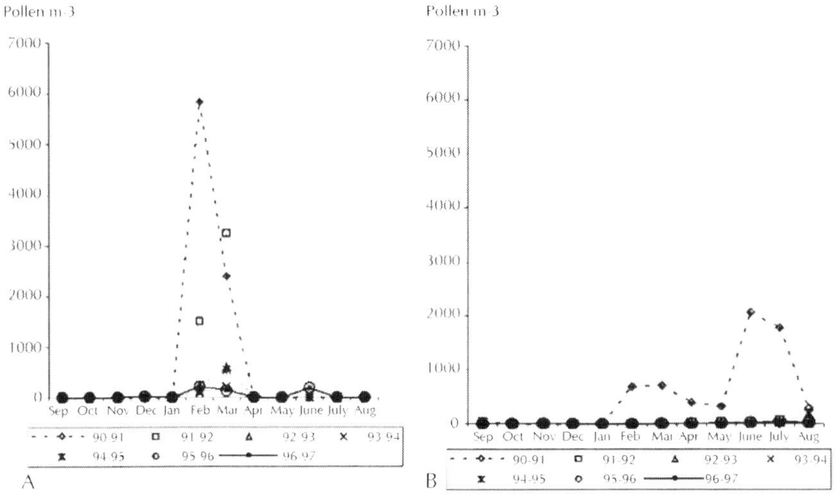

FIGURE 3.7 Monthly total pollen concentration (pollen m^{-3} air) in Delhi during 1990–1997.

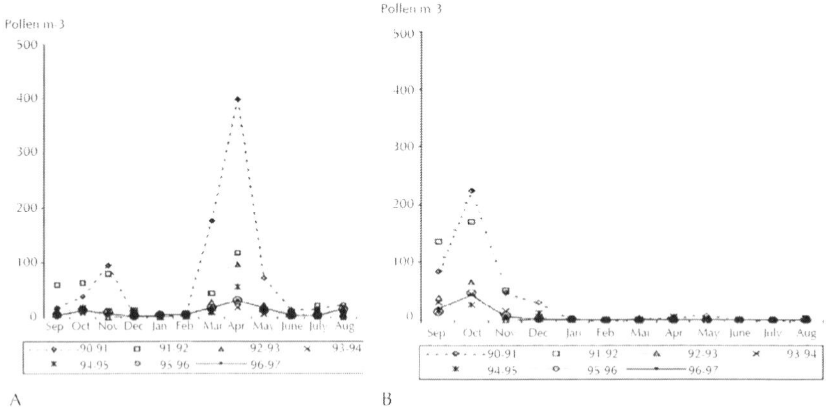

FIGURE 3.8 Monthly total pollen concentration (pollen m^{-3} air) in Delhi during 1990–1997.

etan near Kolkata three species *of Cassia* pollen as *C. tora, C. occidentalis, and C. fistula* were recorded during 2004–2006 (Hussain et al., 2013).

Studies carried out from Southern India, revealed that *Casuarina*, Chenopod/Amaranth, *Cocos*, Cyperaceae, *Eucalyptus*, *Parthenium*, *Peltophorum,* Poaceae and *Spathodia* are dominant pollen types (Anonymous 2000;

Singh and Kumar, 2002). Pollen calendars are very useful for clinicians as well as allergic patients to establish chronological correlation between the concentration of pollen in air and seasonal allergic symptoms. Based on aerobiological data obtained from India, pollen/flowering calendars have been prepared for Calcutta, Sambalpur, Gulberga, Imphal, Kodaikanal by different workers (Chanda, 1973; Pande et al., 1992; Maribhat and Rajasab, 1992; Singh and Devi, 1992; Satheesh et al., 1992). Poaceae, *Cocos*, *Artocarpus*, *Amaranthus*/*Chenopodium* and *Tridax* were the common and dominant pollen types analyzed from four sites studied in Kerala (Nayar and Jothish, 2013).

The Centre for Biochemical Technology now renamed as Institute of Genomics and Integrative Biology (Council for Scientific and Industrial Research) had published a book on pollen calendars of 12 different states in India (Singh et al., 1992), which provides important pollen season for grasses, weeds and trees prevalent in India. The latest information on allergenically important pollen allergens from India has been provided by Singh and Khandelwal on phonological, aerobiological and plant/pollen predominance in different parts of India in the form of a book entitled "An Atlas of Allergenically significant Plants of India" (Singh and Khandelwal, 2016)

3.8.2 FUNGAL AEROBIOLOGY

Fungi are ubiquitous in nature and are reported to be prevalent from different parts of the world, both in indoor and outdoor environments. Airborne surveys of fungal allergens have been reported from different parts of the world including India.

3.8.2.1 Outdoor Survey

In Alaska, *Cladosporium*, and unspecified fungus spores were the dominant aeroallergens (Anderson; 1985). *Cladosporium* has been reported as the most dominant fungal genus on the West Coast in U.S.A as well along with *Alternaria* (Al-Doory et al., 1967; Salvaggio and Seabury, 1971). Fungal spores of Basidiomycota and Ascomycetes are the predominant biological particulate in the atmosphere of Puerto Rico and Northwestern US have been reported for possible role in excaberation of respiratory allergies (Marianai et al., 2011). In a study in northeastern US reported for relative abundance of airborne allergenic fungi from 2.8% to 10.7% of total airborne fungal taxa with majority of allergenic and pathogenic fungi from phylum *Ascomycota*, specifically *Alternaria* and *Epicoccum* (Yamamoto et al., 2012).

An aeromycological study using spore type sampler initiated at La Plata, Argentina reported the most characteristic fungal taxa in the atmosphere as *Cladosporium cladosporioides, Leptosphaeria, Cladosporium herbarum, Coprinus*, and *Agaricus* (Mallo et al., 2011).

In many countries basidiospores have been reported as predominant (Salvaggio and Seabury, 1971; Prince and Meyer, 1976; Tarlo et al., 1979). In Canada, Collins – Williams and Kachyk and Khan observed *Cladosporium*, *Alternaria*, *Penicillium*, *Aspergillus*, yeasts, smuts, rusts occurring most frequently in Canadian air (Collins-Williams et al., 1973; Kachyk and Khan, 1977). In UK, the major fungal forms observed in air are *Cladosporium*, basidiospores, ascospores, *Pullularia*, *Botrytis*, smut, rusts, *Phoma*, *Epicoccum*, *Erisiphe* and *Alternaria* (Hyde, 1969). A study from Derby showed that *Cladosporium* has the highest count followed by *Sporobolomyces*, *Tilletiopsis*, *Botrytis*, *Alternaria*, *Leptoshaeria*, *Ustilago* and basidiospores (Brown and Jackson, 1978).

In Spain and Denmark the dominant types that contributed more than 70% of the total catch were *Cladosporium*, *Alternaria*, *Aspergillus* and *Penicillium* (Calvo et al., 1980; Larsen, 1981). In Almeria (Spain), Sabariego detected spores of *Alternaria* and *Cladosporium* throughout the year on air samples collected. The diurnal patterns of these taxons reflected a similar presence of spores during a 24-hr period. The correlation of meteorological parameters on fungal presence showed a positive association with temperature, hours of sunshine and accumulate rainfall, but negative with daily rainfall (Sabariego et al., 2004). In Germany, Wittmaack studied bioaerosols suspended in ambient air using single-stage impactors at a semiurban site in southern during late summer and early autumn (Wittmaack, 2005). The observed bioaerosols include fungal spores, hyphae, insect scales, hairs of plants and, less commonly, bacteria and epicuticular wax.

Spores of *Cladosporium*, *Alternaria*, *Penicillium*, *Aspergillus* and *Stemphyilum* are chiefly encountered in Israel. Other common types are *Helminthosporium*, *Epicoccum*, *Fusarium*, *Mucor*, *Pullularia*, *Monilia*, *Botrytis*, *Rhizpous* and *Phoma* (Barkai and Glazer, 1962; Barkai et al., 1977).

Ogunlana reported the prevalance of *Cladosporium*, *Curvularia*, *Fusarium*, *Aspergilli*, *Penicilli*, *Pithomyces*, *Aureobasidium*, *Geotrichum*, *Phoma, Rhizopus*, *Epicoccum* and *Neurospora* from Nigeria (Ogunlana, 1975).

From China, the dominant forms reported are yeast, *Aspergilli*, *Penicilli*, *Hormodendron*, *Mucor*, *Curvularia*, *Alternata* and *Fusarium* in order of their prevalance (Chen et al., 1978; Long et al., 1987; Lu et al., 1969). In Australia, *Cladosporium* spp have been found to be a major component of the airspora in Australia (Tilak et al., 1981). It is followed by *Leptosphaeria*, *Epicoccum nigrum*, *Nigrospora*, *Geotrichium*, *Neurospora*, *Penicillium* and *Aureobasidium*. A survey carried on the culturable airborne fungi revealed higher fungal concentrations in the greener area around the Research Center for Eco-Environmental Sciences (RCEES) and Beijing Botanical Garden (BBG) than in the densely urban and highly trafficked area of Xizhimen, however the difference was not significant (Fang et al., 2005). *Penicillium* was the most abundant and *Cladosporium* species were the most dominant fungal group, followed by non-sporing isolates, *Alternaria*, *Pencillium* and *Asperigillus* of the total fungal count. A study conducted to assess spatiotemporal fungal distribution in the Greater Taipei area indicated commercial and residential areas as predictor of *Aspergillus*/*Penicillium* levels and road length as predictor of basidiospores levels (Kallawicha et al., 2015).

From India, many reports provide information of prevalence of fungi in ambient air (Shivpuri et al., 1960; Agarwal and Shivpuri, 1974; Tilak and Kulkarni, 1980). *Alternaria* is reported as the dominant fungal type from Delhi (Sandhu et al., 1964; Agarwal, 1970). A survey conducted for culturable and non-culturable fungi reported 98 fungal forms with *Cladosporium* contributing 25–40% of total airborne fungi followed by *Ustilago* (smuts) (24%) *Aspergillus flavus* (10–13%), *Alternaria* (11%) and *A. niger* (8%) (Gupta et al., 1993). Basidiomycetes contributed 7–13% at different sites.

Airborne surveys for fungi have been reported from different parts of India as well. Dominant forms reported from Vishakhapatnam and Gulberga are *Cladosporium*, *Aspergillus*, *Nigrospora*, *Alternaria*, *Curvularia*, basidiospores, ascospores, *Helminthosporium* and *Periconia*. From Mysore, Ramalingam reported high concentrations of *Cladosporium* spp, smuts and *Epicoccum*.

Studies carried out in Gaya, Gauhati and Kolkata revealed that *Cladosporium*, *Alternaria*, *Aspergillus*, *Penicillium*, *Curvularia*, *Helminthosporium*, *Aureobasidium*, *Neurospora*, *Mucor* and *Nigrospora* are the major types reported recorded from Eastern India. Survey from central India Pune and Kolhapur, the dominant fungal forms isolated are *Cladosporium*, *Alternaria*, *Curvularia*, *Nigrospora*, *Periconia*, *Helminthosporium*, smuts, rust, *Aspergillus* and *Penicillium*.

A volumetric paired assessments of airborne viable and non-viable fungi in five outdoor sampling stations (Adhikari et al., 2004) in a rural agricultural area of India concluded that: (i) a rich fungal airspora existed in the rural study area, (ii) to achieve representative information on the total airborne fungal spores of an area, the monitoring in multiple sampling stations is preferable over a single sampling station; for viable fungi, however, one station can be considered, (iii) the percentage of airborne fungal viability is higher in rural agricultural areas.

3.8.2.2 Indoor Survey

The spectrum of indoor airborne mold spores, such as in homes, offices, and other workplaces, differ from place to place due to the influx of spores from outdoor air through ventilation and air exchanges. Hence, it is difficult to arrive at any significant conclusion on the role of the indoor mold spore in the allergic response. Again, it is not always the quantity but allergenicity of the mold, which determines the overall development of clinical allergy. Sampling methods used to evaluate indoor environments include air sampling for spores, measurement of allergens, and determination of microbial generated volatile organic compounds, ergosterols, glucans, and mycotoxins, as well as environmental conditions that lead to fungal contamination

Ren concluded that presence of fungal propagules in indoor air couldn't be reliably predicted by home characteristics (Ren et al., 2001). Actual measurements are required for fungal exposure assessment, and the use of only one medium to collect samples in one location in a home might be adequate to represent residential levels of fungi in indoor air.

In United States, a large number of reports of airborne indoor and outdoor fungal species and concentrations conducted on fungal air samples from buildings showed that the culturable airborne fungal concentrations in indoor air were lower than those in outdoor air (Shelton et al., 2002). *Stachybotrys chartarum* was identified in the indoor air in 6% of the buildings studied and in the outdoor air of 1% of the buildings studied. In US cities, O'connor examined the spectrum and concentration of fungi in the air inside and outside of the homes mold-sensitive children with asthma in urban communities (O'connor et al., 2004). The concentrations of fungi were higher in homes with dampness problems, cockroach infestation, and cats. In a study conducted in residential properties at Leicestershire, United Kingdom total indoor fungal spore concentrations have been recorded approximately 16% of outdoor concentrations. Abundant indoor fungal genera included *Cladosporium, Sporobolomyces, Tilletiopsis,* and *Didymella.* In contrast, Aspergillus/Penicillium-type (Asp/Pen-type) spores were common indoors and exceeded outdoor levels, with the highest concentrations detected in properties over 90 years old ($P = 0.006$) and terraced properties ($P = 0.003$) (Fairs et al., 2010). In a subsequent study in 2012, fungi were reported for its ubiquitous presence and temporal variability in atmosphere with Basidiomycota spores at higher levels than Ascomycota as identified by microscopy (Pashley et al., 2012).

Hayes analyzed air samples from offices in which DNA from air samples was extracted, DNA amplification of fungi and bacteria was performed. The data showed that fungal fauna other than *A. niger* or *A. flavus* is present in 87.2% of the samples (Hayes et al., 2005). In Havana, Cuba the atmospheric fungal concentration in respect of intradiurnal variation reflected maximum of *Cladosporium spores in* morning, *Coprinus* and *Leptosphaeria peaking in nights* alongwith constant presence for *Aspergillus/Penicillium species throughout the day (Almaguer et al., 2014).* Anamorphic fungal spores of *Cladosporium, Alternaria, Fusarium, Torula,*

Botrytis are predominant in the atmosphere of city of Funchal, Portugal (Sousa et al., 2015).

A comparison of MAS-100 and the Andersen air samplers' performances was made and a similar trend in both instruments was observed in the microbial contamination levels in samples of offices, hospitals, industries, and shopping centers, in Brazil (Rio de Janeiro city). The industries' results showed more important similarity among fungi and total heterotrophs distributions. All indoor air samples distributions were very similar. The temperature and air humidity had no significant influence on the samples dispersion patterns in indoors (Nunes et al., 2005).

3.8.2.2.1 Indoor Survey in India

In India, indoor fungal survey has been reported from several cities across different geographical region. At Vishakhapatnam, a total of 8909 and 9327 CFU/m^3 were recorded in from inside and outside, respectively with 47 types identified. The dominant fungal types were *Cladosporium*, *Penicillium nigricans*, *Aspergillus versicolor*, and *Aspergillus oryzae*. While in Solan in Shimla sampling conducted in a wet house revealed *Penicillium* as the most dominant types contributing 30.7% followed by *Aspergillus* sp. (15.4%), *Alternaria* sp. (10.5%). In the same place sampling conducted in a mud house revealed *Aspergillus* sp. At 35.1% as the most dominant contributor followed by *Penicillium* (26.9%). The other dominant types were *Alternaria*, *Cladosporium*, *Curvularia* and *Fusarium* (Anonymous, 2000). Indoor fungal concentration in homes of allergic childrenin Delhi was recorded to be significantly higher ($p < 0.05$) than outdoors. Important indoor fungi were *Aspergillus species, Alternaris, Cladosporium and Pennicillium* (Sharma et al., 2011).

In West Bengal (Kolkata), the volumetric assessment of airborne culturable and nonculturable fungal spore showed higher frequencies of *Aspergilli /Penicilli, Cladosporium, Alternaria*, and smut spores by Burkard Sampler whereas Andersen Sampler showed the prevalence of *Aspergillus niger, Aspergillus flavus and Cladosporium cladosporioides* in large rural indoor cattle shed (Adhikari et al., 2004).

In Delhi, an indoor survey of fungi in the homes of asthmatic/allergic children (Sharma et al., 2005) revealed highest fungal load in the month of January while the lowest in June in indoors (Figure 3.7). A high viable mold concentration was observed in the homes of asthmatic children in Delhi. The predominant fungal types observed were *Aspergillus niger*, *A. flavus*, *A. fumigatus*, *A. nidulans*, *Alternaria* spp, *Cladosporium* spp, *Penicillium* spp, *Rhizopus* spp, and *Curvularia* spp., etc. The houses in Delhi contain rich and varied concentration of fungi, almost parallel to what is encountered just outside the air.

Besides the outdoor environment, indoor, work environments are also greatly influenced by fungi especially occupational sites employing organic raw materials e.g. granary, poultry, flour mills, bakery, sugar factory etc. Survey conducted at working environments by Singh and his students in bakery, poultry, sugar factory and libraries in Delhi revealed, *Aspergilli-Penicilli* and smut spores as significant contributors in indoor air (Singh et al., 1990; Singh and Singh, 1993; Pandit and Singh, 1994).

3.8.3 POULTRY SHEDS

A total of 17 fungal forms were reported from Guwahati out of which *Cladosporium herbarum* was the most dominant followed by *Aspergillus schari* and *Penicillium* spp. In Gwalior 21 fungal types were reported from the poultry. The most dominant being *Aspergillus niger* (24.6 %) followed by *Cladosporium spp* (22.3%), *Penicillium sp.* (10.7 %), *Aspergillus flavus* (9.1 %), *Botrytis*, *Fusarium*, *Aspergillus glaucus*, *Aspergillus fumigatus* and *Curvularia* were the other dominant species (Singh, 1994). While in Bangalore the *Aspergillus* sp. (531 CFU) were the most dominant contributors the environment followed by *Penicillium* spp. (301 CFU) and *Cladosporium* sp. (169 CFU). *Mucor* and *Rhizopus* were amongst the other dominant types. A total of 14,164 and 12,837 colonies were recorded inside and outside, respectively from a poultry farm in Vishakhapatnam. A total of 54 fungal types were reported out of which majority belonged to *Aspergillus* and *Penicillium* group. The other dominant fungi recorded were *Cladosporium*, *Penicillium nigricans*, *Trichoderma,* etc. (Singh, 1994).

3.8.5 CATTLE SHEDS

A total of 51 fungal types were identified in Vishakhapatnam, out of which 22 species belonged to *Aspergillus* and 2 to *Penicillium* group. *Cladosporoides* was the other dominant type (Singh, 1994).

3.8.6 GARBAGE DUMP

A total of 11,040 and 10,630 col/m^3 were recorded in Vishakhapatnam from inside and outside, respectively. The dominant fungal types were *Aspergillus niger*, *Cladosporium*, *Aspergillus versicolor*, *Aspergillus fumigatus*, *Mucor*, etc. At Pune, colonies of *Cladosporium* (36.6%) were in abundance throughout the year whereas A. fumigatus contributed to 12.2% with highest concentration in month of June. *Cladosporium* spores were recorded throughout the year at Aurangabad. *A. fumigatus*, *A. flavus*, *A. niger* were also dominant among all *Aspergillus* species. From Chennai, a total of 41 species were recorded, among which *A. niger* were more commonly encountered. It was followed by *A. flavus*. From Gorakhpur, *Alternaria alternata* (9.54%) was recorded as dominant fungal colony followed by *Fusarium oxysporium* (7.62%) (Singh, 1994).

3.8.7 JAGGARY GODOWN

A total of 12,855 and 10,570 col/m^3 were recorded in Vishakhapatnam from inside and outside respectively. The dominant fungal types were *Aspergillus niger*, *Cladosporium*, *Aspergillus versicolor*, *Penicillium brefeldianum*, *Curvularia*, etc. (Singh, 1994).

3.8.8 LIBRARY

A survey conducted in a library in Gwalior, *Cladosporium* species (30.3 %) inside and (38.2 %) outside was reported as the most dominant fungal type followed by *Aspergillus niger* (20.5%) inside and (15.2 %) outside. Other dominant typed includes *A. teneus* and *Fusarium sp*. Another survey conducted in Bangalore City library also showed *Cladosporium* species (51.6%). Two libraries surveyed at Pune revealed *Cladosporium* as highest contributor (34.08%) followed by different species if *Aspergillus*. Colonies of *Rhizopus* were also recorded frequently from July to September (Singh, 1994).

3.8.9 DAIRY FARM

A total of 9000 CFU/m3, 8500 CFU/m3, 940 CFU/m3, 10,110 CFU/m3, were recorded from reception, processing area, packaging area, cold storage and outside air, respectively in Vishakhapatnam. The dominant fungal types were *Aspergillus niger*, *Cladosporium*, *Curvularia*, *Aspergillus nigricans* in reception; *Aspergillus niger*, *Cladosporium*, *P. nigricans* in processing area and packaging are; *Aspergillus niger*, *Cladosporium* in outside air. Very few colonies were recorded in the cold storage (Singh, 1994).

3.8.10 SUGAR INDUSTRY

In Modinagar, a total of 91 fungal forms belonging to 67 genera were isolated. 15 species of *Aspegillus* and 11 of *Penicillium* were isolated from the site. The common fungi observed in sugar factory environment were *Cladosporium spp.*, *Aspergillus fumigatus*, *Epicoccum nigrum*, Ustilago spp. (smut spores), *Paecilomyces varioti* and *Saccharomyces cerevisiae* (Singh, 1994).

3.8.11 VEGETABLE MARKET

During the survey in fruit/vegetable market in Delhi, 101 forms, both culturable and non-culturable were identified from vegetable market site. *Cladosporium spp* was the highest contributor (54.8%), followed by *Aspergillus* (21.8%). All the *Penicillium spp* together contributed 10.5% both inside and outside the vegetable market. In a vegetable market from Berhampur, *A. niger* was dominant followed by *A. flavus* contributing 6.84%

to the total fungal load inside the market whereas at Nagpur, spores of Aspergillus spp were dominant among the 30 types identified followed by *Cladosporium*. From Chennai, *A. niger* contributed upto 65% of all C.F.U. It was followed by *A. flavus* and *Rhizopus stolonifer. A. niger* (13.7%) was the dominant fungi among all the types recorded from Market area of Gorakhpur. Second important type identified were *Alternaria alternata* (Singh, 1994).

3.8.12 GRAIN STORAGE

In a two-year study inside the grain storage in Delhi, *Aspergillus flavus* contributed a maximum of 68.9% to the total colony concentration. This was followed by *Cladosporium spp*, (18.5%), *Aspergillus niger* (5.0%) and *Penicillium spp* (3.6%). *Epicoccum*, *Curvularia*, *Nigrospora*, *Periconia*, Basidiospores, etc. were also the dominant contributors. Among the dominant types analyzed *Aspergillus flavus* and *Alternaria spp* had significantly higher concentration in the storage as compared to control air (Singh, 1994).

3.9 CLINICALLY IMPORTANT BIOALLERGENS

3.9.1 POLLEN ALLERGENS

Pollen causing allergy are quite variable in different ecozones which makes it very important to identify pollinosis causing species from every region, and prepare extracts from them for diagnosis and immunotherapy for the benefit of allergy sufferers.

In a study, three hundred seventy-one allergy patients were tested serologically for hypersensitivity towards prevalent tree pollens in the surrounding New York area over the years 1993–2000. It was concluded that in the New York City area, hypersensitivity to tree pollens most often is manifested with allergy to oak, birch, and maple tree pollens (Lin et al., 2002). Latter on, among 158 patients with asthma, rhinitis, or both, 102 had positive skin tests to either Eastern red cedar (*Juniperus virginiana*) or white cedar (*Thuja occidentalis*). Among those, 52 patients (51%) had positive skin tests to at least one of the cedar pollens (Deane, 2005). In Cincinnati, the aeroallergens having a significant impact on asthma hospital visits were ragweed, oak/maple and Pinaceae pollen. Their relative risks on asthma hospital visits with respect to a 100-counts/m^3 increase in concentration were in the range of 1.23–1.54 (Zhong et al., 2006).

The effect of pollen grains on morbidity from childhood conjunctivitis and rhinitis was studied. An increase of 72 ragweed grains per m^3, was associated with an increase of about 10% in visits for conjunctivitis and rhinitis (Cakmak et al., 2002). In a study from the Pacific coast to the Atlantic coast of Canada, changes in outdoor aeroallergens and hospitalizations for asthma was assessed. It was concluded that aeroallergens are an important cause of severe asthma morbidity across Canada, and in some situations there might be a modest synergistic adverse effect of ozone and aeroallergens combined (Dales et al., 2005).

In a study carried out in southern Croatia, 46.7% were sensitized to *Ambrosia elatior*. Thus it is an important cause of seasonal allergic rhinitis and asthma in must be included in the routine diagnostic procedures in southern Croatia (Cvitanovic et al., 2007).

In a population-based random sample of 498 adults aged 26–60 years were tested for 15 common aeroallergens with skin prick tests (SPTs) in Finland, 24% was sensitized to at least four allergens. Sensitization to multiple allergens was associated with a high prevalence of asthma, Allergic Rhinitis or conjunctivitis, and wheeze (Pallasaho et al., 2006).

In Cova da Beira, Portugal, the most representative aeroallergens sensitization were grasses mixture (44.9%), *Olea europea* (27.5%), *Parietaria judaica* (23.4%), *Artemisia vulgaris* (17.6%), *Robinia pseudoacacia* (12.2%), *Platanus acerifolia* (11.4%), *Tilia cordata* (11.4%), *Plantago lanceolata* (10.6%) and *Pinus radiata* (7.5%) (Loureiro et al., 2005).

In a comparison of skin tests to aeroallergens in Ankara and Seoul, grass pollens were found to be major allergens more often in Ankara than in Seoul (74.34% vs. 15.87%, $p < 0.001$). Skin test reactivities in Ankara were significantly lower ($p < 0.001$) than in Seoul to weed (6.91% vs. 37.50%) and tree pollens (4.61% vs. 39.42%) (Sener et al., 2003).

On the basis of the results of an aerobiological survey in the Klang Valley of Malaysia, two local extracts of grass pollens, i.e., Ischaemum and Enilia were recruited for Skin Prick Test. The SPT reactivity was 14.1%

and 5.9%, respectively (Wan et al., 2005). In another study by SPT using eight aeroallergens in 206 asthmatic patients, sensitization was observed in Bermuda grass (7.9%), *Acacia sp.* (7.9%) (Liam et al., 2002).

A cross-sectional retrospective study based on SPT conducted on 226 allergic patients referred to allergic clinic of Karaj city, Tehran showed that the most common aeroallergens were: herbacee II (62%), sycamore (57%), chenopodium (53%), tree mix (50%), herbacee III (47%), grass (43%), ash (40%), herbacee I (37%), cedar (27%) (Farhoudi et al., 2005). In a recent study two important pollen contributing maximally to seasonal allergies are reported to be *Broussonetia papyrifera* and *Cannabis sativa* (Abbas et al., 2012).

3.9.1.1 Pollen Allergens of India

Based on clinico-immunological evaluation of pollen antigens, important allergenic pollen in India has been identified. The work on pollen allergy was initiated in the 1950's by Shivpuri in Delhi. Subsequently, Kasliwal and his colleagues reported important pollen allergens of Jaipur (Kasliwal and Solomon, 1958). Shivpuri and Parkash (Shivpuri and Parkash, 1967) observed *Prosopis juliflora* as a major cause of pollinosis with 12% patients showing a positive skin reaction. Later, important pollen allergens were identified for Delhi by Shivpuri and his colleagues. They were: *Ageratum*, *Ailanthus*, *Amaranthus*, *Anogeissus pendula*, *Artemisia*, *Cassia siamea*, *Cenchrus*, *Chenopodium*, *Cynodon*, *Ipomoea fistulosa*, *Paspalum distichum* and *Poa annua* (Shivpuri et al., 1979; Singh et al., 1987). We recorded positive skin reactions in 16.9% patients to *Pinus roxburghii* from the foothills of Himalayas (Singh et al., 1987).

From Northern India, important allergens identified are: *Prosopis juliflora*, *Ricinus communis*, *Morus*, *Mallotus*, *Alnus*, *Quercus*, *Cedrus*, *Argemone*, *Amaranthus*, *Chenopodium*, *Holoptelea*, and grasses. From Central India the important pollen allergens are: *Argemone*, *Brassica*, *Cannabis*, *Asphoedelus*, *Parthenium*, *Cassia*, *Azadirachta*, grasses, *Alnus*, *Betula*, *Malotus*, *Trewia nudiflora*. From Eastern India, allergenically significant pollen types were found as: *Lantana*, *Cucurbita maxima*, *Cassia fistula*, *Cocos nucifera* and *Calophyllum inophyllum*. Recent studies based on clinical and immunologic parameters reported *Phoenix*, *Ricinus communis* and *Aegle marmelos* as causative agents of allergy in this region (Anonymous, 2000).

From South India *Cassia*, *Ageratum*, *Salvadora*, *Ricinus*, *Albizia lebbeck* and *Artemisia scoparia* have been reported as important aeroallergens (Acharya, 1980; Agashe and Anand, 1982). Subbarao et al. (Subbarao et al., 1985) recorded allergenicity to *Parthenium hysterophorus* pollen extracts in 34% of allergic rhinitis and 12% bronchial asthma patients from Bangalore. Agashe and Soucenadin (Agashe and Soucenadin, 1992) recorded high skin reactivity to *Casuarina equisetifolia* in patients from Bangalore.

Clinical studies undertaken by us recently at various medical centers under the All India Coordinated Project (AICP) on Aeroallergens and Human Health (Anonymous, 2000) sponsored by the Ministry of Environment and Forest, revealed important allergenic pollen for various regions in India. 35 pollen antigens were tested on atopic population. At Chandigarh, skin sensitivity was highest against *Rumex acetosa* and *Ailanthus excelsa* (17.6%), followed by *Trewia nudiflora* (9.7%), *Argemone mexicana* (9.5 %), and *Cedrus deodara* (9.3%). In Delhi, 12.6% of the atopic population was positive to *Amaranthus spinosus*, 8.5% to *Populus deltoides* and 7.5% to *Dodonea viscosa*, *Bauhinia vareigata*. In Calcutta, 28.8% of the patients were sensitive against *Solanum sysimbrifolium*, 21.1% to *Crotalaria juncea* and 18.2% each to *Ricinus communis* and *Ipomea fistulosa*. In Trivandrum, maximum skin reactivity was recorded to *Mallotus phillipensis* (12.1%), followed by *Prosopis juliflora* (6.3%). For the first time, *Cedrus deodara* (Pinaceae) pollen has been recognized as a new allergen from India in the patients from the Himalayan region, where *Cedrus deodara* occurs naturally (Rawat et al., 2000). The common allergenic plants of different seasons in India are mentioned in Table 3.1.

A book entitled "An Atlas of Allergenically Significant Plants of India" by Singh and Khandelwal with details of phonological, aeropalynological and allergological information for more than 100 plants from India has been published. This provides a diagnostic and therapeutic tool to allergy practioners and other personnel's in the field of allergy and allergens to select appropriate allergens for testing and immunotherapy (Singh and Khendalwal, 2016). Major allergens vary from place to place. It is

TABLE 3.1 Common Allergenic Plants of Different Seasons in India

	Spring (Feb–April)	Autumn (Sept–Oct)	Winter (Nov–Jan)
Trees	Ailanthus excelsa	*Anogeissus pendula*	Cassia siamea
	Bauhinia variegata	*Carica papaya*	Cedrus deodara
	Casuarina equisitifolia	*Cedrus deodara*	Mallotus phillipensis
	Holoptelea integrifolia	*Cocus nucifera*	Salvadora persica
	Mallotus phillipensis	*Eucalyptus* sp	Quercus incana
	Prosopis juliflora	*Mallotus phillipensis*	
	Putranjiva roxburghii	*Phoenix sylvestris*	
	Quercus incana	*Prosopis juliflora*	
		Quercus incana	
Weeds	Cannabis sativa	Amaranthus spinosus	Ageratum conyzoides
	Chenopodium murale	Artemisia scoparia	Argemone mexicana
	Parthenium hysterophorous	Cassia occidentalis	Asphodelous tenuifolius
	Plantago major	Ricinus communis	Chenopodium album
	Suaeda fruiticosa	Xanthium strumarium	Ricinus communis
Grasses	Cynodon dactylon	Bothriochloa pertusa	Cynodon dactylon
	Dicanthium annulatum	Cenchrus ciliaris	Eragrostis tenella
	Imperata cylindrica	Hetropogon contortus	Phalaris minor
	Paspalum distichum	Pennisetum typhoides	Poa annua
	Poa annua	Sorghum vulgare	
	Polypogon monspeliensis		

important for clinicians to select only those pollen antigens for skin testing which are prevalent in a particular area in which the patient resides.

3.9.2 FUNGAL ALLERGENS

More than 80 species of fungi are suspected of inducing immunoglobulin E (IgE)-mediated hypersensitivity. The most commonly studied fungal species are *Alternaria alternata*, *Aspergillus fumigatus*, *Cladosporium herbarum*, and *Epicoccum purpurascens*, which are prevalent aeroallergen sources throughout the world, and allergy toward them is a risk factor for allergic rhinitis, asthma and even death (Samir et al., 2014).

The prevalence of respiratory allergy to fungi is estimated at 20 to 30% among atopic individuals and upto 6% in the general population (Gravesen, 1979; Singh et al.,1987; Ren et al., 1999). The major allergic manifestations induced by fungi are asthma, rhinitis, allergic bronchopulmonary mycoses, and hypersensitivity pneumonitis (Kang et al., 1979; Burch and Levetin, 2002).

A total of 701 adults living in the USA or Western Europe having symptoms of allergic respiratory disease were skin prick tested with extracts prepared from eight basidiomycetes species and four Fungi Imperfecti species. *Psilocybe cubensis* was the most potent allergen source in both the USA (12.3% reacted) and Europe (16.0%). *Pleurotus ostreatus* was second overall (10.6%) and in the USA (10.7%), and third in Europe (10.3%). *Pisolithus tinctorius* and *Coprinus quadrifidus* produced the least potent allergens, with only 5.4% of the population reacting (Lehrer et al., 1994). In another study in Seattle, 27% subjects responded to at least one Fungi Imperfecti, reactions were most common to *Aspergillus* sp. (21%), and least common to *Penicillium* sp., which were positive in 6%. Positive responses to basidiospore extracts were observed in 10 of 33 (30%) subjects. The prevalence of basidiospore reactivity was similar to that of Fungi Imperfecti, ranging from 18% for *Scleroderma* sp. to 6% for four different spore extracts (Sprenger et al., 1988).

Alternaria alternata and *Cladosporium herbarum* are common fungi in outdoor environments. However, in the Finnish population with allergic symptoms, IgE-mediated sensitization to 2 common fungal allergens, i.e., *A. alternata* and *C. herbarum* was rare and of minor clinical importance. The prevalence of positive SPT results was low (2.8% and 2.7%, respectively) (Reijula et al., 2003).

In Spain, a retrospective review of 247 clinical files of patient that have responded to the office allergy and immunology since 1990 to 1993 in Monclova, Coah revealed sensitization to *Candida* (3.2%), *Alternaria* (2.7%), *Rhizopus* (3.6%), *Penicillium* (2.1%), *Fusarium* (2.1%), other molds (8.7%) (Morin et al., 1994).

Skin prick tests were applied to a cohort of 4962 respiratory subjects, aged 3–80 years. Nineteen percent of the allergic population reacted to at least one fungal extract by means of the skin test. *Alternaria* sp and *Candida* sp accounted for the largest number of positive tests, and along with *Trichophyton* sp they were the main sensitizers in the subset of patients with an isolated sensitization (Mari et al., 2003).

In a study carried out in Malaysia, *Fusarium* was observed to have the highest prevalence of SPT reactivity (23.5%), followed by *Aspergillus flavum* (21.2%), *Dreselera orysae* (18.8%), *Alternaria* sp (17.6%), *Curvularia eragrostidis* (17.6%), *Penicillium oxalicu,m* (16.5%), *Pestolotriopsis gtuepini* (16.5%), *Rhizopus arrhi* (16.5%), *Aspergillus niger* (15.3%). *Penicillium choy* (12.9%), *Aspergillus fumigatus* (11.8%), and *Cladosporium* sp (4.7%) (Wan et al., 2005).

3.9.2.1 Fungal Allergens of India

Agarwal and Shivpuri (1974) performed intradermal skin tests on 1292 patients in Delhi using 27 fungal extracts. They found 19 fungal extracts to be of allergenic significance. Some of these are *Alternaria, Curvularia, Candida, Monilia, Phoma, Acrothecium, Helminthosporium, Mucor, Aspergillus tamarii.* Shivpuri (1980) further performed skin tests on 300 patients and observed besides above fungi, *Cladosporium herbarum, Aspergillus niger* and *A. fumigatus* were also important allergens.

Acharya (1980) investigated on 300 nasobronchila allergy patients in Andhra Pradesh, important allergenic fungi were *Aspergillus flavus, Helminthosporium, Neurospora, Candida, Cladosporium,* etc. From Bangalore, *Mucor mucedo, Fusarium solani, Curvularia, Nigrospora,* etc. are observed to be important allergens (Agashe and Anand, 1982).

The atmospheric concentration of *Fomes* was recorded. The maximum counts (67 spores/m^3) were observed from the North Delhi site in the month of July 1989, compared with 550 spores/m^3 in the South Delhi site. Marked skin positivity (2+ and above) varied from 9.8% to spore to 22% to whole body of *Fomes pectinatis* (Gupta et al., 1999). In a study by Sharma et al. (2012), a high incidence skin reactivity to fungal allergens *of Alternaria alternata,Aspergillus fumigatus*, and *Penicillium citrinumin* has been reported in asthmatic children of Delhi. A strong relation between skin prick test to fungal allergens and serum IgE antibodies ranging 16.7–69.2% cases was observed (Kocher et al., 2014).

3.10 SIGNIFICANCE OF CROSS-REACTIVE ALLERGENS IN CLINICAL PRACTICE

Allergy is the result of binding between the epitopes on the proteins with the IgE. Because of evolution, certain proteins have remained conserved from the different sources. It is known that allergic patients are frequently co-sensitized against different allergen sources. Progress made in the field of allergen characterization by molecular biological techniques has now revealed that sensitization against different allergen sources can be explained as cross-reactivity of IgE antibodies with structurally and immunologically related components present in these allergen sources. The similarities among allergens may facilitate allergy diagnosis in clinical practice by using a few representative cross-reactive allergens to determine the patient's IgE reactivity profile.

Cross reactivity can only be demonstrated by inhibition experiments demonstrating the degree to which an extract in fluid phase inhibits the IgE bindingts in different solid phase coated extract (Crammery et al., 2006)

3.10.1 CROSS REACTIVE POLLEN ALLERGENS

Studies carried our across the globe suggest cross reactivity among different plants. *Lolium perennea* has been found to be cross reactive with *Acacia*, pineapple, *olea europea,Dactylus glomerata,Ligustrum vulgare, Cyodon dactylon and Pinus radiate. Platanus acerifolia* has been found to cross-react with *Corylus avellana*, *Prunus persica*, *Malus domestica*, *Arachis hypogaea*, *Zea mays*, *Cicer arietinum*, *Lactuca virosa*, *Musa* spp., and *Apium* spp. (Enrique et al., 2002; Miralles et al., 2002). Pollen from Japanese cypress (*Chamaecyparis obtusa*) cross reacts with Japanese cedar (*Cryptomeria japonica*) contributing to prolonged symptoms after the cedar pollen season in March and the following cypress pollen season in April (Sone et al., 2005).

Ricinus communis, commonly grown in India for its oil and abundantly present in wasteland, cross-reacts with *Hevea brasiliensis, Mercurialis annua, Olea europaea, Betula, Zygophyllum fabago, Putranjiva roxburghii*, and *Ricinus* (seed) (Belchi-Hernandez et al., 1998; Palosuo et al., 2002; Singh et al., 1997; Singh et al., 1997).

Areca catechu cross-reacts with *Phoenix sylvestris, Cocos nucifera, Borassus flabelifer*, as reported from India (Chowdhury et al., 1998). *Cynodon dactylons* (common grass) cross-reacts with *Pennisetum clandestinum, Stenotaphrum secundatum, Eragrostis, Brassica napus, Olea europaea, Ligustrum vulgare*, and *Lolium perenne* (Chowdhury et al., 1998; Chang et al., 1994; Kazemi-Shirazi et al., 2000; Potter et al., 1993; Prescott et al., 2001).

Holoptelea integrifolia and *Parietaria judaica* belonging to the family Urticaceae are geographically distantly located. *H. integrifolia* is an important pollen allergen of India cross reacts with *P. judaica*, on the other hand, is a very dominant pollen allergen of the Mediterranean region. *H. integrifolia* and *P. judaica* pollens share cross-reactive as well as unique epitopes (Smith et al., 1997). Some examples of cross-reacting tree pollen allergens with different foods as reported by various workers are described in Table 3.2.

TABLE 3.2 Examples of Cross-Reacting Tree Pollen Allergens with Different Foods Reported by Various Workers

Plants	Foods	Evaluation Method
Ambrosia sp. (Ragweed)	Melon, banana	RAST
Grass	Swiss chard, tomato, peanut	RAST, nasal provocation test, RAST inhibition RAST, skin test
Birch	Tomato, melon, water melon apple, carrot, potato, rosaceae, hazelnuts, apple, cherry, peach, pear	Immunoblot, Immunoassay (IgE)
Birch/mugwort	Celery, carrot	SPT, RAST
Grass and birch	Kiwi fruit	
Artemisia	Rosaceae (peach, apple, chestnut)	

3.10.2 CROSS REACTIVE FUNGAL ALLERGENS

RAST/ELISA and ELISA Inhibition and Immunoblot Inhibition techniques are employed in homologous and heterogenous inhibition experiments to study cross reactivity with different fungal allergens (Huang et al., 1995; Brouer et al., 1996; O'Neil et al., 1988). Unfortunately extensive systematic studies on cross-reactive fungal allergens have been lacking. Allergens can be glycelated or not, raising the question of clinical relevance of cross reactive carbohydrate determinants (CCDs). Skin prick test involving Basidiomycetes and Deuteromycetes extracts showed that, although shared allergenic determinants were present, in vivo cross-reactivity between the species was minimal. In contrast radioimmunosorbent test (RAST) inhibition was significant between some phylogenetically distant fungal species indicating IgE-binding components without clinical relevance. This result is likely to be explained by the presence of CCD in the extracts which are able to bind IgE in vitro, but hardly induce wheal and flare reactions in skin tests (Mari et al., 1999).

3.11 MOLECULAR APPROACH TO ALLERGEN CHARACTERIZATION

Pollen extracts are complex mixtures of several proteins, lectins, complex carbohydrates, lipids, nucleic acids, enzymes etc. Every time an extract is prepared, there is considerable variation in their content within a company, besides inter-company variability. These great differences result in unreliable prick test results, prevents comparison of skin tests world over and in generating a dose response data. Also their use in therapeutics makes it necessary to have an international standard.

The need for standardization of allergenic extracts has been recognized since the advent of immunotherapy (Noon, 1911). The early attempts towards standardization were based on consistency in crude w/v ratio or estimation of PNU content of the extracts. But it was found to be a poor indicator of allergen content.

The standardization of allergenic extracts can be done by biological standardization. The concept of biologic equivalence test was established by Northern Society of Allergology and adopted by European investigators (Ass, 1980). One HEP unit was defined as a positive skin prick test, which gave a wheal diameter equivalent to that given by a prick with 1 mg/mL concentration of histamine hydrochloride. Later on Dirksen et al. (1985) designated 1 HEP as concentration of extract that gives a wheal diameter equivalent to 1 mg/mL of histamine hydrochloride.

Pollen and fungal extracts are also studied for their immunochemical properties, mainly protein and glycoprotein fractions.

3.12 FUTURE TRENDS IN ALLERGEN RESEARCH

Since mid 1980, a fast growth has seen in the information of allergy. A large number of major allergens have been isolated, purified and their amino acid sequencing and epitope mapping have been done. The allergenic epitopes have also been analyzed using Human T cells (Perez et al., 1990).

The introduction of recombinant allergens has undoubtedly allowed better standardization of allergen extracts and affords the opportunity for individualized treatment, which is tailor made according to individual sensitivities (Valenta and Kraft, 2002). However, at present, there are no published trials of recombinant allergens for Immunotherapy.

The use of short T cell peptides for immunotherapy has the potential to stimulate "protective" Th1 and/or T regulatory responses whilst avoiding systemic side effects associated with cross linking of IgE on mast cells and basophils which are the risk associated with conventional whole allergen extracts. Initial studies in cat allergy are encouraging, although, again, further studies are required (Marcotte et al., 1998).

TH_2 to TH_1 shift: It is hypothesized that transit through this critical window, with active minimization of allergen exposure and respiratory syncytial virus infection, will reduce the development of persistent disease. The incidence of occupational asthma in adults and acquisition of allergic diseases in immigrants to westernized countries from countries where protective factors would be expected to operate in infancy. To the extent that allergic responses can develop throughout life, the success of strategies applied in infancy will be limited.

The primary reasons are suggested to lie in sensitization to multiple allergens and the ubiquity of opportunities for exposure at different domestic sites coupled with the partial effectiveness of the interventions.

3.12.1 RECOMMENDATIONS

Important pollen and fungal allergens vary in concentration and prevalence from place to place so it is advisable to measure their concentration and establish relationship with the patient symptoms.

The remedial action depends on the actual problem and conditions prevailing in different occupational sites, however following preventive measures in general are recommended.

3.13. ENVIRONMENTAL MANAGEMENT OF POLLEN ALLERGENS

3.13.1 RECOMMENDATIONS FOR TREE PLANTATIONS

1. All the allergenically significant trees need to be deleted from the list of Recommended tree plantation in gazette of India.
2. Ornamentals, insect/bird pollinated and medicinally important trees or others which can help in controlling pollution, should be encouraged in various tree plantation and afforestation programs.
3. The existing allergenically significant trees need to be replaced with non-allergenic trees in a phased manner.
4. On medical ground, citizens should have the right to cut or demand removal of allergy causing trees in close vicinity. However, these should be replaced with some non-allergenic trees.
5. A genuine beginning needs to be made by sensitizing tree lovers/ horticulturist/foresters/botanist and other associated with tree plantation so that the share of allergenically significant plants could be minimized in the near future. The earlier it is done the better.

3.14 PREVENTION OF FUNGAL ALLERGENS

1. It is important to isolate and identify important airborne fungi that cause allergic disorders.

2. Knowledge of life history of these fungi is essential in identifying their source and environmental conditions that help in getting airborne in significant concentration on which microorganism build up their numbers should be removed from the work place.
3. Reduction of moisture inside the work place.
4. Air quality can be enhanced by periodic maintenance of air treatment plant, fumigation, application of antifungal agents', etc.
5. Personal filter masks of the pore size sufficient to entry of respirable size microbes may be beneficial at the work place.
6. Environmental factors like air pollution and smoking also can aggravate the existing symptoms. These should be controlled.

Allergy has been known for more than a century now, but the subject has suffered due to lack of knowledge about basic mechanisms involved in allergic diseases and poor diagnostic procedures. The rapid development in the field of immunology and clinical diagnosis in the pool of knowledge, is of, direct significance to allergy practitioners. The detailed information on indigenous pollen and fungal allergens will be very useful in diagnosis and management of allergic patients in the country.

3.15 SUMMARY

Allergic diseases such as bronchial asthma, allergic rhinitis and atopic dermatitis are dramatically increasing all over the world including developing countries. Today, more than 30% of the population is known to suffer from one or other allergic ailment. Major causative agents implicated are pollen grains, fungal spores, dust mites, insect debris, animal epithelia, etc. Several aerobiological studies have been conducted in different parts of the world to ascertain aerial concentration and seasonality of pollen grains and fungi.

From medical, especially clinical point of view, it is important to know the details about the occurrence of the pollen load in the atmosphere. The flowering time of higher plants are events that come periodically in each season, but the time of blooming may differ from year to year, in different geographic locations. Based on differences recorded in several years of observations in airborne pollen, pollen calendars are drawn as an aid to allergy diagnosis and management.

In this review, efforts have been made to provide aerobiological aspects of environmental pollen as well as fungi from different parts of the world. The historical development of aerobiology, prevailing airborne pollen flora in different ecogeographical regions and their role in the diagnosis and management allergic diseases has been discussed with particular emphasis on Tropical Allergens from India and neighboring countries.

KEYWORDS

- **aerobiology**
- **allergy**
- **allergens**
- **pollen allergy**
- **fungal allergy**
- **indoor fungi**
- **India**

REFERENCES

Acharya, P. J., Skin test response to some inhalant allegens in patients of nasobronchial allergy from Andhra Pradesh. *Asp Allergy App Immunol.* 1980, 13, 14.

Adhikari, A., Sen, M. M., Gupta Bhattacharya, S., Chanda, S., Volumetric assessment of airborne fungi in two sections of rural indoor dairy cattle shed. *Environ Int* 2004, 1071–1078.

Agarwal, M. K., Shivpuri, D. N., Fungal spores—their role in respiratory allergy. *Adv Pollen-Spore Res.* 1974, 1, 78.

Agarwal, M. K., Jones, R. T., Yunginger, J. W., Shared allergenic and antigenic determinants in *Alternaria* and *Stemphyllum* extracts. *J Allergy Clin Immunol.* 1982, 70, 437.

Agashe, S. N., Anand, P., Immediate type hypersensitivity to common pollen and molds in Bangalore city. *Asp Allergy App Immunol.* 1982, 15, 49–52.

Agashe, S. N., Soucenadin, S., Pollen productivity in some allergenically significant plants in Bangalore. *Ind J Aerobiol.* 1992, (Special Vol), 63–67.

Al Doory, Y., Domson, J. F., Beset, T., Further studies on the airborn fungi and pollen of the Washington D.C. metropolitan area. *Ann Allergy.* 1982, 49, 265.

Almaguer, M., Aira, M. J., Rodríguez-Rajo, F. J., Rojas, T. I., Temporal dynamics of airborne fungi in Havana (Cuba) during dry and rainy seasons: influence of meteorological parameters. *Int J Biometeorol.* 2014, 58, 1459–1470.

Almehdi, A. M., Maraqa, M., Abdulkhalik, S., Aerobiological studies and low allerginicity of date-palm pollen in the UAE. *Int J Environ Health Res.* 2005, 15, 217–224.

Andersen, I., Korsgaard, J., Asthma and indoor environment: Assessment of health implications of high indoor humidity. *Environ Int.* 1986, 12, 121.

Anderson, E. F., Dorsett, C. S., Fleming, E. O., The airborne pollens of Walla Walla, Washington. *Ann Allergy.* 1978, 41, 232–235.

Anderson, J. H., Allergenic airborne pollen and spores in Anchorage, Alaska. *Ann Allergy.* 1985, 54, 390–399.

Anonymous. All India Coordinated Project on Aeroallergens and Human Health. Report. Ministry of Environment and Forests, New Delhi, 2000.

Ass, K., Some variables in skin testing standardisation of clinical (Biological) methods. Workshop No. 4. *Allergy.* 1980, 36, 250.

Baldo, B. A., Panzani, R. C., Bass, D., Zerboni, R., Olive (*Olea europaea*) and privet (*Ligustrum vulgare*) pollen allergens. Identification and cross-reactivity with grass pollen proteins. *Mol Immunol.* 1992, 29, 1209–1218.

Barkai, G. R., Glazer, R. I., Indoor survey of moulds and prevalence of mould atopy in Israel. *Israel J Allergy* 1962, 33, 342–348.

Barkai, G. R., Frank, M., Kantor, D., Karadavid, R., Toshner, D., Atmospheric fungi in the desert town of Arad and in the coastal plain of Israel. Ann. *Allergy.* 1977, 28, 270–274.

Bassett, I. J., Air-borne pollen surveys in. Manitoba and Saskatchewan. *Can. J. Pl. Sci.,* 1964, 44, 7.

Bassett, I. J., Crompton, C. W., Parmalee, J. A., An Atlas of Airborne Pollen Grains and Common Fungus Spores of Canada. Scientific Editing, Research Branch, Ontario, Canada, 1978.

Beaumont, F., Kauffman, H. F., Sluiter, H. J., De Vries, K., A volumetric-aerobiologic study of seasonal fungus prevalence inside and outside dwellings of asthmatic patients living in northeast Netherlands. *Ann Allergy.* 1984, 53, 486–492.

Belchi-Hernandez, J., Moreno-Grau, S., Sanchez-Gascon, F., Bayo, J., Elvira Rendueles, B., Bartolome, B., Moreno, J. M., Martinez Quesada, J., Palacios Pelaez, R., Sensitization to *Zygophyllum fabago* pollen. A clinical and immunologic study. *Allergy.* 1998, 53, 241–248.

Belmonte, J., Roure, J. M., Characteristics of the aeroplane dynamics at several localities in Spain. Grana 1991, 30, 364–372.

Blackley, C. H., Hay Fever: Experimental research on the causes, treatment of catarrhus Aestivus. 1873. Baillere Tindall & Cox, London.

Bostock, J., Case of periodical affection of the eyes and chest. *Medico Chirugical Trans.* 1819, 10, 161.

Breton, M. C., Garneau, M., Fortier, I., Guay, F., Louis, J., Relationship between climate, pollen concentrations of Ambrosia and medical consultations for allergic rhinitis in Montreal, *1994–2002 Sci Total Environ.* 2006, 15, 39–50.

Brouwer, J., Cross-reactivity between Aspergillus fumigatus and Penicillium. Int Arch 27 Allergy Immunol 1996, 110, 166–173.

Brown, H. M., Jackson, F. A., Aerobiological studies based in Derby I. I. Simultaneous pollen and spore sampling at eight sites within a 60 km radius. *Clin Allergy.* 1978, 8, 599–609.

Burch, M., Levetin, E., Effects of meteorological conditions on spore plumes. *Int J Biometeorol.* 2002, 46, 107–117.
Cadman, A., Dames, J. F., Airspora of Durban: a subtropical, coastal South African city, I., Pollen component. *Grana* 1993, 32, 372–375.
Cadman, A., Airspora of Johannesburg and Pretoria, South. Africa, 1987/88. II. Meteorological relationships. *Grana* 1991, 30, 181–183.
Calvo, M. A., Guarro, J., Suarez, G., Ramirez, C., Airborne fungi in the air of Barcelona, Spain. V. The yeasts. *Ann Allergy.* 1980, 45, 115–116.
Celenk, S., Bicakci, A., Aerobiological investigation in Bitlis, Turkey. *Ann Agric Environ Med.* 2005, 12, 87–93.
Chanda, S., Atmospheric pollen flora of Greater Calcutta and Falta. *Asp Allergy Appl Immunol.* 1973, 6, 74.
Chang, Z. N., Liu, C. C., Perng, H. C., Tsai, L. C., Han, S. H., A common allergenic epitope of Bermuda grass pollen shared by other grass pollens. *J Biomed Sci,* 1994, 1, 93–99.
Charpin, D., Hughes, B., Mallea, M., Sutra, J. P., Balansard, G., Vervloet, D., Seasonal allergic symptoms and their relation to pollen exposure in south-east France. *Clin Exp Allergy* 1993, 23, 435–439.
Chen, K., Liao, Y., Zhang, J., The major aeroallergens in Guangxi, China. Blackwell, *Clinical Allergy* 1988, 18, 589–596.
Chen, S. H., Huang, T., Aerobiological study of Taipei Basin, Taiwan. *Grana* 1980, 19, 147–155.
Chen, Z. C., Hsiung, Y. M., Tseng, H. Y., In: *Proc 1st Int Conf on Aerobiology, Munich.* 1978, 148–155.
Chowdhury, I., Chakraborty, P., Gupta-Bhattacharya, S., Chanda, S., Allergenic relationship among four common and dominant airborne palm pollen grains from Eastern India. *Clin Exp Allergy* 1998, 28, 977–983.
Chris Lewis, Patricia, E., Wentz, Marc, C., Swanson and Charles, E., Reed. Immunochemical assay of airborne cat allergen: value in assessing variability of allergen shedding and evaluating human bronchial response. *Aerobiologia.* 1990, 6, 193–196.
Collins Williams, C., Kuo, H. K., Garey, D. N., Davidson, S., Collins Williams, D., Fitch, M., Fischer, J. B., Atmospheric mold counts in Toronto, Canada, 1971. *Ann Allergy.* 1973, 2, 69–71.
Cornford, C. A., Fountain, D. W., Burr, R. G., IgE-binding proteins from pine (*Pinus radiata, D., Don*) pollen: evidence for cross-reactivity with ryegrass (*Lolium perenne*). *Int Arch Allergy Appl Immunol.* 1990, 93, 41–46.
Crameri, R., Molecular cloning of Aspergillus fumigatus allergens and their role in allergic bronchopulmonary aspergillosis. *Immunol* 2002, 81, 73–93.
Cristofori, A., Cristofolini, F., Gottardini, E., Twenty years of aerobiological monitoring in Trentino (Italy), assessment and evaluation of airborne pollen variability. *Aerobiologia* 2010, 26, 253–261.
Cunningham, D. O., *Microscopic Examinations of Air*. Govt. Press Calcutta, 1873.
Cvitanovic, S., Znaor, L., Kanceljak-Macan, B., Macan, J., Gudelj, I., Grbic, D., Allergic rhinitis and asthma in southern Croatia: impact of sensitization to *Ambrosia elatior*. Croat Med, J., 2007, 48, 68–75.
D'Amato, G., Liccardi, G., D'Amato, M., Cazzola, M., Outdoor air pollution, climatic changes and allergic bronchial asthma. *Eur Respir J.,* 2002, 20, 763–776.

Dales, R. E., Cakmak, S., Judek, S., Dann, T., Coates, F., Brook, J. R., Burnett, R. T., Influence of outdoor aeroallergens on hospitalization for asthma in Canada. *J Allergy Clin Immunol*. 2005, 115, 426–427.

Davies, R. R., Smith L P. Weather and the grass pollen content of the air. *Clinical and Experimental Allergy*. 1974, 4, 95–108.

Deane, P. M., Conifer pollen sensitivity in western New York: cedar pollens. *Allergy Asthma Proc*. 2005, 26, 352–355.

Derrick, E., Airborne pollen and spores in Melbourne. *Aust J Bot*. 1965, 14, 49–66.

Dirksen, A., Malling, H. J., Mosbech, H., Soborg, Biering, I., HEP versus PNU standardization of allergen extracts in skin prick testing. *Allergy* 1985, 40, 620.

Durham, O. C., The volumetric incidence of atmospheric allergens, IV. A proposed standard method of gravity sampling, counting and volumetric interpolation of the results. *J Allergy* 1946, 17, 79.

El-Ghazaly, Larsson, G., Kotzamanidou-El-Ghazaly, K. A., Nilsson, P. S., Comparison of airborne pollen grains in Huddinge and Stockholm. *Aerobiologia* 1993, 9, 53–67.

Ellis, M. H., Gallup, J., Aeroallergens of southern California. *Immunol Allergy Clin North America* 1989, 9, 365–380.

Emberlin, J., Norris Hill, Bryant, R. H., A tree pollen calendar for London. *Grana* 1990, 29, 301–309.

Enrique, E., Cistero-Bahima, A., Bartolome, B., Alonso, R., San Miguel-Moncin, M. M., Bartra, J., Martinez, A., *Platanus acerifolia* pollinosis and food allergy. *Allergy*. 2002, 57, 351–356.

Fairs, A., Wardlaw, A. J., Thompson, J. R., Pashley, C. H., Guidelines on Ambient Intramural Airborne Fungal Spores. *J Investig Allergol Clin Immunol* 2010, 20, 490–498.

Fang, Z., Ouyang, Z., Hu, L., Wang, X., Zheng, H., Lin, X., Culturable airborne fungi in outdoor environments in Beijing, China. *Sci. Total Environ*. 2005, 1–3: 47–58.

Farhoudi, A., Razavi, A., Chavoshzadeh, Z., Heidarzadeh, M., Bemanian, M. H., Nabavi, M., Descriptive study of 226 patients with allergic rhinitis and asthma in karaj city. *Iran J Allergy Asthma Immunol*. 2005, 4, 99–101.

Feinberg, S. M., Mold allergy. Its importance in Asthma and Hayfever. *Wisconsin Med J.*, 1935, 34, 254–262.

Floyer, J., Violent asthma after visiting a wine cellar. *A Treatise on Asthma*. 3 rd ed. London, 1726.

Galan, C., Infante, F., Ruiz de Clavijo, E., Guerra, F., Miguel, R., Dominguez, E., Allergy to pollen grains from Amaranthaceae and Chenopodiaceae in Cordoba, Spain. Annual and daily variation of pollen concentration. *Ann Allergy*. 1989, 63, 435–438.

Golberg, C., Buch H., Moseholm, L., Weeke, E., Airborne pollen records in Denmark, 1977–1986. *Grana*. 1988, 30, 201–209.

Gonianakis, M. I., Baritaki, M. A., Neonakis, I. K., Gonianakis, I. M., Kypriotakis, Z., Darivianaki, E., Bouros, D., Kontou-Filli, K., A 10-year aerobiological study (1994–2003) in the Mediterranean island of Crete, Greece: trees, aerobiologic data, and botanical and clinical correlations. *Allergy Asthma Proc*. 2006, 27, 371–377.

Gravesen, S., Fungi as a cause of allergic disease. *Allergy* 1979, 135–154.

Groenewoud, G. C., de Jong, N. W., Burdorf, A., de Groot, H., van Wyk, R. G., Prevalence of occupational allergy to Chrysanthemum pollen in greenhouses in the Netherlands. *Allergy* 2002, 57, 835–840.

Gupta S and Chanda, S., Aeropalynological survey in subtropical Eastrn Himalayas, Kurseong, *Grana* 1989, 28, 219.
Gupta, S. K., Pareira, B. M., Singh, A. B., Survey of airborne culturable and non-culturable fungi at different sites in Delhi metropolis. *Asian Pac J Allergy Immunol.* 1993, 19–28.
Gupta, S. K., Pereira, B. M., Singh, A. B., Fomes pectinatis: an aeroallergen in India. *Asian Pac J Allergy Immunol.* 1999, 17, 1–7.
Hawke, P. R., Meadows, M. E., Winter airspora spectra and. meteorological conditions in Cape Town, South Africa. *Grana.* 1989, 28, 187–192.
Hayes, T., Lopez, S., Montealegre, F., Suarez, E., Employment of a PCR-based monitoring system to detect bacteria and fungi from indoor air samples at indoor work places: a pilot study in Ponce, *Puerto Rico. Ethn Dis.* 2005, 4, 29–30.
Hayward, B. J., Augustin, R., Longbottom, J. L., Separation and characterization of antibodies to moulds in human sera. *Acta Allergol. Suppl. (Copenh).* 1960, 7, 87–93.
Higuchi, K., Nakagawa, S., Katsuda, M., A survey on atmospheric pollen and pollinosis in West Japan. *Jap J Allergol.* 1977, 26, 104.
Hirst, J. M., An automatic volumetric spore trap. *Ann Appl Biol.* 1952, 39, 252–263.
Hjelmroos, M., Long-distance transport of *Betula* pollen grains and allergic symptoms. *Aerobiologia* 1992, 8, 231–236.
Howlett, B. J., Hill, D. J., Knox, R. B., Cross-reactivity between Acacia (wattle) and rye grass pollen allergens. Detection of allergens in Acacia (wattle) pollen. *Clin Allergy* 1982, 12, 259–268.
Huang, X., Johansson, S. G., Zargari, A., Nordvall, S. L., Allergen cross-reactivity between Pityrosporum orbiculare and Candida albicans. *Allergy* 1995, 50, 648–56.
Hussain, M. M., Mandal, J., Bhattacharya, K., Airborne load of Cassia pollen in West Bengal, eastern India: its atmospheric variation and health impact. *Environ Monit Assess* 2013, 185, 2735–2744.
Hyde, H. A., Williams, D. A., Studies in Atmospheric Pollen. I. A Daily Census of Pollens at Cardiff, *1942 New Phytologist* 1944, 43, 49–61.
Hyde, H. A., Aeropalynology in Britain: An Outline. *New Phytologist* 1969, 68, 579–590.
Hyde, H. A., Oncus, a new term in pollen morphology. *New Phytologist.* 1955, 54, 255–256.
Ishizaka, T., Koizumi, K., Ikemori, R., Ishiyama, Y., Kushibiki, E., Studies of prevalence of Japanese cedar pollinosis among the residents in a densely cultivated area. *Ann. Allergy* 1987, 47, 265–270.
Johansen, S., Airborne pollen and spores on the Arctic island of Jan Mayen. *Grana.* 1991, 30, 373–379.
Kachyk SJT and Khan, R. S., Airborn mold survey – Edmanton. *J Asthma Res.* 1977, 14, 103–106.
Kallawicha, K., Tsai, Y. J., Chuang, Y. C., Lung, S. C., Wu, C. D., Chen, T. H., Chen, P. C., Chompuchan, C., Chao, H. J., The spatiotemporal distributions and determinants of ambient fungal spores in the Greater Taipei area. *Environ Pollut.* 2015, 204, 173–80.
Kang, B., Velody, D., Homburger, H., Yuninger, J. W., Analysis of indoor environment and atopic allergy in urban population with bronchial asthma. *J Allergy Clin Immunol.* 1979, 63, 80.

Kantor, S. Z., Frank, M., Hoch-Kantor, D., Barkai-Golan, R., Marian, D., Schachnner, E., Kessler, A., de Vries, A., Airborne allergens and clinical response of asthmatics in Arad, a new town in a desert area in Israel. *J Allergy*. 1966, 37, 65–74.

Käpylä, M., Diurnal variation of tree pollen in the air in Finland. *Grana*. 1984, 23, 167–176.

Kasliwal, R. M., Solomon, S. K., Correlation of respiratory allergy cases with atmosphere pollen concentrations and meteorological factors. *J Ass Physics (India)*, 1958, 6, 180–195.

Kazemi-Shirazi, L., Pauli, G., Purohit, A., Spitzauer, S., Froschl, R., Hoffmann-Sommergruber, K., Breiteneder, H., Scheiner, O., Kraft, D., Valenta, R., Quantitative IgE inhibition experiments with purified recombinant allergens indicate pollen-derived allergens as the sensitizing agents responsible for many forms of plant food allergy. *J Allergy Clin Immunol*. 2000, 105, 116–125.

Kino T and Oshima, S., Allergy to insects in Japan. The reaginic sensitivity to moth and butterfly in patients with bronchial asthma. *J Allergy Clin Immunol*. 1978, 10–16.

Kochar, S., Ahlawat, M., Dahiya, P., Chaudhary, D., Assessment of allergenicity to fungal allergens of Rohtak city, Haryana, India. *Allergy Rhinol* 2014, 5, e56–e65.

Kotzamanidou P and Nilsson, S., On the pollen incidence and. phenology of some trees in Southern and Central Sweden, 1974–1975. A preliminary study. *Grana* 1977, 16, 195–198.

Lacey J and Crook, B., Fungal and actinomycetes spore as pollutants of workplace and occupational allergens. *Ann Occup Hyg*. 1988, 32, 515.

Larsen, L. S., A three-year-survey of microfungi in the air of Copenhagen 1977–79. *Allergy* 1981, 1, 15–22.

Lehrer, S. B., Hughes, J. M., Altman, L. C., Bousquet, J., Davies, R. J., Gell, L., Li, J., Lopez, M., Malling, H. J., Mathison, D. A., et al., Prevalence of basidiomycete allergy in the USA and Europe and its relationship to allergic respiratory symptoms. Investigation on airborne pollen in Basel and Davos (Switzerland) in connection with pollinosis. *Allergy*. 1994, 49, 460–465.

Lewis, W. H., Theory and Practice. Korenblat, P. E., Wender, H. J. (Ed.), Grune and Startton, Orlando, *Allergy*. 1984, 353–369.

Liam, C. K., Loo, K. L., Wong, C. M., Lim, K. H., Lee, T. C., Skin prick test reactivity to common aeroallergens in asthmatic patients with and without rhinitis. *Respirology* 2002, 7, 345–350.

Lin, R. Y., Clauss, A. E., Bennett, E. S., Hypersensitivity to common tree pollens in New York City patients. *Allergy Asthma Proc*. 2002, 23, 253–258.

Long, R., Yin, R., He, H., Li, Z., Liu, D., *J West China Univ Med Sci*. 1987, 18, 60–63.

Loureiro, G., Rabaca, M. A., Blanco, B., Andrade, S., Chieira, C., Pereira, C., Lu, Y. C., Tzeng, J. C., Huang, S. G., Aeroallergens sensitization in an allergic paediatric population of Cova da Beira, Portugal. *Allergol Immunopathol (Madr)* 2005, 33, 192–198.

Lugauskas, A., Krikstaponis, A., Sveistyte, L., Airborne fungi in industrial environments-potential agents of respiratory diseases. *Ann Agric Environ Med*. 2004, 11, 19–25.

Mallo, A. C., Nitiu, D. S., Sambeth MCG. Airborne fungal spore content in the atmosphere of the city of La Plata, Argentina. *Aerobiologia* 2011, 27, 77–84.

Marcotte, G. V., Braun, C. M., Norman, P. S., Nicodemus, C. F., Kagey Sobotka, A., Lichtenstein, L. M., Essayan, D. M., Effects of peptide therapy on ex vivo T-cell responses. *J Allergy Clin Immunol.* 1998, 101, 506–513.

Mari, A., Iacovacci, P., Afferini C et al., Specific IgE to cross-reactive carbohydrate determinants strongly affect the in vitro diagnosis of allergic diseases. *J Allergy Clin Immunol* 1999, 103: 1005–111.

Mari, A., Schneider, P., Wally, V., Breitenbach, M., Simon-Nobbe, B., Sensitization to fungi: epidemiology, comparative skin tests, and IgE reactivity of fungal extracts. *Clin Exp Allergy* 2003, 33, 1429–1438.

Martin, C. J., Platt, S. D., Hunt, S. M., Housing conditions and ill health. *Br Med, J.*, 1987, 294–1125.

Martinez Giron, R., Ribas Barcelo, A., Garcia Miralles, M. T., Lopez Cabanilles, D., Tamargo Maribhat, M., Rajasaab, A. H., Airspora of commercial location at Gulbarga. *In J Aerobiol.* 1988, 59–65.

Masuda, S., Fujisawa, T., Iguchi, K., Atsuta, J., Noma, Y., Nagao, M., Nambu, M., Suehiro, Y., Kamesaki, S., Terada, A., Mizuno, M., Shimizu, S., Tohda, Y., Prevalence of sensitization of Japanese cedar pollen in children from infancy to adolescence. *Arerugi.* 2006, 55, 1312–1320.

Melissa Anne Hart, Richard de Dear, Paul John Beggs. A synoptic climatology of pollen concentrations during the six warmest months in Sydney, Australia. *Int J Biometeorol* 2007, 51, 209–220.

Mercer, F. V., Atmospheric pollen in the city of Adelaide and. *Environs Trans Roy Soc SA* 1941, 63, 373–383.

Michel, F. B., Cour, P., Quet, L., Marty, J. P., Qualitative and quantitative comparison of pollen calendars for plain and mountain areas. *Clin Exp Allergy.* 1976, 6, 383–388.

Miralles, J. C., Caravaca, F., Guillen, F., Lombardero, M., Negro, J. M., Cross-reactivity between Platanus pollen and vegetables. *Allergy*. 2002, 57, 146–149.

Moss, J. E., Airborne pollen in Brisbane. *Aus J Bot.* 1965, 13, 23–27.

Mourad, W., Mecheri, S., Peltre, G., David, B., Hebert, J., Study of the epitope structure of purified. Dac, G. I., and Lol, P. I., the major allergens of *Dactylis glomerata* and *Lolium perenne* pollens, using monoclonal antibodies. *J Immunol.* 1988, 141, 3486–3491.

Mullins, J., Warnock, D. W., Powell, J., Jones, I., Harvey, R., Grass pollen content of the air in the Bristol Channel region in 1976. *Clin Allergy*. 1977, 7, 391–395.

Naranjo, P., Etiological agents of respiratory allergy in tropical countries of Central and South America. *J Allergy* 1958, 362–374.

Noon, L., Prophylactic inoculation against hay fever. *Lancet* 1911, 18, 287.

Nunes, Z. G., Martins, A. S., Altoe, A. L., Nishikawa, M. M., Leite, M. O., Agujar, P. F., Fracalanzza, S. E., Indoor air microbiological evaluation of offices, hospitals, industries, and shopping centers. *Mem. Inst. Oswaldo Cruz.* 2005, 4, 351–357.

O'Connor, G. T., Walter, M., Mitchell, H., Kattan, M., Morgan, W. J., Gruchalla, R. S., Pongracic, J. A., Smartt, E., Stout, J. W., Evans, R., Crain, E. F., Burge, H. A., Airborne fungi in the homes of children with asthma in low-income urban communities: The Inner-City Asthma Study. *J Allergy Clin Immunol.* 2004, 3, 599–606.

O'Neil, C. E., Hughes, J. M., Butcher, B. T., Salvaggio, J. E., Lehrer, S. B., Basidiospore extracts: evidence for common antigenic/allergenic determinants. *Int Arch Allergy Appl Immunol* 1988, 85, 161–166.

Ogunlana, E. O., Fungal air spora at Ibaden, Nigeria. *Appl Microbiol.* 1975, 29, 458–463.

Ordman, D., Seasonal respiratory allergy in Windhoek: the pollen and fungus factors. *S Afr Med.* 1970, 44, 250–253.

Oh, J. W., Lee, H. B., Kang, I. J., Kim, S. W., Park, K. S., Kook, M. H., Kim, B. S., Baek, H. S., Kim, J. H., Kim, J. K., Lee, D. J., Kim, K. R., Choi, Y. J., The Revised Edition of Korean Calendar for Allergenic Pollens. *Allergy Asthma Immunol Res.* 2012, 4, 5–11.

Ozkargoz, K., Pollen, spores and other inhalant as etiologic agents of respiratory allergy in the central part of Turkey. *J Allergy.* 1967, 40, 21–25.

Pallasaho, P., Ronmark, E., Haahtela, T., Sovijarvi, A. R., Lundback, B., Degree and clinical relevance of sensitization to common allergens among adults: a population study in Helsinki, Finland. *Clin Exp Allergy.* 2006, 36, 503–509.

Palmas, F., Murgia, R., Deplano, M., Fadda, M. E., Cosentino, S., Results of an airborne spore study in various regions of southern Sardinia. *Ann Ig.* 1989, 1647–1656.

Palosuo, T., Panzani, R. C., Singh, A. B., Ariano, R., Alenius, H., Turjanmaa, K., Allergen cross-reactivity between proteins of the latex from *Hevea brasiliensis*, seeds and pollen of *Ricinus communis*, and pollen of *Mercurialis annua*, members of the Euphorbiaceae family. *Allergy Asthma Proc.* 2002, 23, 141–147.

Pandit T and Singh, A. B., Saccharomyces cerevisiae (Yeast), A Potential Aeroallergen for the workers of Sugar industry. *Ind J Aerobiol.* 1994, 13–19.

Pepys, J., The role of human precipitins to common fungal antigens in allergic reactions. *Acta Allergol. Suppl, (Copenh).* 1960, 108–111.

Perez, M., Ishioka, G. Y., Walker, L. E., Chestnut, E. R., CDNA cloning and immunological characterization of the rye grass allergen Lol P I. *J. Biol. Chem.* 1990, 265, 162–10.

Perkins, W. A., *The Rotorod Sampler.* The second semiannual report. Aerosl Lab. CML Standford University, Stanford, 1957, 186, 66.

Peterson, P. K., Mcglave, P., Ramsay, N. K., Rhame, F., Cohen, E., Perry, G. S., Goldman, A. I., Kersey, J., A prospective study of infectious diseases following bone marrow transplantation: emergence of Aspergillus and Cytomegalovirus as the major causes of mortality. *Infect Control.* 1983, 81–89.

Pike, R. N., Bagarozzi, D. Jr., Travis, J., Immunological cross-reactivity of the major allergen from perennial ryegrass (*Lolium perenne*), Lol p, I., and the cysteine proteinase, bromelain. *Int Arch Allergy Immunol.* 1997, 112, 412–414.

Port, A., Hein, J., Wolff, A., Bielory, L., Aeroallergen prevalence in the northern New Jersey-New York City metropolitan area: a 15-year summary. *Ann Allergy Asthma Immunol.* 2006, 96, 687–691.

Potter, P. C., Mather, S., Lockey, P., Ainslie, G., Cadman, A., IgE specific immune responses to an African grass (Kikuyu, *Pennisetum clandestinum*). *Clin Exp Allergy.* 1993, 23, 537–541.

Prescott, R. A., Potter, P. C., Allergenicity and cross-reactivity of buffalo grass (*Stenotaphrum secundatum*). *S Afr Med J.*, 2001, 91, 237–243.

Prince, H. E., Meyer, G. H., An up-to-date look at mold allergy. *Ann Allergy.* 1976, 1, 18–25.

Ramfjord, H., Outdoor appearance of aroallergens in Norway. *Grana* 1991, 30, 91–97.
Ramos Morin, C. J., Canseco Gonzalez, C., Hypersensitivity to airborne allergens common in the central region of Coahuila. *Rev Alerg Mex.* 1994, 41, 84–87.
Rawat, A., Singh, A., Roy, I., Kumar, L., Gaur, S. N., Ravindran, P., Bhatnagar, A. K., Singh, A. B., Assessment of allergenicity to *Mallotus phillipensis* pollen in atopic patients in India: a new allergen. *J Investig Allergol Clin Immunol.* 2004, 14, 198–207.
Reijula, K., Leino, M., Mussalo-Rauhamaa, H., Nikulin, M., Alenius, H., Mikkola, J., Elg, P., Kari, O., Makinen-Kiljunen, S., Haahtela, T., IgE-mediated allergy to fungal allergens in Finland with special reference to *Alternaria alternata* and *Cladosporium herbarum*. *Ann Allergy Asthma Immunol.* 2003, 91, 280–287.
Ren, P., Jankun, T. M., Leaderer, B. P., Comparisons of seasonal fungal prevalence in indoor and outdoor air and in house dusts of dwellings in one Northeast American county. *J. Expo. Anal Environ Epidemiol.* 1999, 9, 560–568.
Ritchie, J. C., Modern Pollen Spectra from Dakhleh Oasis, Western Desert, Egypt. *Grana* 1986, 25, 117–187.
Roberts, A. M., Van Ree, R., Cardy, S. M., Bevan, L. J., Walker, M. R., Recombinant pollen allergens from *Dactylis glomerata*: preliminary evidence that human IgE cross-reactivity between Dac g, I. I., Lol p I/II is increased following grass pollen immunotherapy. *Immunology* 1992, 76, 389–396.
Roby, R. R., Sneller, M. R., Incidence of fungal spores at the homes of allergic patients in an agricultural community, II. Correlation of skin test with mould frequency. *Ann Allergy.* 1979, 43, 286.
Rose C S. Bioaerosols: Assessment and Control. In: Macher, J., Ammann, H. A., Burge, D. K., Milton, Morey, P. R. (ed.). *American Conference of Governmental Industrial Hygienists* (www.acgih.org), Cincinnati, OH, Antigens, 1999, 25–11.
Saad, S. I., Studies on atmospheric pollen and fungal spores at Alexandria. *Egypt J Bot.* 1959, 17–22.
Sabariego Ruiz, S., Diaz de la Guardia Guerrero, C., Alba Sanchez, F., Aerobiological study of *Alternaria* and *Cladosporium* conidia in the atmosphere of Almeria (SE Spain). *Rev Iberoam Micol.* 2004, 3, 121–127.
Salvaggio, J., Aukrust, L., Postgraduate course presentations. Mold-induced asthma. *J Allergy Clin Immunol.* 1981, 327–346.
Salvaggio J and Seabury, J., New Orleans asthma. IV. Semiquantitative airborne spore sampling, 1967 and 1968. *J Allergy Clin Immunol.* 1971, 2, 82–95.
Samir, H., Wageh, W., Abd-Elaziz Emam, M. M., Demonstration of aeroallergenicity of fungal hyphae and hyphal fragments among allergic rhinitis patients using a novel immunostaining technique. *Egypt J Otolaryngol* 2014, 30, 17–22.
Sandhu, S. K., Shivpuri, D. N., Sandhu, R. S., Studies on the airborne fungal spores in Delhi. Ann. *Allergy*. 1964, 374–384.
Scheppegrell, W., Hayfever in Southern states. *5th Med J Nashville* 1916, 9, 624.
Sen, M. M., Adhikari, A., Gupta-Bhattacharya, S., Chanda, S., Airborne rice pollen and pollen allergen in an agricultural field: aerobiological and immunochemical evidence. *J Environ Monit.* 2003, 5, 959–962.
Sener, O., Kim, Y. K., Ceylan, S., Ozanguc, N., Yoo, T. J., Comparison of skin tests to aeroallergens in Ankara and Seoul. *J Investig Allergol Clin Immunol.* 2003, 13, 202–208.

Shafiee, A., Studies of atmospheric pollen in Tehran, Iran, 1974–1975. *Annals of Allergy*. 1976, 37, 138–142.

Sharma, R., Deval, R., Priyadarshi, V., Gaur, S. N., Singh, A. B., Indoor survey of fungi in the homes of asthmatic/allergic children in Delhi. *In J Aerobiol.* 2005, 18(2), 69–74.

Sharma, R., Deval, R., Priyadarshi, V., Gaur, S. N., Singh, V. P., Singh, A. B., Indoor fungal concentration in the homes of allergic/asthma children in Delhi, India. *Allergy Rhinol* 2011, 2, 21–32.

Sharma, R., Gaur, S. N., Singh, V. P., Singh, A. B., Association between indoor fungi in Delhi homes and sensitization in children with respiratory allergy. *Med Mycol* 2012, 50, 281–290.

Shelton, B. G., Kirkland, K. H., Flanders, W. D., Morris, G. K., Profiles of airborne fungi in buildings and outdoor environments in the United States. *Appl Environ Microbiol.* 2002, 4, 1743–1753.

Shivpuri, D. N., Singh, A. B., Babu, C. R., New allergenic pollens of Delhi state, India and their clinical significance. *Ann Allergy*. 1979, 42, 49–52.

Shivpuri, D. N., Vishwanathan, R., Dua, L. K., Studies in pollen Allergy in Delhi area I—Pollination calendar. *Ind J Med Res*. 1960, 48, 15–20.

Shivpuri, D. N., Clinically important pollen, fungal and insect allergens for naso bronchial allergy patients in India. *Asp Allergy Appl Immunol.* 1980, 13, 19–23.

Silvers, W. S., Ledoux, R. A., Dolen, W. K., Morrison, M. R., Nelson, H. S., Weber, R. W., Aerobiology of the Colorado Rockies: pollen count comparisons between Vail and Denver, Colorado. *Ann Allergy*. 1992, 69, 421–426.

Singh A B, Khandelwal, A., An Atlas of Allergenically Significant Plants of India. *Pub. Himalaya Pub.* Mumbai, India, 2016.

Singh, A., Panzani, R. C., Singh, A. B., Specific IgE to castor bean (*Ricinus communis*) pollen in the sera of clinically sensitive patients to seeds. *J Investig Allergol Clin Immunol.* 1997, 7, 169–174.

Singh, A. B., Kumar, P., Common environmental allergens causing respiratory allergy in India. *Indian J Pediatr.* 2002, 69, 245–250.

Singh, A. B., Ravi Deval. Aerobiology of Fungi Associated with Allergy. In: Mould Allergy Biology and Pathogenesis; 2005, 105–136, ISBN: 81-308-0050-0, Research Signpost; USA.

Singh, A. B., Singh, A., Pollen Allergy—A Global Scenario. In: *Recent Trends in Aerobiology, Allergy and Immunology*. Agashe, S. N. Eds. 1994, Oxford and IBH, New Delhi.

Singh, A. B., Dahiya, P., Pandit, T., Changes in air borne pollen concentration during a seven-year consecutive survey in Delhi metropolis. Grana. 2003, 42, 168–77.

Singh, A. B., FTR, *Ministry of Environment and Forests*, New Delhi, 1994.

Singh, B. P., Singh, A. B., Gangal, S. V., *Calendars of Different States, India*. CSIR Centre for Biochemicals, Pub., Delhi, India, 1992.

Singh, B. P., Singh, A. B., Parkash, D., Skin reactivity to airborne pollen and fungal antigens in patients of Naso Bronchial Allergy of Hill Regions (India). In: Chandra, N. (Ed.), *Atmospheric Bio Pollution*. 1987, 125–134.

Singh, B. P., Verma, J., Sridhara, S., Rai, D., Makhija, N., Gaur, S. N., Gangal, S. V., Immunobiochemical characterization of *Putranjiva roxburghii* pollen extract and cross-reactivity with *Ricinus communis*. *Int Arch Allergy Immunol.* 1997, 114, 251–257.

Smart, I. J., Knox, R. B., Aerobiology of Grass Pollen in the City Atmosphere of Melbourne: Quantitative Analysis of Seasonal. and Diurnal Changes. *Aust J Bot.* 1979, 27, 317–331.

Smith, P. M., Xu, H., Swoboda, I., Singh, M. B., Identification of Ca2+ binding protein as a new Bermuda grass pollen allergen Cyn d 7, IgE cross reactivity with oilseed rape pollen allergen Bra r 1. *Int Arch Allergy Immunol.* 1997, 114, 265–271.

Solomon, W. R., Sampling airborn allergens. *Ann Allergy* 1984, 52, 140.

Sousa, L., Camacho, I. C., Grinn-Gofroń, A., Camacho, R., Monitoring of anamorphic fungal spores in Madeira region (Portugal), 2003–2008. *Aerobiologia,* 2015. doi: 10.1007/s10453-015-9400-8.

Spieksma FThM. Airborne pollen concentration in Leiden, The Netherlands, 1977–1981. III Herbs and weeds flowering in summer. *Grana*, 1986, 25, 47–54.

Sprenger, J. D., Altman, L. C., O'Neil, C. E., Ayars, G. H., Butcher, B. T., Lehrer, S. B., Prevalence of basidiospore allergy in the Pacific Northwest. *J Allergy Clin Immunol.* 1988, 82, 1076–1080.

Stix, E., Grass pollen-gehalt der luft von muchen. *Munch Med Wschr,* 1977, 119, 1595–1698.

Subbarao, M., Prakash, O., Subbarao, P. V., Reaginic allergy to Parthenium pollen: evaluation by skin test and RAST. *Clin Exp Allergy* 1985, 15, 449–454.

Tarlo, S. M., Bell, B., Srinivasan, J., Dolovich, J., Hargreave, F. E., Human sensitization to Ganoderma antigen. *J Allergy Clin Immunol.* 1979, 1, 43–49.

Tilak, S. T., Kulkarni, R. L., Addition in the fungal flora of the air. *Ind Phytopathol.* 1980, 34, 69–71.

Tilak, S. T., Saibaba, M., Pillai, S. G., Bhasale, S. S., *Proc Nat Conf Env Bio.* 1981, 49–54.

Valenta, R., Kraft, D., From allergen structure to new forms of allergen-specific immunotherapy. *Curr Opin Immunol.* 2002, 6, 718–727.

Vishwanathan, R., Definition, incidence, etiology and natural history of asthma. *Ind J Chest Dis.* 1964, 6, 108.

Waegemaekers, M., Wageningen, N. Van, Brunekeef, B., Boleji, J. S. M. Respiratory symptoms in damp homes: a pilot study. *Allergy.* 1989, 44, 192.

Wan Ishlah L and Gendeh, B. S., Skin prick test reactivity to common airborne pollens and molds in allergic rhinitis patients. *Med J Malaysia* 2005, 60, 194–200.

Wittmaack, K., Wehnes, H., Heinzmann, U., Agerer, R., An overview on bioaerosols viewed by scanning electron microscopy. *Sci Total Environ.* 2005, 346, 244–55.

Yamamoto, N., Bibby, K., Qian, J., Hospodsky, D., Rismani-Yazdi, H., Nazaroff, W. W., Peccia, J., Particle-size distributions and seasonal diversity of allergenic and pathogenic fungi in outdoor air. *The ISME Journal* 2012, 6, 1801–1811.

Zhong, W., Levin, L., Reponen, T., Hershey, G. K., Adhikari, A., Shukla, R., LeMasters, G., Analysis of short-term influences of ambient aeroallergens on pediatric asthma hospital visits. *Sci Total Environ.* 2006 Nov 1, 370(2–3), 330–336. Epub 2006.

CHAPTER 4

METEOROLOGICAL AND CLINICAL ANALYSIS OF AEROALLERGEN DATA: INCREASE IN ALLERGY AND ASTHMA CASES IN THE TEXAS PANHANDLE

NABARUN GHOSH,[1] GRISELDA ESTRADA,[1] MITSY VELOZ,[1] DANIUS BOUYI,[1] JON BENNERT,[2] JEFF BENNERT,[2] CONSTANTINE SAADEH,[3] and CHANDINI REVANNA[4]

[1]*Life, Earth and Environmental Sciences, West Texas A&M University, Canyon, Texas 79015, USA, E-mail: nghosh@wtamu.edu, velozfam6401@yahoo.com; gestrada1@buffs.wtamu.edu, emersonbouyi@hotmail.com*

[2]*Air Oasis, Research and Development, Amarillo, Texas 79118, USA, E-mail: jon@airoasis.com; drj@airoasis.com*

[3]*Allergy A.R.T.S., Amarillo, Texas 79124, USA, E-mail: csaadeh@allergyarts.com*

[4]*Department of Environmental Health and Safety, Texas Tech University, Lubbock, TX 79409, E-mail: c.revanna@ttu.edu*

CONTENTS

ABSTRACT

Regional aerobiology can help in diagnosis and treatment of allergic rhinitis. Environmental factors contribute to a high concentration of aeroallergen that led to the increased allergy cases among the residents of Texas Panhandle. Allergy and Asthma cases have doubled in the Texas Panhandle area since 2007 (Ranaivo, 2011). Aeroallergens cause serious allergic and asthmatic reactions. Analyzing the aeroallergens with a Burkard Spore Trap provided information regarding the onset, duration, and severity of the pollen season that clinicians use to guide allergen selection for skin testing and treatment. We have been investigating the daily aeroallergen concentration in terms of the meteorological conditions such as daily temperature, wind speed and precipitation. We used a Burkard Volumetric Spore Trap to determine the daily aeroallergen index by collecting aeroallergen samples and characterizing them for 15 years. In the Burkard Volumetric Spore Trap the drum rotates while a vacuum pump sucks in the air trapping the aeroallergen onto the tape. Exposed Melinex tape was stained, mounted and observed under a BX-40 Olympus microscope attached to a DP-70 digital camera and a computer with the Image Pro plus software. The aeroallergens were micro-graphed and the monthly aeroallergen data were compared with the incidence of allergy and asthma cases from 2000–2014. Aeroallergens were viewed for fluorescence with FITC and TRITC fluorescent filters, micrographed and analyzed. A high-pressure mercury lamp was used to excite the storage molecules or proteins, which exhibited autofluorescence. SEM proved to be useful for observing ultra-structural details like pores, colpi, sulci and ornamentations on the pollen surface. Pollen grains were measured under SEM using the TM-1000 imaging software that revealed the size of colpi or sulci and the distance between the micro-structures. The aeroallergen data that we collected using a Burkard Spore Trap for 15 years showed a steady increase in aeroallergen concentration in the Texas Panhandle area. A fluctuation and gradual shift in aeroallergen index with the warmer climate and a shift in flowering seasons were noticed that contributed to the increased allergy cases. The characterization and analysis of microscopic aeroallergens was accomplished using Fluorescent and Scanning Electron Microscopy. Aeroallergens that were viewed, recorded, and analyzed with fluorescent microscopy exhibited storage protein, oil granules, and the layer of sporopollenin, along with additional ultra-structural details like concordant pattern, exines, pores, colpi, sulci, and other ornamentations. The SEM provided micro-measurements and additional views of the detailed ultra-structural morphology. Analyzing the aeroallergens collected and sampled with the Burkard Spore Trap provided information regarding the onset, duration, and severity of the pollen season that was compared to the number of patient cases seen over a 15-year period. The data accumulated for these studies can be utilized for the forecasting the types and duration of the pollen season. Temperature was found to have an inverse relationship with mold spore concentration. Rainfall had a direct correlation with the mold count directly, increase in precipitation resulted in subsequent higher mold spore concentrations.

4.1 INTRODUCTION

Allergy is a kind of sensitivity to a normally harmless substance, one that does not bother most people. The allergen (the foreign substance that provokes a reaction) can be a food, dust particles, a drug, insect venom, or mold spores, as well as pollen. Allergic people often have sensitivity to more than one substance. Some of the most common symptoms associated with allergy include swelling, wheezing, itchy eyes, ears, lips, throat and palate and sinus pain, shortness of breath, runny nose, sickness vomiting and diarrhea, coughing and increase in secretions. Normally, the immune system functions as the body's defense against invading agents (bacteria and viruses, for instance). In most allergic reactions, however, the immune system is responding to a false alarm. When allergic persons first come into contact with an allergen, their immune systems treat the allergen as an invader and mobilize to attack. The immune system does this by generating large amounts of a type of antibody *immunoglobulin E*, or IgE. Only small amounts of IgE are produced in non-allergic people.

Each IgE antibody is specific for one particular allergen. In the case of pollen allergy, the antibody is specific for each type of pollen: one antibody may be produced to react against oak pollen and another against ragweed pollen, for example. Among North American plants, weeds are the most prolific producers of allergenic pollen. Ragweed is the major culprit, but others of importance are sagebrush, redroot pigweed *(Amaranthus retroflexus)*, lamb's quarters *(Chenopodium album)*, Russian thistle (tumbleweed), and English plantain. Grasses and trees, too, are important sources of allergenic pollens. Trees that produce allergenic pollen include oak, ash, elm, hickory, pecan, box elder, and mountain cedar (Website of Pollen Allergy).

Allergic Rhinitis is an inflammatory disease of the mucous membranes that affects about 7.8% of people 18 years of age and older in the United States and between 10% and 30% of the population worldwide (Pawankar, 2012). Allergic rhinitis is triggered by air-borne allergens. An "allergen" is defined as a usually harmless substance capable of triggering a response that starts in the immune system of a predisposed individual and results in an allergic reaction (Pawankar, 2012). Some of the most common allergens include pollen, dust mites, animal dander, fungal spores and hyphae, medications, insect venoms and various foods. Some of the common symptoms of allergic rhinitis include: rhinorrhea, nasal congestion, postnasal drainage, nasal itching, sneezing, and watery eyes. Even though there are several allergens that can trigger allergic rhinitis, two of the greatest triggers are airborne plant pollen and fungal spores. Pollen is the male gametophyte of seed plants and is produced by both gymnosperms and angiosperms in order to reproduce.

In gymnosperms, the pollen is produced in cones, while in angiosperms the pollen is produced in the anthers. Most airborne pollens range in size from 12 to 70 μm and can only be properly identified using a microscope (Bush, 1989). Fungi reproduce by fragmenting of the fungus body (mycelium) or by specialized cells called spores that are produced on fruiting branches (Bush, 1989). Air contains a massive amount of different particles. The concentration of different kinds of pollen and fungal spores can be very different from one country to another, in different regions of the same country, and even among different cities mainly because airborne pollen depends much on vegetation and its local environment. Commonly, meteorological factors also have a significant influence on this airborne concentration as well. The airborne pollen and spore concentration is of significance in the medical world because these allergens can be inhaled by predisposed individuals and trigger allergic rhinitis or "hay fever." These individuals may visit allergy clinics in need of allergy diagnosing and treatment of their allergy symptoms. There are two types of allergic rhinitis, seasonal and perennial. Seasonal allergic rhinitis is the most common and typically happens only at certain times of the year as to perennial rhinitis that lasts year round.

Recently, there has been a major increase in the number of individuals suffering from allergic rhinitis all over the world. Interestingly enough, there has also been a major increase in the number of people with asthma. The rate of Amarillo residents suffering from allergy and asthma has increased to 13% since 2007 and is twice that of Texas (6.5%) (Ranaivo, 2011). Global Climate change is prompting many plant species into a sort of species survival mode in which they release more pollen (Angelin and Ghosh, 2014). Many studies around the world have suggested that an increase in air-borne pollen as well as fungal spores have had a huge impact in the increased allergic rhinitis and asthma trend. Even though much research has been done globally, not much has been accomplished in the Texas Panhandle. This study was aimed at examining the concentrations of pollen and fungal spores of the Texas Panhandle throughout recent years that could help in establishing a relationship between aeroallergen concentrations in terms of meteorological conditions. It is with this idea in mind that a Burkard spore trap was placed on the 3rd floor roof top of the

Agriculture and Natural Sciences building, on a flat surface away from any walls or obstacles to obtain an adequate reading of the pollen and fungal spore concentrations.

4.2 AEROALLERGENS AND ALLERGIC RHINITIS

Aeroallergens are often the cause of serious allergic and asthmatic reactions, affecting millions of people each year (Nester, 2001). Aeroallergen sampling provides information regarding the onset, duration, and severity of the pollen season that clinicians use to guide allergen selection for skin testing and treatment (Dvorin et al., 2001). Aeroallergens include pollens, fungal spores, dusts, plant fibers, burnt residues and plant products like gums and resins. All these microscopic objects are captured from an urban locality using a Burkard Spore Trap. The types of pollen that most commonly cause allergic reactions are produced by the plain-looking plants (trees, grasses, and weeds) that do not have showy flowers. These plants manufacture small, light, dry pollen granules that are custom-made for wind transport; for example, samples of ragweed pollen have been collected 400 miles out at sea and 2 miles high in the air. Since airborne pollen is carried for long distances, it does little good to rid an area of an offending plant—the pollen can drift in from many miles away.

4.3 FUNGAL SPORES AS AEROALLERGENS

For decades, airborne fungal spores have been implicated as the causative factors in respiratory allergy. Exposure to high atmospheric spore counts and sensitization to specific fungal allergens have been associated with severe asthma, mainly in young adults (Helbling, 2003). Sensitivity to fungi is a significant cause of allergic diseases, and prolonged exposure to fungi is a growing health concern (Santilli, 2003). Bogacka et al. (2003) considers the allergy to mold allergens as a risk factor for bronchial asthma in patients suffering from allergic rhinitis. Most fungi commonly considered allergenic, such as *Alternaria* spp., *Cladosporium* spp., *Epicoccum nigrum*, *Fusarium* spp., or *Ganoderma* spp. display a seasonal spore release pattern, but this is less well defined than it is for pollens (Beaumont, 1985; Solomon et al., 1988). Warm dry weather conditions promote passive dispersal of dry air spora, including *Alternaria, Cladosporium, Curvularia*, *Pithomyces* and many smut teliospores. Diurnal levels of these spores usually have peaks during the afternoon hours under conditions of low humidity and maximum wind speeds (Webster, 1970). Moist weather conditions promote the active dispersal of moist air spora, such as the explosive release of ascospores from Pezizales, and the expulsion of basidiospores from the gills of the Basidiomycetes. Often, the two most encountered mold spores in atmospheric sampling are ascospores from different species of Pezizales and spores from *Alternaria* sp. (Ogden, 1974). Airborne fungal spores are important allergens. These airborne spores come into contact with the eye or enter the body as the air is breathed. Allergic reactions to fungal spores fall into two distinct groups, based on whether the hypersensitive response is immediate or delayed (Gumowski et al., 1991). Individuals are exposed to fungal spores every day. About 20–30% of the population can develop an allergic response shortly after exposure to dust that contains allergens such as fungal spores (Moore-Landecker, 1996).

Many studies have been reported on the role of fungi in allergic disease, but none that systematically documented such a role for the fungal species that are responsible for allergic rhinitis in the Texas Panhandle. Many case studies were found, but none of these unequivocally document a cause/effect relationship between the increase in the fungal allergens and the incidence of allergic rhinitis in this area. Our previous studies revealed the data on the pollen and spore composition in the air in the Texas Panhandle (Ghosh et al., 2003a,b; 2011a,b).

This investigation covered the survey on the aeroallergen present in the Texas Panhandle. The objective of this study was to collect, identify, enlist and characterize the pollen and spores of the local areas. Our study included the recording of the aeroallergen concentration in the air on a diurnal basis. We also tried to find out the relationship between these concentrations with both the weather on a particular day and the incidence of allergic reactions. The aeroallergen data were used to assess and enumerate the impact of airborne pollen and mold spores on the breathing and causes of allergic rhinitis in the susceptible individuals. This study was aimed to help to aid the diagnosis of allergic rhinitis by documenting the relation of pollen and fungal spore composition and concentration with the incidence of allergic rhinitis recorded in the Allergy A.R.T.S. Clinics at the Amarillo Center for Clinical Research (Website for Allergy ARTS).

4.4 FLUORESCENCE AND SCANNING ELECTRON MICROSCOPY ON POLLEN

Wet mounting for viewing the fluorescence in pollen was done following the technique developed in our laboratory (Ghosh et al., 2006) by using 2–3 drops of deionized water on the slides. On a few slides, we added 1–2 drops of 2% safranin for staining the pollen that improved the visibility of the pollen architecture. Pollen grains were extracted from the anthers of the flowers and half of them were mounted with deionized water and half of them were mounted with 2% safranin. The pollen grains were teased with a clean needle and the debris from the anthers was removed using a forceps. The slides were mounted and observed under the microscope.

During the last two decades the use of SEM has greatly increased our knowledge of the microstructure of pollen. Mature pollen grains are stable in a vacuum: this allows quick preparation for SEM examination. The low level of technical expenditure required, in combination with the high structural diversity exhibited and the intuitive ability to understand the "three dimensional", often aesthetically appealing microstructures visualized, has turned pollen studies into a favorite tool of many taxonomists. We used pollen grains from different species of Asteraceae, Alstroemeriaceae, Liliaceae and Malvaceae to standardize a procedure for identifying pollen through Scanning Electron Microscopy.

4.5 INSTALLING AND PREPARING THE BURKARD VOLUMETRIC SPORE TRAP FOR POLLEN AND SPORE ANALYSIS

The analysis of air was performed through the collection of pollen and spores through the use of the Burkard Volumetric Spore Trap (Burkard

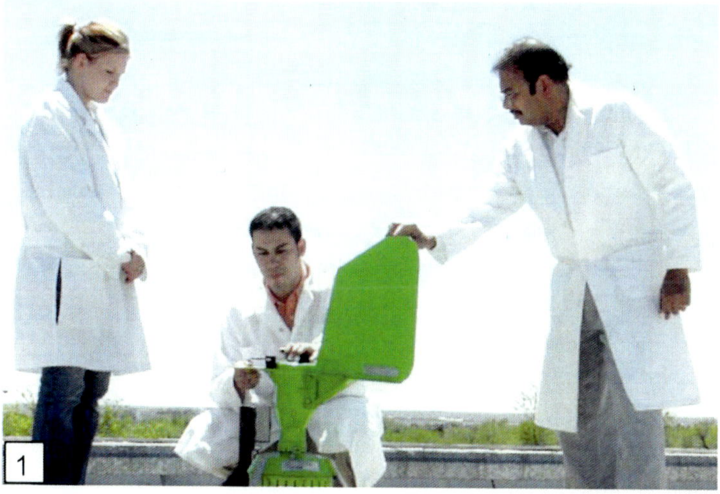

FIGURE 4.1 Working with the Burkard Spore Trap.

Agronomics Division of Burkard Scientific Sales Ltd., UK) (Figure 4.1). We standardized the Burkard Volumetric Spore Trap by using a flowmeter provided by the manufacturer. We mounted the spore trap on the flat roof of the third floor of the Agriculture and Natural Sciences building of West Texas A&M University in Canyon, Texas and standardized it by using a flowmeter provided by the manufacturer. We mounted the spore trap on the flat roof of the Agriculture and Natural Sciences building of West Texas A&M University in Canyon, Texas. This area has adequate exposure to the prevailing winds of West Texas, and is above the trees of the surrounding community. This location is beneficial because it allows adequate sampling of the wind-blown pollen and spores carried to the sampling apparatus on the air currents, while preventing unwanted surface contamination such as excess dirt or sand. In addition, there are no overhanging trees or vegetation to compromise the collection of data.

The spore trap operates on 25 watts of electricity at 240 volts, or 50 watts at 110 volts. Air is suctioned through the trap at a rate of 10 liters per minute. A fan on the ventral portion of the trap rotates at a rate of 2900 rpm to draw air into the trap (Lacey, 1995). Those pollen grains collected by the trap are later analyzed. The trap is driven by a spring located inside the drum, which rotates the drum at a constant speed. This clock is designed to allow one complete rotation of the drum over a seven-day period. Hourly observations can be made because the drum will rotate at a standard rate of 2 mm per hour. The distance from the beginning of the tape designates spore collection time. A template is used to divide the tape into 24-hour periods. To assist in mounting, the template may be coated with a thin film of water to hold the tape in place. Segments of tape are cut from the drum to correspond with a 24-hour interval. These segments are then mounted on individual microscopic slides to be analyzed in 24-hour periods (Figure 4.2). The Melinex tape (a clear plastic tape, Burkard Agronomics, UK) was attached to the drum through the application of double-sided tape at the orifice start position. Once attached, the Melinex tape was coated with a thin layer of paraffin wax (Fisher Scientific cat # 004 S80119WX) to adhere the aerial particles that include fungal spores, pollens, plant debris and carbonated materials from burnt elements. A clean microscopic slide

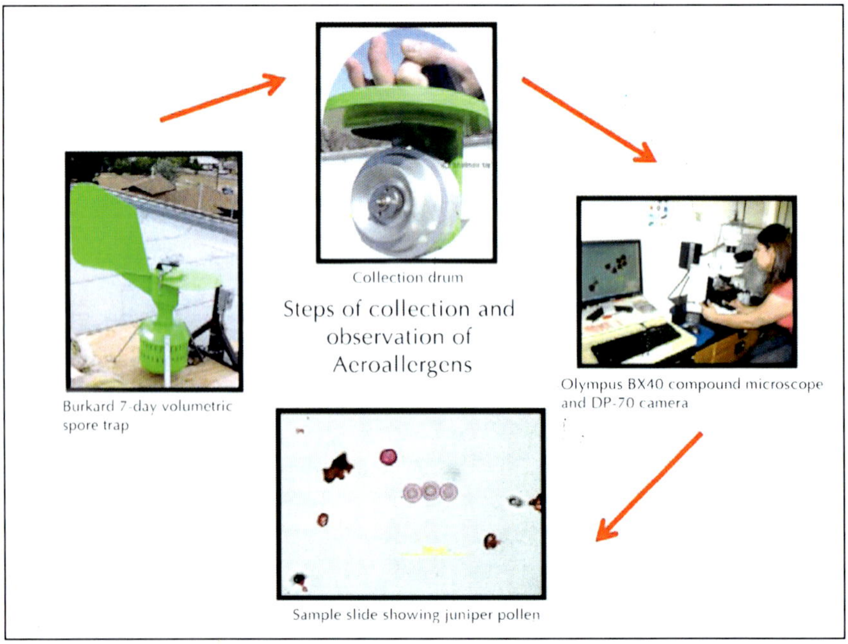

FIGURE 4.2 Steps of collection and observation on aeroallergens.

was coated with a thin layer of water. The segment of tape was then laid upon the microscopic slide with the impregnated surface using forceps so that the long edges of the tape are parallel with the long edges of the slide. Gelvatol, a permanent mountant was applied to the slide using a glass rod. Gelvatol was composed of 35 g Gelvatol powder (Burkard Manufacturing Co Ltd., UK), 50 mL Glycerol, 100 mL distilled water, and 2 g phenol. We prepared Gelvatol by mixing the Gelvatol powder and phenol in water allowing it to sit overnight. Glycerol and distilled water were added to the mixture while heating over a water bath (65°C) and continuous stirring produced the proper emulsion. The Melinex tape was observed under microscope after placing it on a glass slide, staining it with 1% safranin and mounting with Gelvatol (Burkard Agronomics Division of Burkard Scientific Sales Ltd., UK). The addition of few drops of 1% safranin O (Sigma Cat no. 84120, Fluka, Microscopy Grade) to the Gelvatol spread on the exposed Melinex tape enhanced the visibility of the pollen, including their detailed morphology like cell wall patterns, orientation of the pores and colpi.

4.6 DIGITAL MICROSCOPIC ANALYSIS OF COLLECTED AEROALLERGENS

Tapes were analyzed with five latitudinal traverses that correspond to specific hours, and the daily mean concentration was assessed. Daily mean concentration was determined mathematically by taking a sum total of all traverses and multiplying this sum by a correction factor. Correction factor is microscope-objective specific and is determined prior to the counting. It can be expressed as the total area sampled divided by the graticule width (Lacey, 1995). Samples were examined, counted, and photographed using a BX-40 Olympus microscope attached to a DP-70 Digital Camera. We also used an *Image Pro Plus* software to analyze the capture images. This assessment involved the optical counting of pollen grains and fungal spores through a microscope and the use of a micrometer scale and graticule (100 square microns). The graticule is an ocular grid consisting of a square area of 100 square microns. The graticule was calibrated using a stage micrometer. The pollens and fungal spores were identified using standard keys from literature and the websites (Ogden, 1974; Moore et al., 1991; Horner et al., 2002; AAAAI website, website of Palynology, University of Arizona). The diurnal variation in aeroallergen count was determined by counting them from the corresponding traverse of the tape with the specific time period. The time of entrapment of a specific aeroallergen could be determined by placing a scale (Burkard Corporation) beside the slide.

4.7 OBSERVATION ON POLLEN AND SPORES

The most significant aeroallergens recorded were the pollens like grass pollen (Poaceae) (Figure 4.3D), Short Ragweed (*Ambrosia artemisiifolia*) (Figures 4.3D, 4.8A–C, SEM), Pine (*Pinus strobus*) (Figure 4.3C), Common Sunflower *(Helianthus annuus)*, Hairy Sunflower *(Helianthus hirsutus*) (Figure 4.3B), Buffalo Bur *(Solanum rostratum)*, Purple Nightshade (*Solanum elaeagnifolium*) and Lamb's Quarters (*Chenopodium album*) (4F) and the fungal spores like *Alternaria* (Figure 4.3F), ascospores from Pezizales, *Dreschlera*, *Stachybotrys* (Figure 4.3H), *Cladosporium* (Figure 4.3E), *Curvularia*, Teliospores of *Ustilago* sp. (3G).

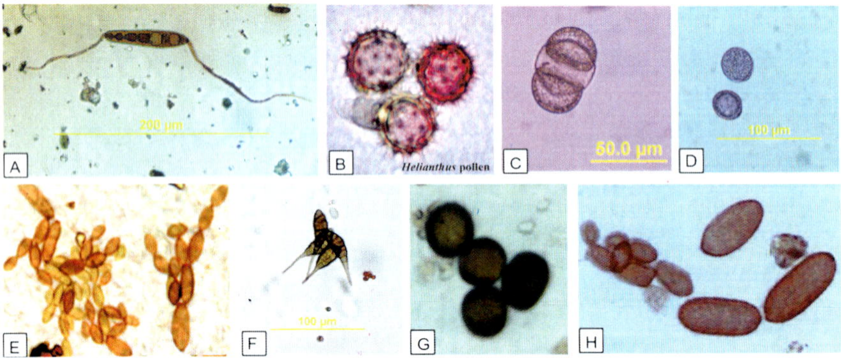

FIGURE 4.3 (A–H) The most frequent aeroallergen of Texas Panhandle. (A) Germinating spore from *Dreschlera*, (B) *Helianthus hirsutus* (hairy sunflower) pollen, (C) *Pinus strobus* (pine) pollen, (D) Grass and Ragweed pollen, (E) *Cladoisporium*, (F) *Alternaria alternata* conidia, (G) Teliospores of *Ustilago* species, (H) *Stachybotrys* spore.

4.8 EFFECT OF METEOROLOGICAL FACTORS ON DISTRIBUTION OF POLLEN AND SPORES

Temperature was found to have an inverse relationship with mold spore concentration. Rainfall was found to affect the mold count directly, with increases in precipitation bringing subsequent higher mold spore concentrations.

Significant increases in fungal spores were observed in late summer following several inches of rain. Fungal spore concentrations did show more susceptibility to meteorological conditions on a daily basis than did pollen concentrations. Of all the airborne pollens observed, most significant was that of annual or short ragweed (*Ambrosia artemisiifolia* L.) pollen. It is characterized by a spherical morphology with a multi-porate surface and 16–27 micrometers in diameter (Figures 4.4A, 6AC). Pores are geometrically arranged about the surface and can be seen easily using phase-contrast microscopy. *A. artemisiifolia* begins its pollination cycle in mid-August and continues until mid-October in the Texas Panhandle. Ragweed pollen is arguably the largest single seasonal allergen in North America (Knox, 1979).

Grass (*Poaceae*) pollen was constant component of the pollen count throughout the study, having peaks in mid-July and then again in late-August. We observed different types of grass pollens. Most grass pollens were similar in morphology. Grass pollen has an ovate morphology with a single pore (Figure 4.3D). Sizes range from 7 micrometers to over 75 micrometers, as in the case of corn (*Zea maize*) pollen. Significant smooth cell walls were observed on grass pollen, with little ornamentation being present on the surface (Figure 4.5A).

Specifically, the mean concentration of tree pollen over the study period was 2 grains/cubic meter of air. The mean concentration of grass pollen was 6.0 grains/cubic meter of air, and of weeds the mean concentration was 33.2 grains/cubic meter of air. For molds, the mean was 713.7 spores/cubic meter of air over the study period. Mold spore concentration varied the most, followed by weed pollen. Tree pollen did not make up a significant amount of the overall pollen count, and was present only in the beginning of summer to any great amount. Weed pollen increased

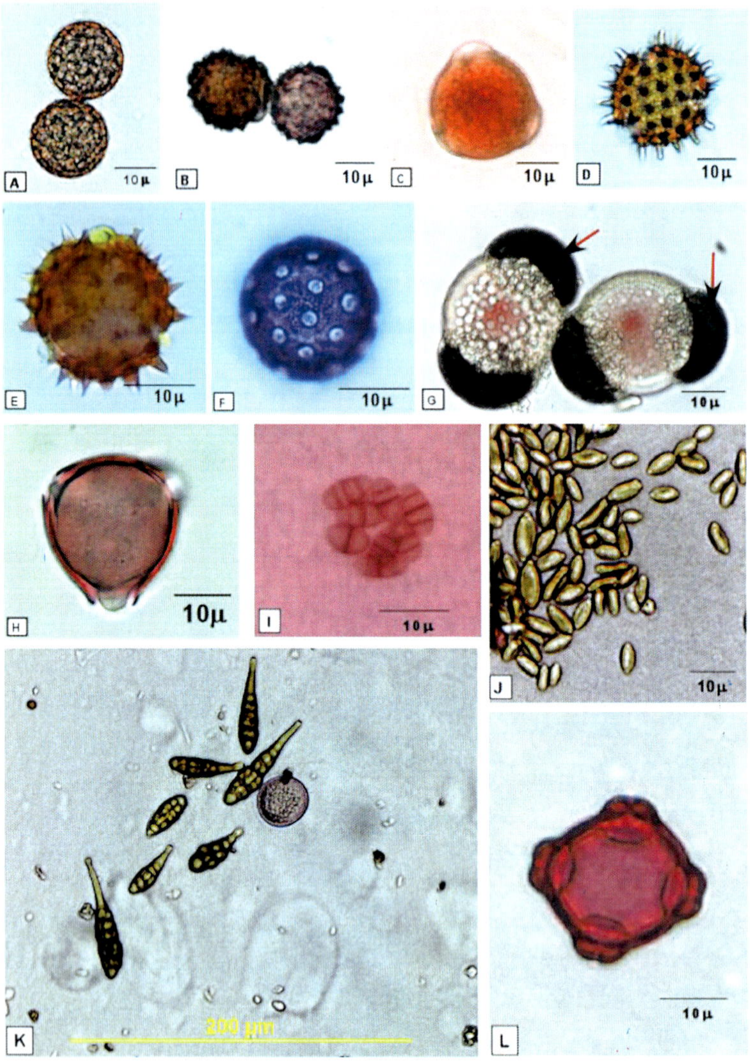

FIGURE 4.4 A–H showing most frequent allergens of Texas Panhandle: Pollens. (A) *Ambrosia artemisiifolia* (Short Ragweed), (B) *Helianthus ciliaris* (Texas Blueweed), (C) *Solanum rostratum* (Buffalo Bur), (D) *Helianthus hirsutus* (Hairy Sunflower), E. *Helianthus annuus* (Common Sunflower), (F) *Chenopodium album* (Lamb's Quarters), (G) *Pinus sylvestris* (Scot's Pine), (H) *Solanum elaeagnifolium* (Purple Nightshade), Fungal spores, (I) *Curvularia* sp., (J) *Cladosporium* sp., teliospore, (K) A group of *Alternaria alternata* conidia trapped in the spore trap, (L) *Alnus serrulata* (Smooth Alder) pollen was recorded once in 12 years as the effect of a tornado.

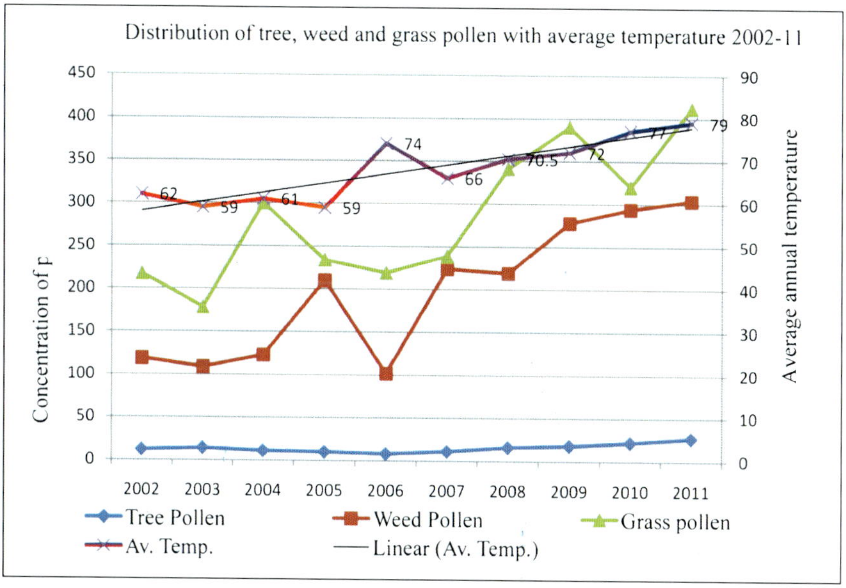

FIGURE 4.5A Graph showing the distribution of tree, weeds and grass pollen with variation of temperature.

drastically in mid-August. Grass pollen concentrations remained steady throughout the season.

The comparative collected pollen and spore data and the weather information revealed that specific weather variants could influence dispersal and concentration of a specific aeroallergen. The mean maximum temperature for this survey was 31.4°C, and the mean minimum temperature was 18.2°C. Temperature was found to have an inverse relationship with mold spores. As the temperature rose, mold spore concentrations would decrease to a great extent. We observed a significant reduction in the ascospore concentration with the increase in temperature. The count of ascospores during the wet weather could surpass the total concentration of dry conidia measured on a typical summer day.

There was a great variation in the occurrence of spore species in different times of the day. Ascospores, although observed throughout the day, were in greater concentration in the early morning hours. *Alternaria* conidia were present in greater quantities during the warmer, dryer afternoon and evening hours. The effect of temperature on pollen concentration is not as clear, though there does appear to be a long-term relationship. Temperature variations as they relate to seasonal changes have been shown to affect primarily the types of pollens observed, not necessarily the concentrations.

It was observed that precipitation increased the number of mold spores, but there was no direct correlation between number of spores and amount of rainfall. As noted earlier, certain genera of fungi, such as the Ascomycetes, require raindrops to initiate their active dispersal mechanism. Corresponding to this knowledge, it was found that the concentrations of the Ascomyceteous fungi increased significantly in the hours just following a rain shower. Precipitation in general affected mold spore concentrations directly by increasing the daily concentrations, due to an increased relative humidity and to the availability of moisture. It was noted that in the hours just following precipitation, pollen concentrations were observed to drop drastically, as the particles were washed from the atmosphere.

In the Texas Panhandle wind speed is an important factor that controls the aeroallergen concentration. Peak wind speed showed some direct correlation with mold spore or pollen concentrations. The mean peak wind speed over the study period was 5.4 m/s. It was observed that sustained windy or windless periods did have an effect on pollen and spore concentrations. Wind speeds over 8.0 m/s increased pollen and spore concentrations on average. Due to smaller size and less mass, mold spores were more directly influenced by wind speeds. Possibly a more representative comparison would be to compare average daily wind speed to the concentration of aeroallergens. Overall, the most prevalent aeroallergens present during the summer months were *Alternaria*, short ragweed (*Ambrosia artemisiifolia*) and grass (*Poaceae*) pollen. During the summer months the most dominant pollen was the grass (*Poaceae*) pollen, which peaked in July and then dropped off in August. In mid-August, the dominant pollen changed to ragweed (*Ambrosia artemisiifolia.*), corresponding to the beginning of the flowering season for short ragweed (Muilenberg et al., 1996). A very remarkable observation was encountered during this study on April 4, 2012. A pollen grain not normally found in the Texas Panhandle area was recorded on the slide prepared for the pollen count. The pollen was identified as *Alnus serrulata* (Ait.) Willd. (Figure 4.4L) using the standard key provided by the AAAAI (American Academy of Allergy Asthma and Immunology). The pollen belonged to the plant species of *Alnus serrulata* (Ait.) Willd. or most commonly known as smooth alder,

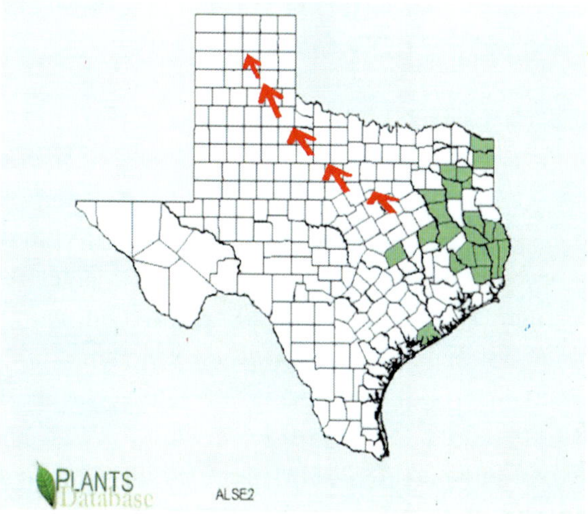

FIGURE 4.5B Path of *Alnus serrulata* pollen from East Texas.

a type of alder only found in the East Texas area (USDA plant database). The pollen grain was trapped in the Burkard Spore Trap on the following evening when a tornado hit the Dallas Fort-Worth area of Texas on April 3, 2012. The pollen grain is thought to have been carried with the heavy wind generated by the tornado through the path marked with the red arrows on Figure 4.5B. Pollen grains of the particular species of alder, *Alnus serrulata* (Ait.) Willd. was never recorded in the last twelve years from the Texas Panhandle area since the vegetation is completely absent in this locality (Estrada, 2012).

The effect of aeroallergens on clinical patients was apparent. The number of reported cases of rhino sinusitis increased directly to the increases in overall allergen counts as reported by the other workers (Narita 2001, 2002; Skoner, 2001; Ito, 2002). There was an increased incidence of pollinosis in Hakodate of Japan with allergic rhinitis caused by house dust and mite and pollens from *Artemisia*, grass (Poaceae) and *Cryptomeria japonica* (Narita et al., 2002). The most significant correlation that was revealed in this study was the increase in patients with that of the increases in mold and *A. artemisiifolia* counts. Grass pollen was not as influential in cases presented to the clinic as weed pollen.

4.9 OBSERVATION ON POLLEN WITH FLUORESCENCE AND SCANNING ELECTRON MICROSCOPY

During the last two decades the use of SEM has greatly increased our knowledge of the microstructure of pollen. Mature pollen grains are stable in a vacuum: this allows quick preparation for SEM examination. The low level of technical expenditure required, in combination with the high structural diversity exhibited and the intuitive ability to understand the "three dimensional", often aesthetically appealing micro-structures visualized, has turned pollen studies into a favorite tool of many taxonomists. We used pollen grains from different species of Asteraceae and Liliaceae and standardized a procedure for identifying pollen through Scanning Electron Microscopy (Ghosh et al., 2011a). Temperature was found to have an inverse relationship with mold spore concentration. Rainfall was found to affect the mold count directly, with increases in precipitation bringing subsequent higher mold spore concentrations. Significant increases in fungal spores were observed in late summer following several inches of rain. Fungal spore concentrations did show more susceptibility to meteorological conditions on a daily basis than did pollen concentrations. Of all the airborne pollens observed, the most significant was that of annual or short ragweed (*Ambrosia artemisiifolia* L.) pollen is characterized by a spherical morphology with a multi-porate surface and 16–27 micrometers in diameter (Figures 4.4A and 4.8A-C). Pores are geometrically arranged about the surface and can be seen easily using fluorescence and Scanning Electron Microscopy (Figures 4.8A-L). *A. artemisiifolia* begins its pollination cycle in mid-August and continues until mid-October in the Texas Panhandle. Ragweed pollen is arguably the largest single seasonal allergen in North America.

Grass (*Poaceae*) pollen was constant component of the pollen count throughout the study, having peaks in mid-July and then again in late August. We observed different types of grass pollens. Most grass pollens were similar in morphology. Grass pollen has an ovate morphology with a single pore. Sizes range from 7 micrometers to over 75 micrometers, as in the case of corn (*Zea maize*) pollen. Significant smooth cell walls were observed on grass pollen, with little ornamentation being present on the surface. In the Texas Panhandle wind speed is an important factor that

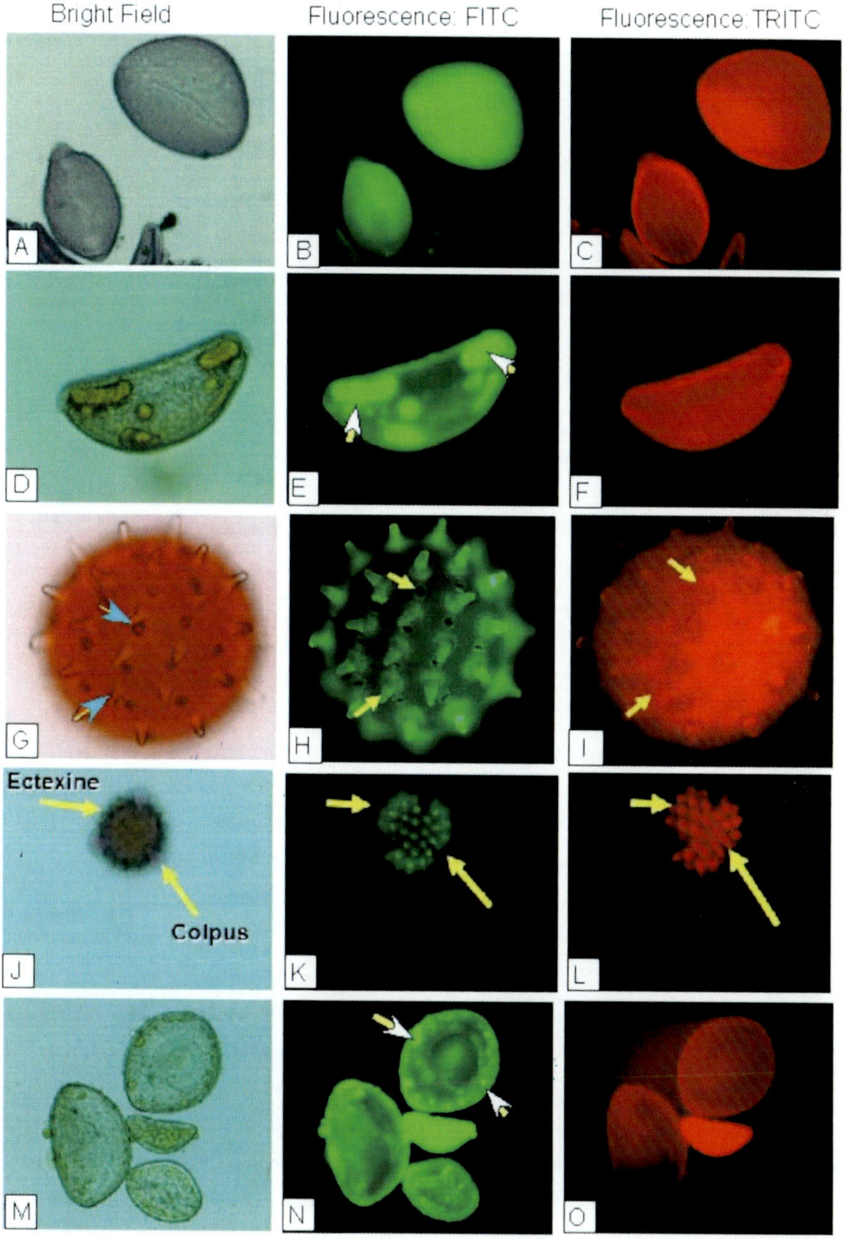

FIGURE 4.6 A-O showing the pollen grains from the plants species of the three families, Asteraceae, Alstroemeriaceae, Liliaceae and Malvaceae that were studied using bright field, TRITC, and FITC filters.

controls the aeroallergen concentration. The highest in number of pollen that we recorded were grass and weed pollen. The grass pollen showed significant increase in number at warmer temperature, especially the Tall Fescue (*Festuca pratensis*) and *Festuca elatior* L.

Figure 4.6A shows *Alstroemeria* (Alstroemeriaceae) (Easter lily) under bright field, Figure 4.4.B with FITC fluorescent filter, Figure 4.4.C with TRITC fluorescent filter (Top view), 4.4D-F Bottom view. Figure 4.4.G shows the pollen from *Hibiscus rosa-sinensis* L. (Malvaceae) (China rose) under bright field, Figure 4.4.H with FITC fluorescent filter, Figure 4.4.I with TRITC fluorescent filter. Figure 4.4.J shows *Bellis perennis* L. (Asteraceae) (Common Daisy) under bright field, Figure 4.4.K with FITC fluorescent filter and Figure 4.4.L with TRITC fluorescent filter. The pollen grains were collected from the stamens of the fresh flower and were teased with a needle for a uniform spreading and were stained with Fluorol Yellow 88. This is an azo dye, which is derived chemically from anthraquinone. The spectral transmittance is determined on solutions of this dye in mineral spirit. Use of fluorescent stains increase the fluorescence helping in visualizing the architecture on pollen ectexine. The *Hibiscus* pollen revealed its concordant pattern and pores on the ectexine on using fluoresce with a TRITC filter. The *Lilium* pollen revealed the Heterobrochate pattern (Lattice like pattern). Both in the *Hibiscus* and *Bellis* pollen the colpi and spiny projections on ectexine became conspicuous after using fluorescence from FITC and TRITC. The micrographs were taken using a BX 40 Olympus microscope attached with DP-70 digital camera and Image Pro Plus software.

As noted earlier, certain genera of fungi, such as the Ascomycetes, require raindrops to initiate their active dispersal mechanism. Corresponding to this knowledge, it was found that Ascomycetes concentrations significantly increased in the hours just following a rain shower. Precipitation in general affected mold spore concentrations directly by increasing the daily concentrations, due to an increased relative humidity and to the availability of moisture. It was noted that in the hours just following precipitation, pollen concentrations were observed to drop drastically, as the particles were washed from the atmosphere. From the analysis of the ten years aeroallergen data from Texas Panhandle region it can be concluded that there was a gradual shift in the aeroallergen index and that caused the increased cases of allergic rhinitis (Figure 4.5A).

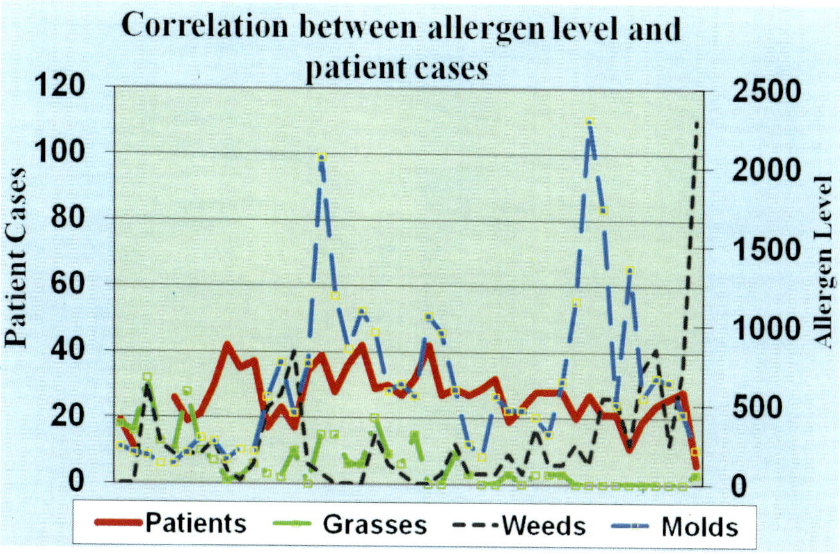

FIGURE 4.7 Correlation between allergen level and cases of allergy and asthma (data analyzed from Allergy A.R.T.S Clinic, 2001–2014).

A gradual shift was noticed in the aeroallergen concentrations with the increase in temperature (Figure 4.5A). Even this slight change reflects the impact of global warming amongst the aeroallergens. From the analysis of aeroallergen data it is very clear that the concentration of pollen from the trees, grass and weeds have a significant correlation with the number of patients suffering from allergy and asthma. The peaks in pollen and mold concentration match with the peak of the number of patients visited the allergy clinics. Figure 4.7 shows the graphical representation of the aeroallergen and patients' data analyzed from Allergy A.R.T.S Clinic, for the period of 2001–2014 (Figure 4.7).

4.10 CONCLUDING REMARKS

Allergy and Asthma cases have been doubled in the Texas Panhandle area since 2007. The aeroallergen data that we collected using a Burkard Spore Trap for 15 years showed a steady increase in aeroallergen concentration in the Texas Panhandle area. A fluctuation and gradual shift in aeroallergen index with the warmer climate and a shift in flowering seasons

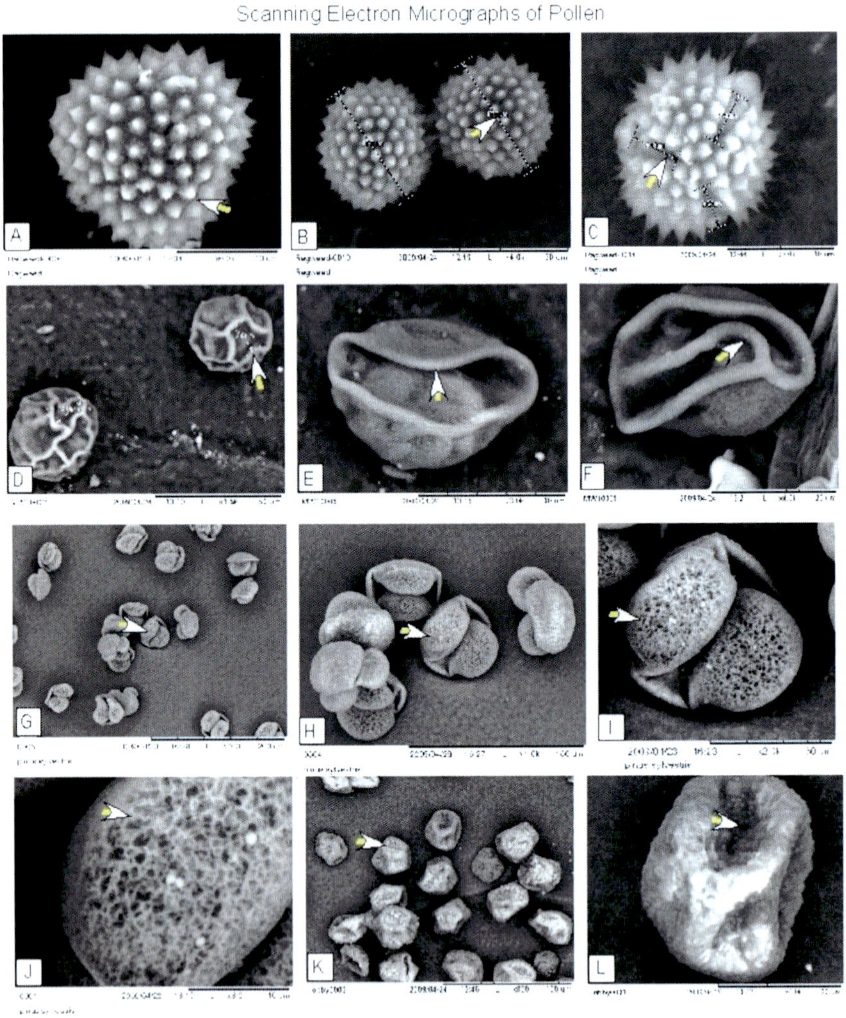

FIGURE 4.8 Figures A–L showing Scanning Electron Micrographs of pollen. Figures A-C showing pollen from *Ambrosia artemisiifolia* (Ragweed) Figures B and C showing the lines measuring the diameter of the pollen and colpi using the software with TM-1000. Figures D, E and F SEM view of *Quercus robur* (Oak) pollen at low (D) and E and F at High magnifications. Figures G-J showing pollen from *Pinus sylvestris* at low and high magnifications. Figures K-L showing pollen from *Lagerstroemia sp.*

were noticed that contributed to the increased allergy cases. Analysis of aeroallergen can help in diagnosis and treatment of allergic rhinitis. Analyzing the aeroallergens with a Burkard Spore Trap provided information regarding the onset, duration, and severity of the pollen season that clinicians use to guide allergen selection for skin testing and treatment. We have been investigating the daily aeroallergen concentration in terms of the meteorological conditions such as daily temperature, wind speed and precipitation. We used a Burkard Volumetric Spore Trap to determine the daily aeroallergen index by collecting aeroallergen samples and characterizing them with digital, fluorescence and Scanning Electron Microscopy for 15 years. The most significant aeroallergens recorded were the pollens from Asteraceae, Chenopodiaceae, Poaceae and spores from *Alternaria, Stachybotrys, Aspergillus* and *Curvularia*. The characterization and analysis of microscopic aeroallergens was accomplished using Fluorescent and Scanning Electron Microscopy. Aeroallergens were viewed, recorded, and analyzed with fluorescent microscopy exhibited storage protein, oil granules, and the layer of sporopollenin, along with additional ultra-structural details like concordant pattern, exines, pores, colpi, sulci, and other ornamentations. The SEM provided micro-measurements and additional views of the detailed ultra-structural morphology. Analyzing the aeroallergens collected and sampled with the Burkard Spore Trap provided information regarding the onset, duration, and severity of the pollen season that was compared to the number of patient cases seen over a 15-year period. The data accumulated from these studies can be utilized for the forecasting the types and duration of the pollen season. Temperature was found to have an inverse relationship with mold spore concentration. Rainfall had a direct correlation with the mold count directly, increase in precipitation resulted in subsequent higher mold spore concentrations.

ACKNOWLEDGEMENTS

The authors are thankful to the researchers at the Pollen Research Laboratory of the West Texas A&M University, Canyon, Texas and the clinical personnel at the Amarillo Center for Clinical Research/Allergy A.R.T.S., Amarillo, Texas for collecting the clinical data.

KEYWORDS

- **aeroallergen**
- **allergic rhinitis patient cases**
- **allergy index in Texas Panhandle**
- **fluorescent microscopy**
- **Scanning Electron Microscopy**

REFERENCES

Air Oasis Research and Development: Air Oasis website: http://www.airoasis.com/.

Allergy ARTS: http://www.allergyarts.com/

American Academy of Allergy Asthma and Immunology: http://www.aaaai.org/

Anglin, R., Ghosh, N. "Experts: High pollen count increases medical dangers." Amarillo Globe-News. 10 Dec. 2014. Web link: http://amarillo.com/news/local-news/2013-10-12/experts-high-pollen-count-increases-medical-dangers.

Beaumont, F., Kauffman, H. F., Sluiter, H. J., De Vries, K., Sequential sampling of fungal air spores inside and outside the homes of mold-sensitive, asthmatic patients: a search for a relationship to obstructive reactions. *Ann. Allergy* 1985, 55, 740–746.

Bogacka, E., Nittner-Marszalska, M., Fal, A. M., Kuzniar, J., Nikiel, E., Malolepszy, J., Allergy to mould allergens as a risk factor for bronchial asthma in patients suffering from allergic rhinitis. *Pol Merkuriusz Lek.* 2003 May, 14(83), 388–392.

Bush, R. Aerobiology of pollen and fungal allergens. Journal of Allergy and Clinical Immunology. 1989, 64, 1120–1124.

Dvorin, D. J., Lee, J. J., Belecanech, G. A., Goldstein, M. F., Dunsky, E. H., A comparative, volumetric survey of airborne pollen in Philadelphia, Pennsylvania (1991–1997) and Cherry Hill, New Jersey (1995–1997). *Ann Allergy Asthma Immunol.* 2001, Nov, 87(5), 394–404.

Estrada, Griselda. Effect of Meteorological Factors on Aeroallergens of Texas Panhandle, and a Comparative Account with Albuquerque, NM. MS Thesis, West Texas A&M University, 2014, 33.

Ghosh, N., Patten, B.. Lewellen, G. T., Saadeh, C., Gaylor, M., Aeroallergen survey of the Texas Panhandle using a Burkard Volumetric Spore Trap. *The Journal of Allergy and Clinical Immunology.* 2003b, 111(2), S91.

Ghosh, N., Camacho, R., Schniederjan, E., Saadeh, C., Gaylor, M. Correlation between the meteorological conditions with the aeroallergen concentration in the Texas Panhandle. *Texas Journal of Microscopy.* 2003a, 34(1), 12–13.

Ghosh, N., Saadeh, C., Gaylor, M. Quantification and characterizing the Aeroallergen by scanning and analyzing the tapes from the Burkard Spore-trap, *Journal of Scanning Microscopies*, 2006, 28(2), 127–128.

Ghosh, N., Silva, J., Vazquez, A., Das, A. B., Smith, D. W. Use of fluorescence and scanning electron microscopy as tools in teaching biology. *Scanning Microscopies 2011: Advanced Microscopy Technologies for Defense, Homeland Security, Forensic, Life, Environmental, and Industrial Sciences*, edited by Michael, T., Postek, Dale, E., Newbury, S. Frank Platek, David, C., Joy, Tim, K., Maugel, Proceedings of SPIE Vol. 8036 (SPIE, Bellingham, WA 2011) 2011a, 13, 1–11.

Ghosh, N., Whiteside, M. Fluorescent Microscopy in Characterizing Some Biological Specimens. *Journal of Scanning Microscopies*, 2006, 28(2), 129–130.

Ghosh, N., Wylie, D., Caraway, E., Bennert, J., Bennert, J., Saadeh, C., Bringing Biotechnology into Business: Application of AHPCO Nanotechnology to Market a Novel Filter-Less Air Purifier. *International Journal of the Computer, the Internet and Management*, 2013, 21(2) (May–August, 2013), 51–55.

Ghosh. N., Aranda, A., Bennert, J. (2011b). Photo-Catalytic Oxidation Nanotechnology Used in Luna Improved the Air Quality by Reducing Volatile Organic Compounds and Airborne Pathogens (2011) *International Journal of the Computer, the Internet and Management*, Vol. 19 No. SP1, 2011, 2.1–2.5.

Gumowski, P. I., Latge, J.-P., Paris, S., Fungal Allergy. In: Arora, D. K., Ajello, L. K., Mukerji, G., Eds. *Handbook of Applied Mycology. Vol. 2, Humans, Animals and Insects. Marcel* Dekker Inc. NY, 1991, 163–204.

Helbling, A., Reimers, Immunotherapy in fungal allergy. *Current Allergy Asthma Rep.* 2003 Sep., 3(5), 447–453.

Horner, E., Levetin, E., Shane, J. D., Solomon, W., *Advanced Aeroallergen*: 58th AAAAI Annual Meeting, March 2, 2002, 1–68.

Ito, Y., Kimura, T., Miyamura, T., Gramineae pollen dispersal and pollinosis in the city of Hisai in Mie Prefecture. A 14-year study of Gramineae pollen dispersal and cases of sensitization to Gamineae experienced at an allergy clinic over a 15-year period. *Arerugi* 2002 Jan, 51(1), 9–14.

Knox, B. R. *Pollen and Allergy*. University Park Press: Baltimore, 1979, 3–57.

Lacey, J. *Airborne Pollens and Spores. A Guide to Trapping and Counting*. The British Aerobiology Federation, U.K. 1995, 1–59.

Lewellen, G. T., Ghosh, N., Saadeh, C., Gaylor, M. (2002). Assessment of Pollen Concentration in the atmosphere of Texas Panhandle through the use of a Burkard Volumetric Spore Trap. *Texas Journal of Microscopy*. 2002, 33(2), 39.

Moore-Landecker, E. *Fundamentals of the Fungi*, 4th edition, Prentice Hall, NJ 07458, 1996, 342–343, 400–401, 464.

Moore, P. D. Pollen Analysis, Second Ed. Blackwell Scientific Publications. Oxford, 1991, 62–166.

Muilenberg, M., Burge, H. *Aerobiology*. Lewis Publishers: Boca Raton, Florida, 1996, 18–26.

Narita, S., Chin, S., Shirasaki, H., Takano, Y., Kurose, M., Kobayashi, K., Kisikawa, R., Koto, E., Himi, T., A study on the nasal and eye symptoms of pollinosis in Hakodate. *Arerugi* 2002 Nov; 51(11), 1103–1112.

Narita, S., Shirasaki, H., Yamaya, H., Mitsuzawa, H., Kikuchi, K., Kishikawa, R., Kobayashi, K., Himi, T., The pollen survey and dynamic statistics of patients with allergic rhinitis in Hakodate. *Arerugi,* 2001, May, 50(5), 473–480.

Nester, E. W. *Microbiology: A Human Perspective,* Third Ed. McGraw-Hill, NY, 2001, 1–15.

Ogden, Eugene, C. *Manual for Sampling Airborne Pollen*, Hafner Press, NY, 1974, 146–157.

Pawankar, R., Canonica, G. W., Holgate, S. T., Lockey, R. F., White Book on Allergy 2011–2012 Executive Summary. World Health Organization. American Academy of Allergy, Asthma, and Immunology. http://www.aaaai.org/about-the-aaaai/newsroom/allergy-statistics.aspx

Pollen Allergy: http://www.niaid.nih.gov/publications/allergens/pollen.htm

Ranaivo, Y. An Increasing Trend. Study: More Amarilloans Battle Asthma's Effects. Amarillo Globe-News. August 28, 2011. Weblink: http://amarillo.com/news/local-news/2011-08-28/increasing-trend.

Santilli, J., Rockwell, W., Fungal contamination of elementary schools: a new environmental hazard. *Ann Allergy Asthma Immunology*. 2003 Feb, 90(2), 175.

Skoner, D. P., Allergic rhinitis: definition, epidemiology, pathophysiology, detection, and diagnosis, J Allergy Clin Immunol. 2001 Jul, 108(1 Suppl.), S2–8.

Solomon, W. R., Matthews, K. P. Aerobiology and inhalant allergens, In: E. Middleton, C. E. Reed, E. F. Ellis, N. F. Adkinson, J. W. Yunginger (eds.), Allergy: Principles and Practices, 3rd ed. The C.V. Mosby Co., St. Louis, 1988, 312–372.

University of Arizona: http://www.geo.arizona.edu/palynology/polonweb.html

USDA Plant Database: http://plants.usda.gov/java/

Webster, John. Introduction to Fungi University Press: Cambridge, 1970, 68.

CHAPTER 5

AIRBORNE POLLEN IN EUROPE

C. GALÁN,[1] A. DAHL,[2] G. FRENGUELLI,[3] and R. GEHRIG[4]

[1]*Department of Botany, Ecology and Plant Physiology, University of Córdoba, Spain*

[2]*Department of Biological Environmental Science, University of Gothenburg, Gothenburg, Sweden*

[3]*Department of Agriculture, Food and Environmental Sciences, University of Perugia, Italy*

[4]*Federal Office of Meteorology and Climatology MeteoSwiss, Zurich, Switzerland*

CONTENTS

5.1 INTRODUCTION TO MODERN PHENOLOGY

Schwartz (2013) defines this science in *Phenology: An Integrative Environmental Science* as the study of recurring animals and plants life cycle stages, especially their timing and relationships with weather and climate; presenting "seasonality" as a related term when referring to non-biological events.

Human knowledge about phenology was probably originated with the sedentary agriculture, which emerged with changes on climate associated with the retreat of the glaciers at the end of the last Ice Age. The original objective would be to detect changes in the distribution and growing patterns of different plants. The oldest phenological monitoring records are from cherry in Japan for about 1300 years, but phenology in China is at least 3000 years old (Koch et al., 2007). In Europe, Carl Linnaeus is presented as father of modern phenological networks in Sweden, during the middle of the 18th century, presenting methodology for annual plant calendars in the *Philosophia Botanica* (Linnaeus, 1751). However, continuous and spatial systematic records started recently, from mid-20 overall century in Europe.

These recent historical databases point out the response of species to climate change under different genotypic and phenotypic plasticity adaptation degrees, i.e., plastic changes on phenology. Depending on their response, it can be observed as impacts on biodiversity and phenology at different levels of individual, population, species or ecosystems. During the last decades changes in geographical distribution of different species in response to warming have been observed, changes in land use and habitat fragmentation, among others, generating possible extinctions or appearing new invasive species.

It is widely recognized that plant phenology in the temperate zone is adapted to local climate. On the other hand, inter-annual variation on temperature in a determined area, and the high plasticity degree of the plant, probably support that the genetic variation among different populations can be insignificant regarding the reproductive phenology pattern in different taxonomic groups (Chuine and Belmonte, 2004). Some studies have observed a high gene flow in forest trees (Chuine et al., 2000).

Today studies on plant and animal physiology, phenology and distributions are considered as one of the best tools to trace the role of global warming on living organisms (Menzel et al., 2006). Phenology is considered as an ideal climate indicator and the length of the growing season and timing of spring events have been proposed as global change indicators by the *European Environment Agency* (Menzel, 2013). On the other hand, the 4º Assessment Report (AR4) of the *Intergovernmental Panel of Climate Change* dedicated a chapter on the role of phenology for fingerprinting climate change (Rosenzweig et al., 2007) and the recent AR5 states that there is a *high confidence* in attributing many observed changes in phenology to changing climate (Cramer et al., 2014), but because the magnitude of these phenological changes depends on the species, this report tries to convey the importance in defining set of limits.

Some papers evidence the role of increasing temperature during the last decades on phenology, from a clearer seasonal advance in early spring to unclear trends during autumn (Menzel et al., 2006). However, Peñuelas et al. (2004) also pays special attention to changes on rainfall and water availability as an important driver of climate change affecting plant phenology in the Mediterranean Region.

Regarding reproductive phenology, it has been presented as particularly vulnerable to the effects of global warming on plants (Hedhly et al., 2009). Today there is an emerging interest in studies on airborne pollen as phenological indicator of both flowering timing and intensity in anemophilous species (Dahl et al., 2013). These studies also evidence the role of increasing temperature on pollen season advance in spring woody species (García-Mozo et al., 2006; Emberlin et al., 2007), and a higher dependency of water availability for herbs and grasses, with not clear trends in South of Europe (Alcázar et al., 2009; Cariñanos et al., 2013). Other studies have observed a link between the timing and intensity of flowering and NAO index in Europe (Smith et al., 2009). However, in the case of flowering intensity, a general increase on airborne pollen in Europe has been also attributed to interaction with other components of global changes, i.e., an increase in anthropogenic CO_2 emissions (Ziello et al., 2012).

Airborne pollen represents one of the main causes of allergic disease. Pollen allergy in Europe has recently increased with population suffering rhinitis, conjunctivitis and/or asthma (D'Amato et al., 2007). Studies on airborne pollen have a high social and economic relevance at different levels. On one hand, this information is important for the repercussion of using preventive medicine on pollen allergies, allowing mitigation measures, *i.e.,* avoid massive use of allergenic pollen plants when designing green urban spaces. Further examples are the use of pollen calendars and forecasts which allow a better planning of the medication by allergologists and of recreation activities by people that suffer from allergy (D'Amato et al., 2007).

Furthermore, these studies provide an understanding not only of flowering timing, but also for the intensity, generating crop forecasting models for both, species with an agricultural interest, such as the olive tree, or forestry in the case of oak or birch, with several months in advance, as an important planning tool when designing economic strategies for agricultural and/or forestry.

5.1.1 BIO-MONITORING NETWORKS IN EUROPE

Bio-monitoring networks provide information on changes over time on different ecosystems, caused by nature or by human activities. Some biological events can be measured as qualitative variables, i.e., phenological observations; and some others as quantitative variables, i.e., flowering intensity or fruit production.

In the case of phenological networks, different national or regional networks are running in Europe during the last decades, and weather services frequently operate phenological networks as additional or integrated climate information (Menzel, 2013). An important requirement is the use of a standardized protocol by all members involved in the network, and in this context, training, quality assurance and quality control programs play an important role. On the other hand, it is also important to note that the variety on phenological changes depends on the species, topography and local climate; however when working with long datasets the results will directly depend on the studied period with a particular climate pattern.

As mentioned before, today airborne pollen is considered as an important variable for studying flowering phenology of wind pollinated plants. For this reason, phenology and aerobiology are considered as highly related and complementary sciences: airborne pollen allows quantifying flowering phenological changes in anemophilous plants and field phenology offer important qualitative information to predict and interpret airborne pollen in a determined area.

Recently two EU COST Actions were taking place, COST 725 (2004–09) *Towards A Pan European Phenology, Establishing a European Phenological Data Platform for Climatological Applications*, that generated the *Pan European Phenology Project* PEP725 http://www.pep725.eu/; and

ES0603 EUPOL (2007–11), *Assessment of production, release, distribution at health impact of allergy pollen in Europe* http:// www.costeupol.unifi.it/.

5.1.1.1 European Phenological Networks

Recent phenological networks are running from mid-last century in Europe at national, regional and European level. The *International Phenological Gardens* (IPG) (http://ipg.hu-berlin.de/) was founded in 1957 by F. Schnelle and E. Volkert as a recommendation from the Commission for AgroMeteorology (CAgM) of the World Meteorological Organization (WMO). This network is coordinated by the Humboldt-University of Berlin. The novelty of this network is to obtain comparable phenological data across Europe by observing clones of different trees. Humboldt-University also coordinates the *Global Phenological Programme* (GPM) http://gpm.hu-berlin.de/, as an initiative of the *Phenology Study Group* of the *International Society of Biometeorology*, with the main goal of generating a "standard observation programme" (Bruns & Vliet, 2003).

In Europe Phenological observations are also made in the *International Cooperative Programme on Assessment and Monitoring of Air Pollution Effects on Forests* (ICP Forest), at level II from mid-90s (http://www.unece.org/) (Menzel, 2013).

Trying to obtain comparable phenological data growth stages observations are based on the BBCH scale and some requirements (Meier, 1997). More information can be found in Meier et al. (2009) about publications with BBCH system, history and publications.

5.1.1.2 European Aerobiology Networks

Today different aerobiology networks exist in Europe at national, regional and European level. The *European Aeroallergen Network* (EAN, https://ean.polleninfo.eu/Ean/en/start, www.polleninfo.org) was established in the late 1980s and provides a valuable service supplying pollen information to a variety of end users, including pollen allergy sufferers and health care professionals. All data suppliers follow a standardized methodology based on the *Minimum Requirements* described by Jäger et al. (1995). The ability to produce comparable data provides opportunities to construct models for predicting airborne pollen over large geographical areas. Today EAN is considered as a technical network in the frame of the *European Aerobiology Society* (EAS). EAS was founded on 2008 and one of the main goals, in the frame of the QC working group, has been to formulate an updated *Minimum Requirements Report* for all members involved in the EAN and ensure data quality, carrying out an external QC exercise for staff involved in pollen counting, in order to examine between analysts reproducibility (Galán et al., 2014).

The MEDAERONET (http://www.pollens.fr/medaeronet/medaeronet.php) is a network gathering the information about allergy risk due to pollen in the Mediterranean Basin. This network is coordinated by the *Réseau National de Surveillance Aérobiologique*, Lyon, France.

5.2 POLLEN SOURCES

5.2.1 BIOGEOGRAPHICAL REGIONS IN EUROPE AND MAIN ALLERGENIC PLANTS

In Europe 13 pollen types are considered of interest from allergological point of view: *Alnus* (alder), *Ambrosia* (ragweed), *Artemisia* (mugwort), *Betula* (birch), *Amaranthaceae* (goosefoot and others), *Corylus* (hazel), *Cupressaceae/Taxaceae* (cypress and others), *Fraxinus* (ash), *Olea* (olive), *Platanus* (plane tree), *Poaceae* (grasses), *Quercus* (oak and others) and *Urticaceae* (wall pellitory and nettle) (D'Amato et al., 2007 and references therein). As can be observed in this list different genera or species sometimes share similar morphological characteristics under light microscopy, i.e., they are stenopalynous. This is the case of some botanical families, i.e., Poaceae, or some genera, i.e., *Quercus*. In other occasions a pollen type represents only one species, i.e., *Olea europaea*. For this reason, biogeographical regions generated by land cover inventories, pollen production per plant and flowering field phenology provide important information on the relative contribution of each species to the airborne pollen concentration, enabling to estimate the potential pollen emission.

Bioclimatic maps have been usually produced following the global vegetation patterns (i.e., Köppen, 1918) and recent high spatial resolution climate data sets offer to develop a detailed region-specific approach for environmental stratification in Europe, e.g., Metzger et al. (2005) based on biodiversity, landscape and land use. These biogeographical distribution maps are based on experts without rules, and for this reason, maps should be designed depending on the main goal of the study but with logical limits in the distribution map between different units. This figure represents the biogeographical regions of European Countries at small scale, each region with its own characteristic blend of vegetation, climate and geology (Natura, 2000) https://en.wikipedia.org/wiki/Biogeography#/media/File:Europe_biogeography_countries.svg. The more species are included in the classification analysis, the smaller the resulting regions with specific characteristics.

5.2.1.1 Biological Inventories

Biological inventories, and especially species inventories, are the most elementary data in biogeography. In the case of pollen sources, Bottom-Up inventories can be considered as a good tool for better understanding the airborne pollen source. Skjoth et al. (2013) proposes using forest inventories and crop databases, or land cover information to a larger geographical domain, or use satellite images for developing source maps of allergenic plants. However, as they has pointed out, in aerobiology we are also interested in species used as ornamentals, without available statistic distribution, and on herbs and grasses that usually are cut and therefore do not flower. In this case, it is easier for working with species of special interest in Europe, i.e., the olive crop. In the case of Top-Down inventories for anemophilous species, Skjoth et al. (2013) propose to use pollen calendars or airborne pollen networks, i.e., EAN. However, some limitations are related to gaps in the network, due to the lack of information about some pollen types in some places or the absence of monitoring sites, or to the detection of medium or long distant pollen transport. For this reason, this study proposes by using Top-Down and Bottom-Up information, when available, and also considering the ecological references published in the *Flora Europaea* (Tutin, 1964, 1980). Skjoth et al. (2008) have published a detailed tree species inventory covering Europe, including important species relevant for pollen dispersion: *Alnus*, *Betula* and *Quercus*, and the possibility to compare Top-Down and Bottom-Up information for these trees.

5.2.1.2 Flowering Intensity Measurement

Even with the limitations mentioned before for Top-Down inventories, in Aerobiology the Annual Pollen Index (API) is considered as an important measure for flowering intensity in anemophilous plants. In networks where there are enough monitoring stations as to adequately represent the relevant region, API can be considered to be a good index for plant distribution and pollen source location at different scales, i.e., to create Top-Down inventories for forest distribution and crop extension in a determined biogeographical area. This index is also considered as an important tool for studies related on ornamental species in green urban spaces that highly contribute to airborne pollen and possible pollinosis. In the case of grasses and other herbaceous species, even when they are cut in some urban spaces for aesthetic and recreational purposes, API can offer information about the different ecological requirements for some species, i.e., while woody plants respond more to temperature in temperate climate, grasses and other herbs also respond to water availability, being an special requirement in the Mediterranean climate (Dahl et al., 2013).

However, since API is a measure for a pollen type, which can group different species or genera with similar morphological characteristic, the knowledge on pollen production per plant and surface unit is useful for estimating the proportion of the contribution of each species to the airborne pollen concentrations.

5.2.2 POLLEN PRODUCTION PER PLANT

Almost all airborne pollen grains are emitted by anemophilous (i.e., wind-pollinated) plants. The wind-pollination syndrome include plants that produce inconspicuous flowers, usually aggregated in inflorescences; no need to attract pollinators, they do not possess a scent, neither do they produce nectar; but they invest all their energy in producing very high numbers of pollen grains. Anemophilous plants usually produce small and very lightweight pollen grains, or larger pollens but with air-sacs in some Gymnosperms.

Regarding anemophilous tree species, Tormo-Molina et al. (1996) have reported that there is a constant value of pollen production for each species. These species show a tendency to compensate different sexual characteristics by increasing some of them or reducing others, so that the result generally lies within defined margins. Even more, anemophilous shrubs probably try to increase the number of some sexual characteristics to compensate their smaller size. It has been observed in *Quercus coccifera* (kermes oak) with highest pollen per anther and higher inflorescences per m^2 of the crown than other *Quercus* species, with a final pollen production similar to *Quercus* trees species (Gómez-Casero et al., 2004).

In the case of Poaceae (grasses), Prieto-Baena et al. (2003) studied 38 species and found no substantial intra-generic variation in pollen *per* anther in most cases; the number of spikelet *per* inflorescence seems to be the most variable value among species. In general, a tendency to compensate different sexual characteristics was also observed, i.e., a lower production of pollen per anther can be compensated with a large number of flowers *per* inflorescence (*Polypogon monspeliensis*) and a lower number of flowers with a larger production of pollen *per* anther (*Arrhenatherum album*). However, in some cases, a high pollen production *per* anther is associated with a larger number of flowers *per* inflorescence, i.e., *Piptatherum miliaceum*, *Sorghum halepense* and *Trisetaria panicea*. Higher differences have been observed between perennial and annual species; pollen production *per* inflorescence in perennial grasses was up to 3.5 times higher than in annual, as a tendency to guarantee cross-fertilization in perennial plants, since most perennial plants display marked self-incompatibility.

When comparing pollen production per anther in trees and herbs, mean pollen production per anther in grasses is approximately 2,000–2,500 (Prieto Baena et al., 2003) and in anemophilous trees is approximately 25,000 pollen grains (Tormo-Molina et al., 1996). This difference may be also understood as a way to increase the probability for pollen reaching distant individuals (Prieto Baena et al., 2003).

5.3 FLOWERING PHENOLOGY

The life cycle of the plants is influenced both by the biotic characteristics of the species and by the climate of the plant's environment. It is easy to deduce that not only geographical and ecological conditions determine the composition of various vegetations, but also meteorological factors, which are important for the reproductive phase of the plants. The weather conditions directly influence pollination by determining the time of onset of flowering, the number of pollen grains produced, and by controlling the amount of pollen that is discharged into the air from day to day.

It should also be noted that meteorological factors can have different effects because the various parameters are not only interdependent among themselves but act on the plants not only singularly but also through interaction among themselves (Comtois and Sherknies, 1987).

5.3.1 PRE-FLOWERING AND CLIMATE INTERACTIONS

Woody species from temperate climate have two clear annual alternative growth periods, an active growth period during spring and summer and a dormancy period during autumn and winter, trying to survive unfavorable environmental conditions during these last seasons, i.e., low temperature stress (Dahl et al., 2013). During autumn and winter these plants are under two dormancy processes: the endodormant process, under innate agents; and ecodormant process, under environmental stress agents, usually provoked by low temperatures. However, these processes, without morphological evidences, usually occur simultaneously and are triggered by decreasing day lengths and low temperature (Arora et al., 2003).

Chilling during winter, under a determined threshold, is a special requirement to prevent a too early release of dormancy for evading risk of freezing damage and to initiate bud break and anthesis. After chilling, heating requirements during early spring are needed; forcing accumulation of heat above a threshold to induce bud break and continuing the anthesis. Timing period and amount, under determined thresholds, of both chilling and forcing unit requirements depend on the species and the populations in different climates, e.g., chilling requirements are usually lower in the Mediterranean Basin and also depend on the latitude and altitude in this region (Aguilera et al., 2013). On the other hand, in some occasions a dynamic relationship between chilling and heat accumulation period before flowering start was observed (Emberlin et al., 2007).

In the case of late successional trees, grasses and other herbaceous plants, they also respond to temperature, but also photoperiod and water availability are considered as primary factors that influence plant growth and development (Deen et al., 1998; Basler and Körner, 2012). Garcia-Mozo et al. (2009) have proposed the use of process-based models under different bioclimatic factors, combining the effect of temperature, photoperiod and rainfall for forecasting the start of the grass pollen season, following prior modeling proposed by Chuine and Belmonte (2004). These results showed the possibility to propose a single model parameter set for forecasting the start of grass pollen season in the Iberian Peninsula, based on different bioclimatic factors.

For this reason, the basic factors governing the seasonal plant development are: (i) chilling temperature; (ii) forcing temperature; (iii) photoperiod; and (iv) water availability. In general, early successional trees respond better to temperature than herbaceous plants and late successional trees, and phenological models are based on only one or on a combination of these four factors (Scheifinger et al., 2013).

Once the plant is ready to flower other local environmental factors determine pollen release, e.g., irradiation and humidity for anther opening.

5.3.2 AIRBORNE POLLEN SEASON

The release of pollen from the anther depends on the phenological phases of the plant. It occurs gradually in the period between the flowering of the first flowers and the fading of the last flowers, and reaches a maximum at the central phase of flowering, although there are significant fluctuation in relation to meteorological episodes and circadian rhythms.

A phenological survey is essential to know the activity of the pollen source, in that phenology deals with the timing of biological events and their relationship to seasonal climatic changes and the interrelation among phases of the same or different species.

Aerobiology is used to study the phenology of many plants with anemophilous pollination, because the monitoring of airborne pollen is the same as registering the flowering phenophase of various species. In this field aerobiological monitoring does not only provide information about the timing and the trend of the phenophase, but can also constitute a measure of the size of the phenomenon.

Normally the accumulated pollen curve has the same pattern as the floral development and this indicates that the aerobiological data coincide well with the phenological curves. Moreover, the pollen in the atmosphere indicates precisely the beginning and the maximum of the anemophilous flowering phase (Latorre, 1997) and the dates of flowering measured by the pollen peaks represent the mean date of flowering of the population living around the sampling station. This is an advantage compared to traditional observations of plant individuals, which may not lead to the characteristics of the population (Chuine and Cour, 1998).

Airborne pollen grains do not clearly indicate the length of flowering period and in particular do not indicate the final phase of flowering directly or explicitly. The prolonging of the season can be due to the fact that the pollen grains can stay in the atmosphere even after flowering has finished, or they can be transported from distant or nearby sources (O'Rourke, 1990; Latorre, 1999).

Measured airborne pollen data are a result of different aerobiological processes: emission, transport and/or dispersion, and deposition, and possible resuspension. In these processes different meteorological parameters play an important role, i.e., temperature, humidity and irradiation for pollen emission. For pollen transport and dispersion different meteorological processes at micro and meso-scale affect airborne pollen concentrations, such as frontal zones, see-breezes, foehn or föhn effects, atmospheric stability, convection and topographical forced air flow (Skjoth, 2015). In the case of deposition, it will depend on a dry deposition, by sedimentation or impact, or on humid deposition, by washout or rainout. All these parameters are important for short term forecasting and modeling.

Flowering phenology and aerobiology are considered as highly related and complementary sciences. Airborne pollen allows the quantification of flowering phenological changes in anemophilous plants, and field phenology prediction and interpretation of airborne pollen concetration.

However, taking into account all these limitations, pollen calendars based on historical datasets can be considered as a guide to common airborne pollen in a local area (Martínez-Bracero et al., 2015) and it is considered as a useful tool for allergologists for planning treatments and for and to allergy sufferers for planning their work and recreational activities (D'Amato et al 2007).

5.3.3 PHENOLOGICAL MODELS FOR POLLEN FORECASTING

To forecast the flowering date is a very important objective for phenological research. The flowering periods of different taxa follow each other in a chronological order characteristic in an area. In agriculture it is common to forecast the date of a particular phase from an earlier phenophase, both for the same species or in other species during the same year. The phenological forecasting models can be applied to aerobiology and results from aerobiological monitoring can be used to elaborate a forecast on the beginning of the flowering of many species.

One of the methods is the use of a "phenological model" or "indicator species" (or predictor variables) which is very useful in all those cases in which forecasting must be carried out in climatically heterogeneous regions (Puppi Branzi, 1989; Norris-Hill, 1998; Linkosalo, 2000). This model is a purely statistical model which does not involve meteorological factors, but which uses the correlations between the occurrences of the flowering phenophase in various species. A phenological model could be formulated in the following way:

$$Tf1x = Tf2y + K$$

where $Tf1x$ is the date of the beginning of flowering in the "x" species, while $Tf2y$ is the date of the beginning of flowering in the indicator species "y" which occurs before the flowering f1, and K is a constant. The pollination of a species can give information to predict the pollination of a second species if we know the K-value as warning days calculated after many years of observation in a defined area.

The timing of pollen release of in hazel (*Corylus*), alder (*Alnus*), elm (*Ulmus*), poplar (*Populus*) and willow (*Salix*) have been employed to forecast the beginning of the pollen season of the later-flowering species, assuming that the beginning of pollen release in one species corresponds to a specific moment of phenological development for another species with later pollen emission. This model relies on the fact that the phenological development of some species can be used as "indicator" to predict phenophases occurrence in others (Frenguelli & Bricchi, 1998; Frenguelli et al., 2015). They showed how, starting from the correlation existing in the flowering dates of some taxa, these can be forecasted using a statistical model based on linear regression. A most efficient method to predict the beginning date of the pollen season of some trees, such as birch *(Betula)*, oak *(Quercus)* and plane tree *(Platanus)*, is to use a combination of several indicator species, such as *Corylus* and *Taxus*, which seem to be the most precise and, flowering in the winter, they can provide very early indications (Norris-Hill, 1998). The forecasting model here proposed is simple and purely statistic: it does not involve meteorological parameters, using instead the significant correlation existing between the occurrences of the flowering phenophase in various species. These models are site and species-specific and cannot be applied to a wide range of species and climatic condition (Ruml and Vuliæ, 2005).

A multiple regression approach, involving other variables like temperature, photoperiod and rainfall, would surely produce a better fitting and precise model, but would not be as fast and easy to develop. But such models are necessary in all those cases in which forecasting must be carried out in climatically heterogeneous areas and to foresee the shifts in the timing of different phenological phases in climate change scenarios.

Many papers report air temperature as a dominant factor controlling the timing of flowering and other phenological phases (i.e., Frenguelli et al., 2014; Galan et al., 2001; Kramer, 1994) therefore, one of the widespread phenol-climatic models uses the air temperature as a most relevant environmental parameter influencing the flowering process. Some of them consider only the heat requirements, while others take chilling requirements into account (Richardson et al., 1974; Galan et al., 2001; Garcia-Mozo et al., 2008; Scheifinger et al., 2013; Frenguelli et al., 2014; Fu et al., 2014).

The dates of the beginning of flowering of trees with winter flowering or flowering at the beginning of spring are very variable, above all in temperate zones. As mentioned before, to predict the beginning of pollination it is necessary to model when the plant has satisfied the chilling requirement in order to complete dormancy and when the heat necessary for flowering begins to accumulate. The timing of the pollen season is due to these important and successive temperature requirements, and delays on the onset of flowering are caused either by high temperature during chilling requirement and/or low temperature during heat accumulation (Frenguelli, 1999; Chuine et al., 2003; Linkosalo et al., 2006).

The one most widely used is the accumulation of daily mean temperature above a base temperature, known as "thermal time" (°C days) or Growing Degree Day (GDD) (Monteith, 1984; Linkosalo et al., 2008). The standard calculation of the thermal time between two flowering periods (1 and 2) can be summarized:

$$T_t = [(T_{max} - T_{min}) \times 0.5] - T_b$$

where T_t is the thermal time between periods 1 and 2, T_{max} and T_{min} are the daily maximum and minimum temperatures, respectively, and T_b is the base temperature.

The linear approach consists of the claim that the product remains constant between the duration in days of a phenological phase and the efficacious temperature, defined as the difference between the air temperature and a value of the base temperature considered a real constant which is characteristic of the species or the variety. Physiologically the base temperature is the lowest temperature at which phenological development stops.

This proposed forecast method allows a good prediction of the beginning of pollen season in many arboreal plants, like oak (Frenguelli et al., 1999; Garcia-Mozo et al., 2008), birch (Myking, 1997; Kalvans et al., 2015), ash (Peeters, 1998; Pauling et al., 2014), alder and poplar (Frenguelli and Bricchi, 1998), olive (Galan et al., 2001; 2005; Aguilera et al., 2013), plane (Tedeschini et al., 2006). The thermal time could be calculated considering the beginning of pollination of an indicator species, assuming the existence of a linear relationship between the phenological development rate and air temperature in the time interval separating the flowering dates of one species, assumed as indicator, and a second one flowering later on. When the indicator species flowers, the predicted one has reached an unknown but fixed fraction of its own phenological development (Marletto et al., 1992).

The response of trees depends largely on the species, the latitude and the intensity of change (Taiz and Zeiger, 1998). The thermal time models are also limited and sometimes do not offer constant values but present variation due to various causes. Among these there is the temperature during various stages of development, when the heat accumulation starts and the base temperature, which varies according to the different genera and species.

In some regions and species, such as in Spain for oak, the percentages of variance explained by local models are on average greater than those explained by regional and national models. Nevertheless, acceptable results were also found obtained using regional models. This suggests that regional models may be sufficiently effective, and thus that local models are not necessary (Garcia-Mozo et al., 2008).

Moreover, in Japan and Korea, in some tree species, the responses to temperature can vary significantly among sites, suggesting that phenological changes at one location may not always be good indicators of changes at other locations (Ibanez et al., 2010).

Beside temperature, photoperiod, alone or together with temperature, is the major environmental determinant of plant phenology and it interactively modulates plant development. Floral initiation in most herbaceous plants is much more sensitive to day length that it is in many woody plants. For herbaceous crops, many models simulate plant phenology based on temperature and photoperiod: the model simulates the rate of development (R) using a function of temperature multiplied by a function of photoperiod (Yan and Wallace, 1998):

$$R = f(T)f(P)$$

A high predictive capability of these models is shown for many crops in different area. In soybean, the temperature in a constant photoperiod greatly influences the time to flowering with cool temperatures causing delayed flowering; the longer daylengths inhibit the development rate to flowering in many cultivars, and there is a strong inhibitory effect of longer daylengths on development rate as the photoperiod approaches the critical photoperiod. That is, the time to flowering is greatly lengthened when the soybeans are exposed to longer daylengths (Sinclair et al., 1991).

Under long daylength the time to flowering of short-day plant like beans is delayed by higher temperature; for long-day plant like pea under short day length, higher temperatures delayed the development. Ragweed has a not sensitive period during juvenile phase, but following this phase, sensitivity to photoperiod is constant and continues until the beginning of pollination. A photoperiod of 14 hours or less is optimal, and results in a maximal rate of development (Deen et al., 1998). However, the role of photoperiod and its interaction with chilling and forcing temperatures is complex, i.e., for *Betula* short-day conditions stabilize dormancy, whereas long days promote dormancy release (Myking, 1999).

5.4 CHANGES IN THE PAST AND EXPECTED CHANGES IN THE FUTURE

5.4.1 OBSERVED CHANGES IN THE PAST

5.4.1.1 Climate Influence on Airborne Pollen Trends

Over the period 1880–2012 the globally averaged combined land and ocean surface temperature data show a linear warming trend of 0.85°C (0.65 to 1.06) (IPPC, 2014). It is extremely likely that more than half of the observed increase in global average surface temperature from 1951 to 2010 was caused by the anthropogenic increase in greenhouse gas concentrations and other anthropogenic forcings together. In Europe, the average temperature has continued to increase, with regionally and seasonally different rates of warming (Kovats et al., 2014). Three independent records show long-term warming trends of average annual temperature since the end of the 19th century, with most rapid increases in recent decades (EEA, 2012). The last decade (2002–2011) was the warmest on record globally and in Europe. Annual average temperature across European land areas has warmed more than global average temperature, and slightly more than global land temperature. The average temperature for the European land area for the last decade (2002–2011) is 1.3°C (± 0.11°C) above the pre-industrial level. The interannual temperature variability over Europe is generally much higher in winter than in summer. The relatively rapid warming trend since the 1980s is most clearly evident in the summer. Particularly large warming has been observed in the past 50 years over the Iberian Peninsula, across Central and North-Eastern Europe, and in mountainous regions. Over the past 30 years, warming was the strongest over Scandinavia, especially in winter, whereas the Iberian Peninsula warmed mostly in summer (EEA, 2012).

Precipitation changes across Europe show more spatial and temporal variability than temperature. Since the mid-20th century, annual precipitation has been generally increasing across most of northern Europe, most notably in winter, but decreasing in parts of southern Europe (EEA, 2012).

The observed climate change has already led to a wide range of impacts on the environment including vegetation and pollen. A meta-analysis of an European wide phenological dataset of time series from several plant species for onset dates of flowering, leaf unfolding and fruit maturation showed that the majority of these phases advanced between 1971 and 2000 (Menzel et al., 2006). It was demonstrated that plant species phenology is responsive to temperature of the preceding months. An advance of spring/summer of 2.5 days/decade was detected in the period 1971–2000 and matches the increasing temperature trend. Earlier species were more sensitive than later species and spring phases in warmer countries exhibited a stronger response to temperature. Like phenological phases also the start dates of the pollen season of allergenic species are mainly dependent on temperatures in the preceding months (Frenguelli, 2002; Emberlin et al., 2007; Pauling et al., 2014). A higher dependency on temperature has been observed in plants that flower in spring and early summer, whereas species that flower in late summer and fall generally are more correlated with photoperiod. Consequently, the former species are more affected by warmer winters and springs, showing an earlier flowering in recent years (Levetin and Van de Water, 2008). Due to increasing temperatures earlier pollen seasons were observed in Europe, especially for long pollen data series starting earlier than 1990 (Emberlin et al., 2002; Clot, 2003; Galán et al., 2005; García-Mozo et al., 2006). Since temperature trends are not linear, the slopes of the pollen trends in Europe show important variations depending on the covered time period of the trend analysis. Especially in the analysis of shorter data series the advance of the pollen season is frequently not significant. Smith et al. (2014) calculated regional trends for different pollen species across Europe starting in 1990 to 2003 and all ending 2009. During this time period no consistent changes were observed in the start or duration of the pollen season. Also in studies from Italy or

Hungary the start dates did not significantly change (Makra et al., 2011; Ugolotti et al., 2015). Many of the pollen data series are still not long enough to show stable, significant advancing trends. According to Menzel et al. (2001), at least 20 years of data should be used for getting reliable trend results. In addition to robust multi-decadal warming, the globally averaged surface temperature exhibits substantial decadal and interannual variability. Due to this natural variability, trends based on short records are very sensitive to the beginning and end dates and do not in general reflect long-term climate trends. As one example, the rate of warming over the past 15 years (1998–2012; 0.05 [–0.05 to 0.15] °C per decade), which begins with a strong El Niño, is smaller than the rate calculated since 1951 (1951–2012; 0.12 [0.08 to 0.14] °C per decade) (IPCC, 2014). This smaller warming rate in the last years influences the pollen trend results in the way that slopes of trends get smaller. Even a tendency for later start dates, although not significant, was observed for *Platanus* pollen in Andalusia, Spain (Alcázar et al., 2011). The influence of precipitation on start dates of the grass pollen season is seen in the long term trend of grass pollen in Cordoba 1982–2008 (Spain), which shows a weak but significant trend towards earlier start dates (García-Mozo et al., 2010). Years with earliest start dates had warm and wet early springs, while years with late start dates usually had cooler and drier early springs.

Climate has also an impact on the pollen season intensity. Several studies demonstrate increasing trends in the annual pollen index (API) (Damialis et al., 2007; Ziello et al., 2012). In Europe most of the allergenic tree species show trends to higher API, especially Cupressaceae, *Platanus*, *Corylus*, *Fraxinus*, *Alnus* and *Betula* pollen. In the herbaceous pollen species *Ambrosia* show increasing API, while *Artemisia* and Amaranthaceae significantly decrease. The API of Poaceae does not change significantly throughout Europe (Ziello et al., 2012). In this study 14% of all analyzed API data series (in total, 1221) increased significantly and 8% decreased significantly. Regional differences showed that Greece, Hungary, Poland Switzerland and Germany showed more increasing trends, while Spain had more significantly decreasing trends. On the other hand in the European wide study of Smith et al. (2014) very few consistent trends were actually observed, apart from a trend towards decreased exposure to Asteraceae pollen at 8 of 13 sites (including three significant trends). The influencing factors for the pollens season intensity are manifold: temperature, precipitation, CO_2, changes in land use, urban green space management, urbanization, deposition of nitrogenous compounds, plant diseases and others (Dahl et al., 2013). Temperature, sunshine hours and precipitation in the preceding year and a system of resource allocation among years determine *Betula* season intensity (Dahl and Strandhede, 1996; Ranta et al., 2005; Dahl et al., 2013). *Quercus* pollens season intensity in Spain is influenced by temperature and in Mediterranean climate also by rainfall prior to flowering (Garcia-Mozo et al., 2006). Precipitation in the preceding year or during the same year before flowering affects the Poaceae pollen season intensity positively (Gonzales Minero et al., 1998; Schäppi et al., 1998; García-Mozo et al., 2010). The hot summer 2003 with unusual drought in Central Europe led to an intense grass pollen season in Switzerland, which ended remarkably earlier than normal and favored the pollen production of drought resistant herbs (Gehrig, 2003). Similar observations were made in southern Spain where Amaranthaceae plants react rapidly to rainfall after drought and tolerate high temperatures. Although their API shows a decreasing trend from 1991–2011, they have a potential to increase their distribution, which can lead to higher airborne pollen counts in drier conditions (Cariñanos et al., 2014). Higher temperatures in spring can lead to earlier germination of *Ambrosia artemisiifolia* so that a greater biomass, a higher average weight per inflorescence, and a larger number of inflorescences are produced which results in earlier flowering and increased pollen production (Rogers et al., 2006).

Increased atmospheric carbon dioxide is one of the most important drivers of climate change. Carbon dioxide also directly affects carbon availability for plants as the primary carbon resource obtained through photosynthesis (Levetin and Van de Water, 2008). Greenhouse experiments have demonstrated that higher CO_2 concentrations have a positive effect on the growth, pollen production and flowering intensity of *Ambrosia artemisiifolia* (Ziska and Caulifield, 2000; Rogers et al., 2006). A significant portion of allergenic pollen is produced by larger perennial plants, shrubs, and trees. These large plants are harder to study, as their size and the time needed to reach fecundity necessitate a significant investment to realize results (Levetin and Van de Water, 2008). Free air CO_2 experiments (FACE) still shows contradictory results. Generally, the effect of high CO_2

levels shows a strong initial effect on growth, which diminishes over time (Adams, 2010). Nevertheless an experiment with *Pinus taeda* showed increased stand-level pollen production after more than 5 years of growth at heightened CO_2 concentrations (Ladeau and Clark, 2006).

5.4.1.2 Invasive Species

In all populated parts of the world, humans put their mark on vegetation. In Europe, men and women manipulated the landscape at least since Neolithicum, and there is hardly any place outside the Artic and Alpine regions that is not affected. Therefore, the typical pollen flora in the ambient air is also the result of human activities. We use promote the abundance of plant species with certain strategies, involving a high reproductive output.

In nature, ecosystems undergo predictable changes in a constant flux, called succession. Each plant species performs best during a certain stage during this process, and becomes temporarily more prominent while other species fade out of existence. Plant cover and biomass increase over time, as the first low-growing colonists of bare ground are replaced by larger herbs and grasses, which in turn are followed by shrubs and trees. The late stages of succession are characterized by long-lived species. The course of succession can be broken by disturbance; an impact that partially or totally destroys plant biomass in the ecosystem. Natural forces bringing disturbance are, e.g., wildfires, flooding, drought, land-slides, hurricanes, and insect plagues. In landscapes modified by people, recurrent artificial disturbance interrupting the natural course of succession is the rule, caused by trampling, mowing, ploughing, clear-cutting, road and building construction, fertilization, pollution, and pesticide application. The result is a dominance of plant species belonging to the earliest or intermediate stages of succession. They especially occur in the ruderal and unkempt areas that are common around human settlements, not least in cities. But they are also in the abandoned agricultural and pastoral land, that since the last 60–70 years is common it their surroundings. And here, the conditions are optimal for many of the species that are the main offenders in pollen allergy.

Among these plants, some are classified as competitive ruderals (Grime, 1977) and others as competitors, able to assert themselves in fertile, derelict environments. These plants are quick to tap into available resources, have fast growth rates, are often comparatively large, and they tend to be dominating in the ecosystem. Since their optimal stage in succession is ephemeral, they are also favoured by a large seed production. There are generally more pollen grains than there are ovules, and if dispersed in the wind, they contribute significantly to the local pollen load. Competitive ruderals thrive when there is some competition from other plants, but when it still not is overwhelming, as in roadsides and verges that now and then are subject to disturbance, or in agricultural fields. They use resources for ample biomass production before flowers are even initiated, but then, they afford a large reproductive output. Among these plants are *Artemisia vulgaris*, *Parietaria judaica,* and *Hordeum murinum.* Also several invasive, alien species belong to this group, e.g., *Ambrosia artemisiifolia*, *Amaranthus* spp., *Chenopodium ambrosioides*, and *Panicum* spp. Members of the other group, competitors sensu Grime (1977) dominate the sera of incipient vegetation closure which initially are characterized by fast-growing, large herbs and grasses, later by pioneer tree species. Although this stage is transient, it may last for several decades and from the perspective of a human life, during a long time. *Dactylis glomerata*, *Hyparrhenia hirta*, *Arrhenatherrum* spp, are examples of competitors, as well as trees and shrubs, e.g., within the genera *Salix*, *Betula*, *Fraxinus*, and *Ulmus*, and the invaders *Ailanthus altissima* and *Acer negundo*. *Ailanthus altissima*, originating from China, and *Acer negundo* from North America, are now found in many kinds of habitats, including forests, in the European continents. They combine a prolific vegetative growth with abundant flowering, and are potent competitors. *Acer negundo* is a well-known offender of pollen allergy sufferers; there are reports of sensitisation to pollen of *Ailanthus* (Ballero et al., 2003), which is pollinated by small insects but has open flowers with some pollen grains escaping into the air.

Some of the tree species are able to persist during later successional stages, if the opportunity to establish during an early stage was there. Competitive species in both groups often respond to atmospheric pollution, such as nitrogen deposition mainly emanating from traffic exhausts, and increased carbon dioxide concentration (Ziska et al., 2003).

5.4.2 EXPECTED CHANGES IN THE FUTURE: CLIMATE SCENARIOS FOR EUROPE, EXPECTED CHANGES FOR ALLERGENIC PLANTS (DUE TO CLIMATE, CO_2, HUMAN INFLUENCE, AIR POLLUTION)

5.4.2.1 Climate Influence on Airborne Pollen Trends

According to EEA Report (2012) the average temperature over Europe is projected to continue increasing throughout the 21st century, more than global land temperature. The annual temperature for Europe is projected to increase by 1.0°C to 2.5°C (between periods 2021–2050 and 1961–1990) and 2.5°C to 4.0°C (between periods 2071–2100 and 1961–1990). The warming is projected to be the greatest in northeastern Europe and Scandinavia in winter and over southern Europe in summer. Annual precipitation is projected to increase in northern Europe and decrease in southern Europe. The change in annual mean between 1961–1990 and 2071–2100 varies between 10% and 20% in northern Europe and between –5 and –20% in southern Europe and the Mediterranean. Projections for summer precipitation show a decrease over southern, central and northwest Europe, which can reach of up to 60% in parts of southern Europe. Precipitation is projected to remain constant or to increase slightly in northeast Europe. The number of consecutive dry days is projected to increase significantly in southern and central Europe, in particular in summer, and to decrease in northern Europe, in particular in winter.

Due to the timing and the intensity of pollen season is expected to change in future. Chilling and forcing temperature, precipitation and day length (photoperiod) are the most dominant climate factors triggering the development of plants until the start of the pollen season and belong also to the important factors for pollen release. Due to this close relationship, the timing and the intensity of pollen season is expected to change in future. An early start of the pollen release is likely, especially in regions with sufficient water availability. This can be expected to be associated with an earlier appearance of symptoms of allergic diseases (Cecchi et al., 2010). In Spain scenarios for the end of the 21st century indicate that *Quercus* pollination season could start on average one month earlier and airborne pollen concentrations will increase by 50% with respect to current levels, with higher values in Mediterranean inland areas (Garcia-Mozo et al., 2006).

However, winter chilling conditions can have a significant impact on the timing of bud burst. If trees receive insufficient chilling, there may be a delay in bud burst even if spring temperatures rise. Therefore, it is important to understand the effect of chilling on spring phenology of trees (Myking, 1999; Dahl et al., 2013; Pietsers et al., 2015). Pietsers et al. (2015) demonstrate that inadequate chilling has the potential to slow both the rate and speed of bud burst of *Betula pubescens* and *Populus tremula*. The range of chilling and forcing intervals is not yet satisfactorily known, nor is it clarified when and how chilling and forcing temperatures act on bud growth (Dahl et al., 2013). Also the role of photoperiod in forecast models needs further research, since its interaction with chilling and forcing temperatures is not yet understood totally.

Climatic change will influence the distribution of plant species in Europe and there will be a distinct change in the potential ranges of European trees (Hanewinkel et al., 2013). Deciduous oak is projected to spread in central Europe and to almost double its area, while spruce loses important parts of its present range. Mediterranean oak forest type will cover many parts of European forests, while the area of birch trees is decreasing. Changes in biomes of major tree species are gradual changes, but forests are likely to be more and more exposed to extreme events such as the increased risk of fire and drought and, partly linked to that, the spread of pests and diseases (Lindner et al., 2012). These changes in vegetation distribution will have important impacts on the pollen season. Sorkey et al. (2014) used a process-based model of weed growth, competition and population dynamics to predict the future distribution of *Ambrosia artemisiifolia* in Europe. The model predicted a northward shift in the available climatic niche for populations to establish and persist due to more favorable growing conditions and delayed frost, creating a risk of increased health problems.

Projections for future pollen loads and the impact on allergies in a changing climate are still in a preliminary stage. More research is needed to establish physiological plant models which model the interaction of the plant development and their environmental conditions for better understanding the processes (D'Amato et al 2015). There is also a limited availability of long time series of data of airborne pollen and spore concentrations (Cecchi et al., 2010). Additionally, current knowledge shows that the magnitude and characteristics of climate change varies by different geographic areas. Thus, projections on climate change in general and on the effects on plants at continental scale are speculative (Cecchi et al., 2010; D'Amato et al 2015).

5.4.2.2 Invasions: Challenges for Routine Aerobiology and for Modelers

Global change involves increasing trade and travel, followed by transport of plants across borders beyond their own dispersal ability. This is not a new phenomenon. Humans have moved thousands of organisms from one area to another since prehistory, with migration, spread of agriculture, colonization, trade and warfare. The difference to earlier times is the scale of this international exchange, and the impact they could have on native ecosystems and society, as an effect of the ongoing climate change.

Alien plants are often found around railways stations, harbors, motorways, large industrial areas and rubbish dumps which are situated along import routes and provide favorable conditions for establishment (Kowarik, 2000; Walter et al., 2003). They may escape to be casual oddities in the local flora, or perhaps to be more successful weeds. Their effect is not always detrimental, or their negative impact may be limited. But a fraction of aliens becomes invasive, i.e., they are species that disperse and grow to a scale as to damage the ecosystems, biodiversity, and/or society, where they establish. Humans also import alien plants to use as ornamentals in gardens and parks. There is a concern that exotic ornamentals which produce allergenic pollen are potent sensitizers of the urban population (D'Amato et al., 2007; Cariñanos and Casares-Porcel, 2011), as they often are planted *en masse*. Since they usually are selected to thrive in the local climate, competitive ornamentals with efficient propagule dispersal are prone to naturalize.

There is not an universal explanation for the evolution of invasiveness, but 10 key traits have been identified as to be involved, viz. (1) high growth rate, (2) wide climatic or environmental tolerance, (3) short generation time, (4) prolific or consistent reproduction, (5) small seed size, (6) efficient dispersal, (7) high capacity for uniparental reproduction, (8) absence of specialized germination (9) high competitive ability, and (10) ability to escape or survive natural enemies (Whitney & Gabler, 2008).

Although native plants can have invasive behavior not least due to environmental change, an invasive plant is by definition of alien origin. In wind-pollinated plants, invasiveness can be a concern to health, since invasive plants often are very competitive, tending to dominate the sites where they grow, and since they often produce a lot of pollen that may be allergenic. Moreover, when they spread to new regions, their pollen may be especially aggressive, since people tend to be more easily sensitized towards allergens they did not meet with during their infancy (Lombardi et al., 2011). Because of the considerable negative impact, it would desirable to predict what alien species will be transformed from precious garden joys, or from curiosities pleasing floristic inventors, into monster plants.

One could imagine that if only the suitable habitat is there in the non-native area, the non-native species just can invade. But the effects of evolutionary processes in the new environments are often underestimated. There is a lack of a shared history with other organisms in the new ecosystem, and there will be latitudinal and longitudinal differences (Hellman et al., 2008). Selection pressures are not the same. Thus, the ecological niche in the native range is generally a poor predictor of the future invaded range.

The genetic composition of the introduced populations is important for their capacity to adapt to new circumstances, and it is different to that of their ancestral ones. A single introduction is often a genetic bottleneck, where stochastic forces determine what traits will survive. In order to respond to selection, a population must contain the necessary genetic variation for the traits that promote survival, such as emergence time, growth rate, phenology, and resistance towards hostile organisms. Many genes in concert, each with a small but additive effect, usually govern such traits. Therefore, a background of multiple introduction events, followed by a mixture between the introduced populations, is a common feature for several invasive plants, just as described for the prime example of *Ambrosia artemisiifolia*. Originating in North America, it was repeatedly introduced to Europe with American soldiers during the two World Wars and with import of contaminated cereal and forage seed. Ornamental species are also likely to have been introduced several times. Also interspecific hybridization, possible in many plant genera, may promote adaption to the new area. *Rhododendron ponticum* has a disjunct distribution in the area of Black Sea and in the Iberian Peninsula. It is generally not frost-resistant, but turned invasive in Britain, even in Scotland, after multiple introductions since the 18th century, and after introgression of genes from the popular ornamentals *R. maximum* and *R. catawbiense* (Milne and Abbott, 2000). Chromosomal mutations like polyploidization or translocations in the hybrid progeny may result in permanent heterozygosity, resulting in a wider ecological amplitude than that of the parental species. Tetraploid *Dactylis glomerata* subsp. *glomerata*, albeit native in Europe but with an invasive behavior on overgrown ground, is at least partly result of hybridization between different subspecies (Lumaret and Borrill, 1998).

There is widespread evidence of rapid evolutionary change in invading populations as they expand along latitudinal and longitudinal gradients (Whitney and Gabler, 2008; Alexander and Edwards, 2010). These changes apparently evolve in situ, and in parallel to similar adaptations in their native range, as was found in, e.g., *Hypericum perforatum*, *Solidago* spp, and in *Ambrosia artemisiifolia* (Weber and Schmid, 1998; Hodgins and Rieseberg, 2011). The selected traits are those mentioned above, related to emergence, phenology, growth and dispersal. Introduced European populations of *A. artemisiifolia* exhibited improved competitively and reproduction in a range of stressful environments, as compared to native American conspecifics (Hodgins and Rieseberg, 2011). In European common ragweed populations, growth and flowering phenology were correlated both to latitude and to longitude (Leiblein-Wild and Tackenberg, 2014). *Cynodon dactylon* is one of the most important allergen sources in tropical and subtropical climates. It is reported as naturalized in several European countries within the temperate region, and even as invasive in Czechia and Belgium (Pysek et al., 2012; DAISIE, 2015). It could be assumed that some kind of selection for survival in the comparatively cold climate in these countries took place. Invasive species are often characterized by a degree of phenotypic plasticity, i.e., the capacity of a given genotype to develop one of several phenotypic states, depending on the environment. This capacity facilitates establishment in varying sites. Which is the most important for invasiveness, local selection or plasticity, is not resolved. Plasticity itself is a heritable trait and could therefore also be a target for selection in the non-native area. It has been argued that assessment of the risk of invasive species owing to changing climate must incorporate evolutionary potential (Richardson and Pyšek, 2006; Clements and DiTommaso, 2011).

The evolution towards invasiveness is a time-consuming process of several stages, i.e., introduction, naturalization, spread and "explosion." When an alien species is identified as invasive, it was usually a resident for considerable time, decades or rather centuries (Weber, 1998; Pyšek et al., 2012). There is no universal explanation for this time lag. It was suggested that it is due to the fact that evolutionary adaption takes time (Ellstrand and Schierenbeck, 2000; Holt et al., 2005). In some cases, "sudden" invasiveness may be due to changing environmental conditions, as is suggested for walnuts in East Europe in from 1960's and onwards, after 700 years of cultivation. The combination of milder winters, abandonment of agricultural land and decreased hunting of rooks, who disperse the walnuts, promotes the establishment of the trees in seminatural ecosystems (Lenda et al., 2012). Since urban areas often are warmer than their rural surroundings, species that turn invasive due to climate change may first be observed there, as reported from Central European cities (Sukopp and Wurzel, 2003).

KEYWORDS

- **aerobiology**
- **airborne pollen**
- **climate change**
- **modeling**
- **phenology**
- **pollen allergy**

REFERENCES

Adams, J. 2010. *Vegetation-Climate Interaction. How Plants make the Global Environment.* Springer, 2010. Aguilera, F., Ruiz, L., Fornaciari, M., Romano, B., Galán, C., Oteros, J., Ben Dhiab, A., Msallem, M., Orlandi, F., Heat accumulation period in the Mediterranean region: phenological response of the olive in different climate areas (Spain, Italy and Tunisia) *Int J Biometeorol* 2013, 58, 867–876.

Alcázar, P., Garcia-Mozo, H., Trigo, M. M., Ruiz, L., Gonzalez-Minero, F. J., Hidalgo, P., Diaz de la Guardia, C., Galan, C., *Platanus* pollen season in Andalusia (southern Spain): trends and modeling, *J., Environ. Monit*, 2011, 13, 2502–2510.

Alcázar, P., Stach, A., Nowak, M., Galán, C., Comparison of airborne herb pollen types in Córdoba (South-western Spain) and Poznan (Western Poland). *Aerobiologia* 2009, 25, 55–63.

Alexander, J. M., Edwards, P. J., Limits to the niche and range margins of alien species. *Oikos* 2010, 119, 1377–1386.

Arora, R., Rowland, L. J., Tanino, K., Induction and release of bud dormancy in woody perennials: A science comes of age. *HortScience* 2003, 38, 911–921.

Ballero, M., Ariu, A., Falagiani Piu, P. G., Allergy to *Ailanthus altissima* (tree of heaven) pollen. *Allergy* 2003, 58, 532–533.

Basler, D., Körner, C., Photoperiod sensitivity of bud burst in 14 temperate forest tree species. *Agricultural and Forest Meteorology*, 2012, 165, 73–81.

Bellard, C., Bertelsmeier, C., Leadley, P., Thuiller, W., Courchamp, F., Impacts of climate change on the future of biodiversity. *Ecology Letters* 2012, 15, 365–377.

Bruns, E., Vliet, A. V., *Standardization of Phenological Monitoring in Europe*. Wageningen University and Deutscher Wetterdienst, 2003.

Cariñanos, P., Alcázar, P., Galán, C., Domínguez, E., Environmental behavior of airborne Amaranthaceae pollen in the southern part of the Iberian Peninsula, and its role in future climate scenarios. *Science of the Total Environment* 2014, 470–471, 480–487.

Cariñanos, P., Casares-Porcel, M., Urban green zones and related pollen allergy: A review. Some guidelines for designing spaces with low allergy impact. *Landscape Urban Plann* 2011, 101, 205–214.

Cecchi, L., D'Amato, G., Ayres, J. G., Galan, C., Forastiere, F., Forsberg B., Gerritsen, J., Nunes, C., Behrendt, H., Akdis, C., Dahl, R. & Annesi-Maesano I. Projections of the effects of climate change on allergic asthma: the contribution of aerobiology. Allergy 2010, 65, 1073–1081.

Chuine, I., Belmonte, J., Improving prophylaxis for pollen allergies: Predicting the time course of the pollen load of the atmosphere of major allergenic plants in France and Spain. *Grana* 2004, 43, 65–80.

Chuine, I., Cour, P., Advantages of aerobiological data for phenology modelling and studies. Abs. *6th Internat.Congress on Aerobiology*, Perugia, 1998, p. 103.

Chuine, I., Kramer, K., Hänninen, H., Plant development models. In: M. D. Schwartz (ed.), *Phenology: An Integrative Environmental Science*. Dordrecht/Boston/London: Kluwer Academic Publishers, 2003, p. 564.

Chuine, I., Mignot, A., Belmonte, J., A modeling analysis of the genetic variation of phenology between tree populations. *Journal of Ecology* 2000, 88, 1–12.

Clements, D. R., DiTommaso, A., Climate change and weed adaptation: can evolution of invasive plants lead to greater range expansion than forecasted? *Weed Research* 2011, 51, 227–240.

Comtois, P., Sherknies, D., An aerobiological model for pollen forecasting. *18th Conference on Agricultural and Forest Meteorology and 8th Conference on Biometeorology and Aerobiology*. 1987, Sep. 14–18.

Cramer, W., Yohe, G. W., Auffhammer, M., Huggel, C., Molau, U., da Silva Dias, M. A. F., Solow, A., Stone, D. A., Tibig, L., *Detection and attribution of observed impacts*. In: *Climate Change 2014: Impacts, Adaptation, and Vulnerability. Part A: Global and Sectoral Aspects*. Contribution of Working Group II to the Fifth Assessment Report of the Intergovernmental Panel on Climate Change Field, C. B., Barros, V. R., Dokken, D. J., Mach, K. J., Mastrandrea, M. D., Bilir, T. E., Chatterjee, M., Ebi, K. L.,

Estrada, Y. O., Genova, R. C., Girma, B., Kissel, E. S., Levy, A. N., MacCracken, S., Mastrandrea, P. R., White, L. L. (Eds.). Cambridge University Press, Cambridge, United Kingdom and NY, USA, 2014, pp. 979–1037.

D'Amato, G., Cecchi, L., Bonini, S., Nunes, C., Annesi-Maesano, I., Behrendt, H., Liccardi, G., Popov, T., Van Cauwenberge, P. Allergenic pollen and pollen allergy in Europe. Allergy 2007, 62, 976–990.

D'Amato, G., Holgate, S.T., Pawankar, R., et al. Meteorological conditions, climate change, new emerging factors, and asthma and related allergic disorders. A statement of the World Allergy Organization. A statement of the World Allergy Organization, World Allergy Organization Journal (2015) 8, 25. doi: 10.1186/s40413-015-0073-02.

Dahl, A., Galán, C., Hajkova, L., Pauling, A., Sikoparija, B., Smith, M., Vokou, D., *The Onset, Course and Intensity of the Pollen Season*. InL *Allergenic Pollen: A Review of the Production, Release, Distribution and Health Impact*. Sofiev, M., Bergmann, K. Eds. Springer, Netherland, 2013.

Dahl, Å., Strandhede, S. O., Predicting the intensity of the birch pollen season. *Aerobiologia* 1996, 12, 97–106.

DAISIE. *Delivering Alien Invasive Species in Europe*. Database at http//:www.europe-aliens.org. Accessed at 30/08/2015, 2015.

Deen, W., Hunt, T., Swanton, C. J., Influence of temperature, photoperiod, and irradiance on the phenological development of common ragweed (*Ambrosia artemisiifolia*). *Weed Science* 1998, 46, 555–560.

EEA, 2012. *Climate Change, Impacts and Vulnerability in Europe 2012*, an Indicator-Based Report. EEA Report No. 12/2012, European Environment Agency (EEA), Copenhagen, Denmark, 304 pp.

Ellstrand, N. C., Schierenbeck, K. A., Hybridization as a stimulus for the evolution of invasiveness in plants. *Proceedings of the National Academy of Sciences USA*, 2000, 97, 7043–7050.

Emberlin, J., Detandt, M., Gehrig, R., Jaeger, S., Nolard, N., Rantio-Lehtimaki, A., Responses in the start of *Betula* (birch) pollen seasons to recent changes in spring temperatures across Europe. *International Journal of Biometeorology* 2002, 46, 159–170.

Emberlin, J., Smith, M., Close, R., Adams-Groom, B., Changes in the pollen seasons of the early flowering trees *Alnus* spp. and *Corylus* spp. in Worcester United Kingdom 1996–2005. *International Journal of Biometeorology*, 2007, 51, 181–191.

Frenguelli, G., Spieksma FThM, Bricchi, E., Romano, B., Mincigrucci, G., Nikkels, A. H., Dankaart, W., Ferranti, F., The influence of air temperature on the starting dates of the pollen season of *Alnus* and *Populus*. *Grana* 1991, 30, 196–200.

Frenguelli, G., Bricchi, E., The use of the pheno-climatic model for forecasting the pollination of some arboreal taxa. *Aerobiologia* 1998, 14, 39–44.

Frenguelli, G., Jato, M. V., Andreutti, R., Rodriguez, F. J., Aira, M. J., The influence of air temperature on the starting dates of *Quercus* pollination. Abs. *IV Symposium International de Palynologie Africaine*, Sousse, 1999, 59.

Frenguelli, G., Interactions between climatic changes and allergenic plants. *Arch. Chest. Dis.* 2002, 57(2), 141–143.

Frenguelli, G., Ghitarrini, S., Tedeschini, E., Climatic change in Mediterranean area and pollen monitoring. *Fl. Medit.* 2014, 24, 99–107.

Frenguelli, G., Ghitarrini, S., Tedeschini, E., Time linkages between pollination onsets of different taxa in Perugia, Central Italy: an update. *Agric. Environ. Med.*, 2015, 23, 92–96.

Fu, Y., Zhang, H., Dong, W., Yuan, W., Comparison of Phenology Models for Predicting the Onset of Growing Season over the Northern Hemisphere. *PLoS One*, 2014, 9(10), e109544.

Galán, C., Garcia-Mozo, H., Vazquez, L., Ruiz-Valenzuela, L., Díaz de la Guardia, C., Trigo-Perez, M., Heat requirement for the onset of the Olea europaea, L., Pollen season in several places of Andalusia region and the effect of the expected future climate change. *International Journal of Biometeorology* 2005, 49(3), 184–188.

Galan, C., García-Mozo, H., Cariñanos, P., Alcazar, P., Dominguez-Vilches, E., The role of temperature in the onset of the Olea europaea, L., pollen season in southwestern *Spain. Int. J. Biometeorol.* 2001, 45, 8–12.

Galan, C., Tormo, R., Cuevas, J., Infante, F., Dominguez, E., Theoretical daily variation patterns of airborne pollen in the South-West of Spain. *Grana* 1991, 30, 201–209.

Galán, C., Smith, M., Thibaudon, M., Frenguelli, G., Oteros, J., Gehrig, R., Berger, U., Clot, B., Brandao, R., EAS QC Working Group (2014) Pollen monitoring: minimum requirements and reproducibility of analysis. *Aerobiologia* 2014, 30, 385–395.

García-Mozo, H., Chuine, I., Aira, M. J., Belmonte, J., Bermejo, D., Diaz de la Guardia, C., Elvira, B., Gutierrez, M., Rodriguez-Rajo, J., Ruiz, L., Trigo, M. M., Tormo, R., Valencia, R., Galan, C., Regional phenological models for forecasting the start and peak of the *Quercus* pollen season in Spain. *Agricultural and Forest Meteorology* 2008, 148, 372 –380.

García-Mozo, H., Galán, C., Belmonte, J., Bermejo, D., Candau, P., de la Guardia, C. D., Elvira, B., Gutiérrez, M., Jato, V., Silva, I., Trigo, M., Valencia, R., Chuine, I., Predicting the start and peak dates of the Poaceae pollen season in Spain using process-based models. *Agricultural and Forest Meteorology*, 2009, 149, 256–262.

García-Mozo, H., Galán, C., Alcázar, P., de la Guardia, C., Nieto-Lugilde, D., Recio, M., Hidalgo, P., Gónzalez-Minero, F., Ruiz, L., Domínguez-Vilches, E., Trends in grass pollen season in southern Spain *Aerobiologia*, 2010, 26, 157–169.

García-Mozo, H., Galán, C., Jato, V., Belmonte, J., Díaz de la Guardia, C., Fernández, D., Gutiérrez, M., Aira, M. J., Roure, J. M., Ruiz, L., Trigo, M. M., Domínguez-Vilches, E., *Quercus* pollen season dynamics in the Iberian Peninsula: response to meteorological parameters and possible consequences of Climate Change. *Annals Agriculture and Environmental Medicine* 2006, 13, 209–224.

Gehrig, R., The influence of the hot and dry summer 2003 on the pollen season in Switzerland *Aerobiologia* 2006, 22, 27–34.

Gómez-Casero, M. T., Hidalgo, P. J., García-Mozo, H., Domínguez, E., Galán, C., Pollen biology in four Mediterranean *Quercus* species. *Grana* 2004, 43, 22–30.

Gonzales Minero FJ; Candau, P., Tomás, C., Morales, J., Airborne grass (Poaceae) pollen in southern Spain. Results of a 10-year study (1987–96). *Allergy*, 1998, 53, 266–274.

Grime, J. P., Evidence for the existence of three primary strategies in plants and its relevance to ecological and evolutionary theory. *American Naturalist* 1977, 111, 1169–1194.

Hanewinkel, M., Cullmann, D. A., Schelhaas, M. J., Nabuurs, G. J., Zimmermann, N. E., Climate change may cause severe loss in the economic value of European forest land. *Nature Climate Change* 2013, 3, 203–207.

Hedhly, A., Hormaza, J. I., Herrero, M., Global warming and sexual plant reproduction. *Trends in Plant Science*, 2009, 14, 30–36.

Hellman, J. J., Byers, J. E., Bierwagen, B. G., Dukes, J. S., Five potential consequences of climate change for invasive species. *Conservation Biology* 2008, 22, 534–543.

Hodgins, K. A., Rieseberg, L., Genetic differentiation in life-history traits of introduced and native common ragweed (*Ambrosia artemisiifolia*) populations. *Journal of Evolutionary Ecology* 2011, 24, 2731–2749.

Holt, J., Barfield, M., Gomulkiewicz, R., *Theories of niche conservatism and evolution: could exotic species be potential pests?* In: *Species Invasions: Insights into Ecology, Evolution, and Biogeography*. Sax, D. F., Stachowicz, J. J., Gaines, S. D., Eds. Sinauer, Sunderland, MA, USA.2005, pp. 259–290.

Ibanez, I., Primack, R. B., Miller-Rushing, A. J., Ellwood, E., Higuchi, H., Lee, S. D., Kobori, H., Silander JA.2010. Forecasting phenology under global warming. *Phil. Trans. R. Soc. B* 365, 3247–3260.

IPCC, *Climate Change 2014: Synthesis Report. Contribution of Working Groups, I, II and III to the Fifth Assessment Report of the Intergovernmental Panel on Climate Change*. Core Writing Team, R.K. Pachauri, L. A. Meyer (eds.). IPCC, Geneva, Switzerland, 2014, 151 pp.

Jäger, S., Mandroli, P., Spieksma, F., Emberlin, J., Hjelmroos, M., Rantio-Lehtimak, A., Dominguez-Vilches, E., Ickovic, M. R., News. *Aerobiologia*, 1995, 11, 69–70.

Kalvâns, A., Bitâne, M., Kalvâne, G., Forecasting plant phenology: evaluating the phenological models for *Betula pendula* and *Padus racemosa* spring phases, Latvia. *Int J Biometeorol* 2015, 59, 165–179

Koch, E., Bruns, E., Chmielewski, F. M., Defila, C., Lipa, W., Menzel, A., 2007, *Guidelines for plant phenological observations*. WMO Technical Commission for Climatology, Open Program Area Group on Monitoring and Analysis of Climate Variability and Change (OPAG2).

Köppen, W., Klassifikation der Klimate nach Temperatur, Niederschlag und Jahresablauf (Classification of climates according to temperature, precipitation and seasonal cycle). *Petermanns Geogr. Mitt.* 1918, 64, 193–203, 243–248, map 1 and map 2.

Kovats, R. S., Valentini, R., Bouwer, L. M., Georgopoulou, E., Jacob, D., Martin, E., Rounsevell, M., Soussana, J. F., *Europe*. In: *Climate Change 2014: Impacts, Adaptation, and Vulnerability. Part A: Global and Sectoral Aspects*. Contribution Galán, C., Dahl, A., Frenguelli, G., and Gehrig of Working Group II to the Fifth Assessment Report of the Intergovernmental Panel on Climate Change Field, C. B., Barros, V. R., Dokken, D. J., Mach, K. J., Mastrandrea, M. D., Bilir, T. E., Chatterjee, M., Ebi, K. L., Estrada, Y. O., Genova, R. C., Girma, B., Kissel, E. S., Levy, A. N., MacCracken, S., Mastrandrea, P. R., White, L. L. Eds. Cambridge University Press, Cambridge, United Kingdom and NY, USA, 2014, pp. 979–1037.

Kowarik, I., *Some Responses of Flora and Vegetation to Urbanization in Central Europe*. In: *Plants and Plant Communities in the Urban Environment*. Sukopp, H., Hejny, S., Kowarik, I., Eds. SPB Academic Publishing, 1990.

Kramer, K., Selecting a model to predict the onset of growth of Fagus sylvatica. *J. Appl. Ecol* 1994, 31, 172–181.

Ladeau, S. L., Clark, J. S., Pollen production by *Pinus taeda* growing in elevated atmospheric CO2. *Functional Ecology*, 2006, 20, 541–547.

Latorre, F., Comparison between phenological and aerobiological patterns of some arboreal species of Mar del Plata (Argentina). *Aerobiologia*, 1997, 13, 49–59.

Latorre, F., Differences between airborne pollen and flowering phenology of urban trees with reference to production, dispersal and interannual climate variability. *Aerobiologia*, 1999, 15, 131–141.

Lee, C. E., Evolutionary genetics of invasive species. *Trends in Ecology and Evolution* 2002, 17, 386–391.

Leiblein-Wild, M. C., Tackenberg, O., Phenotypic variation of 38 European *Ambrosia artemisiifolia* populations measured in a common garden experiment. *Biological Invasions* 2014, 16, 2003–2015.

Lindner, M., Fitzgerald, J. B., Zimmermann, N. E., Reyer, C., Delzon, S., van der Maaten, E., Schelhaas, M. J., Lasch, P, Eggers, J., van der Maaten-Theunissen, M., Suckow, F., Psomas, A., Poulter, B., Hanewinkel, M., Climate change and European forests: What do we know, what are the uncertainties, and what are the implications for forest management? *Journal of Environmental Management* 2012, 146, 69–83.

Lenda, M., Skórka, P., Knops JMH, Moroñ, D., Tworek, S., Woyciechowski, M. Plant establishment and invasions: an increase in a seed disperser combined with land abandonment causes an invasion of the non-native walnut in Europe 2012. *Proceedings of the Royal Society B: Biological Sciences,* 2012, 22, 1491–1497.

Levetin, E., Van de Water, P., Changing pollen types/concentrations/distribution in the United States: fact or fiction? *Curr Allergy Asthma Rep*2008, 8, 418–424.

Linkosalo T., Häkkinen, R., Hänninen, H., Models of the spring phenology of boreal and temperate trees: Is there something missing? *Tree Physiology* 2006, 26, 1165–1172.

Linkosalo T., Lappalainen, H. K., Hari, P., A comparison of phenological models of leaf bud burst and flowering of boreal trees using independent observations. *Tree Physiology* 2008, 28, 1873–1882.

Linkosalo, T., Mutual regularity of spring phenology of some boreal tree species: predicting with other species and phenological models. *Can. J. For. Res.* 2000, 30, 667–673.

Lombardi, C., Canonica, G. W., Passalacqua, G., The possible influence of the environment on respiratory allergy: a survey on immigrants to Italy. *Annals of Allergy, Asthma and Immunology* 2011, 106(5), 407–411.

Lumaret, R., Borrill, M., Cytology, genetics, and evolution in the genus *Dactylis*. *Critical Reviews in Plant Sciences*, 1988, 7, 55–91.

Marletto, V., Puppi Branzi, G., Sirotti, M., Forecasting flowering dates of lawn species with air temperature: application boundaries of the linear approach. *Aerobiologia* 1992, 8, 75–83.

Meier, U., *Growth Stages of Mono- and Dicotyledonous Plants*. BBCH Monograph. Federal Biological Research Centre for Agriculture and Forestry. Berlin, 1997.

Meier, U., Bleiholder, H., Buhr, L., Feller, C., Hack, H., Heß, M., Lancashire, P. D., Schnock, U., Stauß, R., van den Boom, T., Weber, E., Zwerger, P., The BBCH system to coding the phenological growth stages of plants – history and publications. *Journal Für Kulturpflanzen* 2009, 61(2), 41–52.

Menzel, A., Plant phenological anomalies in Germany and their relation to air temperature and NAO. *Climatic Change*, 2003, 57, 243–263.

Menzel, A., *Europe*. In: *Phenology: An Integrative Environmental Science*, Second Edition. Schwartz MD Ed. Springer, Netherland, 2013.

Menzel, A., *Plant phenology "fingerprints."* In: *Phenology: An Integrative Environmental Science*, second Edition. Schwartz MD Ed. Springer, Netherland, 2013.

Menzel, A., Estrella, N., Fabian, P., Spatial and temporal variability of the phenological season in Germany from 1951 to 1996. *Global Change Biology*, 2001, 7, 657–666.

Menzel, A., Sparks, T. H., Estrella, N., Koch, E., Aasa, A., Ahas, R., Alm-Kübler, K., Bissolli, P., Braslavska, O., Briede, A., Chmielewski, F. M., Crepinsek, Z., Curnel, Y., Dahl, A., Defila, C., Donnelly, A., Filella, Y., Jatczak, K., Mage, F., Mestre, A., Nordli, Ø., Peñuelas, J., Pirinen, P., Remišová, V., Scheifinger, H., Striz, M., Susnik, A., Van Vliet, A. J. H., Wielgolaski, F. E., Zach, S., Zust, A., European phenological response to climate change matches the warming pattern. *Global Change Biology* 2006, 12(10), 1969–1976.

Metzger, M. J., Bunce RGH, Jongman RHG, Mücher, C. A., Watkins, J. W., A climatic stratification of the environment of Europe. *Global Ecology and Biogeography* 2005, 14, 549–563.

Milne, R. I., Abbott, R. J., Origin and evolution of invasive naturalized material of *Rhododendron ponticum*, L., in the British Isles. *Molecular Ecology* 2000, 9, 541–556.

Monteith, J. L., Consistency and convenience in the choice of units for agricultural science. *Experimental Agriculture* 1984, 20, 125–137.

Myking, T., Dormancy, budburst and impacts of climatic warming in coastal-inland and altitudinal *Betula pendula* and, *B. pubescens ecotypes*. In: *Phenology in Seasonal Climates*, I. Lieth, H., Schwartz, M. D., Eds. Backuys Publ., Leiden 1997, pp. 51–66.

Natura, *Habitats Directive Sites according to Biogeographical Regions*. 2000. http://ec.europa.eu/environment/nature/ natura2000/sites_hab/biogeog_regions/index_en.htm

Norris-Hill, J., A method to forecast the start of the Betula, Platanus and Quercus pollen seasons in North London. *Aerobiologia* 1998, 14, 165–170.

O'Rourke, M. K., Comparative pollen calendars from Tucson, Arizona: Durham vs. Burkard samplers. *Aerobiologia* 1990, 6, 136–140.

Parmesan, C., Influences of species, latitudes and methodologies on estimates of phenological response to global warming. *Global Change Biology* 2007, 13, 1860–1872.

Pauling, A., Gehrig, R., Clot, B., Toward optimized temperature sum parameterizations for forecasting the start of the pollen season. *Aerobiologia* 2014, 30, 45–57.

Peñuelas, P., Filella, I., Zhang, X., Llorens, L., Ogaya, R., Lloret, F., Comas, P., Estiarte, M., Terradas, J., Complex spatiotemporal phenological shifts as a response to rainfall changes. *New Phytologist* 2004, 161, 837–846.

Peeters, A. G., Cumulative temperatures for prediction of the beginning of ash (*Fraxinus excelsior* L.) pollen season. *Aerobiologia* 1998, 14, 375–382.

Puppi Branzi, G., *Rilevamenti fenologici su piante della flora spontanea*. In: *Schirone, B., edtor: Metodi di rilievo e di rappresentazione degli stadi fenologici*. CNR-IPRA, Roma, 1989, 9–38.

Pyšek, P., Danihelka, J., Sádlo, J., Chrtek, J., Jr, Chytrý, M., Jarošík, V., Kaplan, Z., Krahulec, F., Moravcová, L., Pergl, J., Štajerová, K., Tichý, L., Catalogue of alien plants of the Czech Republic (2nd Edition): checklist update, taxonomic diversity and invasion patterns. *Preslia* 2012, 84, 155–255.

Prieto-Baena, J. C., Hidalgo, P. J., Domínguez, Galán, C., Pollen production in the Poaceae family. *Grana*, 2003, 42, 153–160.

Ranta, H., Oksanen, A., Hokkanen, T., Bondestam, K., Heino, S., Masting by Betula-species; applying the resource budget model to north European data sets. *International Journal of Biometeorology* 2005, 49, 146–151.

Ribeiro, H., Oliveira, M., Ribeiro, N., Cruz, A., Ferreira, A., Machado, H., Reis, A., Abreu, I., Pollen allergenic potential nature of some trees species: a multidisciplinary approach using aerobiological, immunochemical and hospital admissions data. *Environmental Research* 2009, 109, 328–333.

Richardson, D. M., Pyšek, P., Naturalization of introduced plants: ecological drivers of biogeographical patterns. *New Phytologist* 2012, 196, 383–396.

Richardson, E. A., Seeley, S. D., Walker, D. R., A model for estimating the completion of rest for "Red-haven" and "Elberta" peach trees. *Hortic. Sci.* 1974, 9, 331–332.

Rosenzweig, C., Casassa, G., Karoly, D. J., Imeson, A., Liu, C., Menzel, A., Rawlins, S., Root, T. L., Seguin, B., Tryjanowski, P., Hanson, C. E., *Assessment of observed changes and responses in natural and managed systems*. In: *Climate Change 2007: Impacts, Adaptation and Vulnerability. Contribution of Working Group II to the Fourth Assessment Report of the Intergovernmental Panel on Climate Change*. Parry, M. L., Canziani, O. F., Palutikof, J. P., van der Linden PJ Eds. Cambridge University Press, Cambridge, United Kingdom and NY, USA, 2007, 79–131.

Rogers, C. A., Wayne, P. M., Macklin, E. A., Muilenber, M. L., Wagner, C. J., Epstein, P. R., Bazzaz, F. A., Interaction of the onset of spring and elevated atmospheric CO_2 on ragweed (*Ambrosia artemisiifolia* L.) pollen production. *Environ Health Perspect* 2006, 114, 865–869.

Ruml, M., Vuliæ, T., Importance of phenological observations and predictions in agriculture. *Journal of Agricultural Sciences* 2005, 50(2), 217–225.

Schäppi, G., Taylor, P., Kenrick, J., Staff, I., Suphioglu, C., Predicting the grass pollen count from meteorological data with regard to estimating the severity of hayfever symptoms in Melbourne (Australia) *Aerobiologia*, 1998, 14, 29–37.

Scheifinger, H., Belmonte, J., Celenk, S., Damialis, A., Dechamp, C., Garcia-Mozo, H., Gehrig, R., Grewling, L., Halley, J. M., Hogda, K. A., Jäger, S., Karatzas, K., Karlsen, S. R., Koch, E., Pauling, A., Peel, R., Sikoparija, B., Smith, M., Galán-Soldevilla, C., Thibaudon, M., Vokou, D., de Weger, L., Monitoring, modeling and forecasting of the pollen season. In: *Allergenic Pollen: a review of the Production, Release, Distribution and Health Impact*. Sofiev, M., Bergmann, K., Eds. Springer, Netherland, 2013.

Schwartz, M. D., Ed. *Phenology: An Integrative Environmental Science*, second Edition. Springer, Netherland, 2013.

Sinclair, T. R., Kitani, S., Hinson, K., Bruniard, J., Horie, T., Soybean flowering date: linear and logistic models based on temperature and phoperiod. *Crop Sci.* 1991, 31, 786–790.

Skjoth, C. A. *Meteorological aspects of pollen dispersal*. Manual for Aerobiology. 12th European Course on Basic Aerobiology. Wydawnictwo Uniwersytetu Rzeszowskiego. Rzeszòw, Poland, 2015.

Skjoth, C. A., Sikoparija, B., Jäger, S., EAN-Network. *Pollen Sources*. In *Allergenic Pollen: a review of the Production, Release, Distribution and Health Impact*. Sofiev, M., and Bergmann K Eds. Springer, Netherland, 2013.

Skjoth, C. A., Geels, C., Hvidberg, M., Ole, H., Brandt, J., Frohn, L. M., Hedegaard, G. B., Christensen, J. H., Moseholm, L., An inventory of tree species in Europe-An essential data input for air pollution modeling. *Ecological Modeling* 2008, 217, 292–304.

Smith, M., Emberli, J., Stach, A., Rantio-Lehtimäki, A., Caulton, E., Thibaudon, M., Sindt, C., Jäger, S., Gehrig, R., Frenguelli, G., Jato, V., Rodríguez Rajo, F. J., Alcázar, P., Galán, C., Influence of the North Atlantic Oscillation on grass pollen counts in Europe. *Aerobiologia* 2009, 25, 321–332.

Sukopp, H., Wurzel, A., The effects of Climate Change on the vegetation of Central European cities. *Urban Habitats* 2003.

Taiz, L., Zeiger, E., *Plant Physiology*. Sinauer Ass., Inc., Sunderland, USA, 1998.

Tedeschini, E., Rodriguez-Rajo, F. J., Caramiello, R., Jato, V., Frenguelli, G., The influence of climatic changes in *Platanus* spp. pollination in Spain and Italy. *Grana* 2006, 45(3), 222–229.

Tormo-Molina, R., Muñoz Rodríguez, A., Silva Palacios, I., Gallardo López, F., Pollen production in anemophilous trees. *Grana* 1996, 20, 38–46.

Tutin, T. G., *Flora Europaea*. Cambridge University Press, 1964–1980.

Turner, K. G., Fréville, H., Rieseberg, L. H., Adaptive plasticity and niche expansion in an invasive thistle. *Ecology and Evolution* 2015, 5, 3183–3197.

Ugolotti, M., Pasquarella, C., Vitali, P., Smith, M., Albertini, R., Characteristics and trends of selected pollen seasons recorded in Parma (Northern Italy) from 1994 to 2011; *Aerobiologia*, 2015, 1–12, doi: 10.1007/s10453-015-9368-4.

Walter, J., Essl, F., Englisch, T., Kiehn, M., *Neophytes in Austria*. In: *Biological Invasions: From Ecology to Control*. Nentwig, E., et al. Eds. *Neobiota* 2005, 6, 13–25.

Weber, E., The dynamics of plant invasions: a case study of three exotic goldenrod species (*Solidago* L.) in Europe. *Journal of Biogeography* 1998, 25, 147–154.

Weber, E., Schmid, B., Latitudinal population differentiation in two species of Solidago (Asteraceae) introduced into Europe. *American Journal of Botany* 1998, 85, 1110–1121.

Whitney, K. D., Gabler, C. A., Rapid evolution in introduced species, invasive traits, and recipient communities: challenges for predicting invasive potential. *Diversity and Distributions* 2008, 14, 569–580.

Wolfe, L. M., Why alien invaders succeed: support for the escape-from-enemy hypothesis. *American Naturalist*, 2002, 160, 705–711.

Yan, W. K., Wallace, D. H., Simulation and prediction of plant phenology for five crops based on photoperiod x temperature interaction. *Annals of Botany* 1998, 81, 705–716.

Ziello, C., Sparks, T. H., Estrella, N., Belmonte, J., Bergmann, K. C., Bucher, E., Brighetti, M. A., Damialis, A., Detandt, M., Galán, C., Gehrig, R., Grewling, L., Bustillo, A. M. G., Hallsdottir, M., Kockhans-Bieda, M. C., De Linares, C., Myszkowska, D., Pàldy, A., Sánchez, A., Smith, M., Thibaudon, M., Travaglini, A., Uruska, A., Valencia-Barrera, R. M., Vokou, D., Wachter, R., de Weger, L. A., Menze, A., Changes to Airborne Pollen Counts across Europe. PlosOne 2012, 7, 1–8.

Ziska, L. H., Caulfield, F. A., Rising CO_2 and pollen production of common ragweed (*Ambrosia artemisiifolia*), a known allergy-inducing species: implications for public health. *Aust J Plant Physiol*, 2000, 27, 893–898.

Ziska, L. H., Gebhard, D. E., Frenz, D. A., Faulkner, S., Singer, B. D., Straka, J. G., Cities as harbingers of climate change: common ragweed, urbanization, and public health. *Journal of Allergy and Clinical Immunology* 2003, 111, 290–295.

CHAPTER 6

INDOOR POLLUTANTS WITH SPECIAL REFERENCE TO HEALTH AND HYGIENE

RAJIV R. SAHAY and ALAN L. WOZNIAK

Environmental Diagnostics Laboratory at Pure Air Control Services, Inc. 4911-C Creekside Drive Clearwater, FL, 33760, USA

CONTENTS

ABSTRACT

Understanding indoor pollution has become more important and challenging in recent years. The associated risks of pollutants pose a serious challenge on health, wealth, and hygiene. The quality of indoor environments is defiled considerably in absence of proper management of contaminants that adversely impact the living space. In this chapter, relevant information on evaluating indoor pollutants is provided for improving the quality of indoor environments. The suggested, straightforward practices not only minimize the risk associated with health and hygiene of inhabitance, but insure increasing comfort and productivity. A numerical reference for the indoor environment assessment has been compiled by pooling findings with common a-biogenic and biogenic pollutants of indoor environments along with some important, influential parameters such as temperature, relative humidity, and others. We have reported 439 types of bacteria, 353 forms of fungi, and 91 categories of pollen grains besides other contaminants/allergens from indoor environments after examining and/or appraising 248,500 specimens obtained from 60,000 environmental samples.

6.1 INTRODUCTION

Pollution is generally understood as any adverse change in the natural environment that impacts ecological cycles. However, when the term pollution is used, things like automobile exhaust, smoke, obnoxious gases, bad odors/smells, excessive noise, nuisance dusts, etc. come to mind and are some commonly associated examples of outdoor pollution. Contrary to outdoor environments, indoor environments also deal with pollutants, which are real and more dangerous, especially from a health and hygiene point of view. Due to confined/defined spaces, indoor pollutants are generally more concentrated and many fold higher than that of outdoor pollutants. Poorly ventilated, dark, hot and humid conditions allow these pollutants to thrive rapidly. Indoor pollutants that have a biological origin are termed as biogenic (bio-pollutants) and those without a biogenic source are referred to as a-biogenic (physical, chemical and environmental pollutants; or PCEP). Some common examples of bio-pollutants include, but are not limited to, viruses, mycoplasma, protozoa, fungi, pollen grains, insects/their particulates, dust mites, animal hair/dander, plant fibers/trichomes, and other plant or animal particulates along with other organic entities. Volatile organic compounds, suspended particulate matters, fibers (such as fiberglass, asbestos, etc.), metals, rust particulates, obnoxious and toxic gases are excellent examples of a-biogenic pollutants in the indoor environment. Substances like mycotoxins, endotoxins, and other microbiological volatile compounds (MVOC) are biological in origin, but they may be active by themselves or in association with their source. Both a-biogenic as well as biogenic pollutants may be capable of influencing the natural habitat and throwing it off balance. The quality of indoor environments is directly proportional to the existing pollutants in that specific surrounding area. It has been observed that environmental pollutants are associated with three matrices: air, surface, and liquid. Therefore, transmission of these pollutants in indoor environments is mainly carried out by a number of sources that come in contact with contaminated air, surface and liquid/water. Dispersal of indoor pollution is a complex phenomenon and depends on various factors such as the prevailing environmental conditions, besides physical, chemical and biological factors. Although dispersal of these pollutants in indoor environments is mainly carried out due to aerosolization, surface infestation, and liquid/water contamination, the activities of occupants may also be listed as a contributing factor for spreading these nuisance particulates.

The impact of pollutants within closed structures is on the rise. It adversely affects both health and hygiene. According to the World Health Organization (Gobal Health Observatory data, 2012), 4.3 million people a year die from exposure to household air pollution. People start noticing health based symptoms either immediately or after several hours of exposure to these pollutants. Allergies, asthma and other ailments are common amongst the elderly, infant, children and other immune-compromised individuals due to indoor pollutants. Hypersensitivity, headache, fatigue, shortness of breath, sinus congestion, coughing, sneezing, dizziness, nausea, and other nonspecific symptoms may be common due to extraneous adulteration of indoor environments.

Building related symptoms (BRS), Building Related Illness (BRI), Mold Associated Conditions (MAC), Dirty Duct Syndromes (DDS) and other issues may adversely impact the economy and well-being of occupants. Understanding the factors responsible for influencing the above mentioned conditions within closed structures are very complex (Gregory, 1973; Burge, 1996). These factors may be physical, chemical, biological or environmental in nature (Mandrioli et al., 1998). The lack of information on the above factors is often an obstacle in addressing BRS (Baker, 1989). There is no universally accepted indoor environmental reference index/guideline to evaluate indoor air/environments for pollutant load. Increasing evidence suggests that specific risk factors need to be established in order to respond to an indoor environmental concern (Macher et al., 1999) that occurs due to indoor pollutants. The lack of a universal protocol, uncertainty about what to measure, and how to measure the factors responsible for indoor environment related issues makes it very difficult and poses a serious challenge in evaluating the indoor air/environments for abnormalities (Flanning et al., 2001; NIOSH, 2005).

In order to successfully manage the issues associated with the above challenges, it is essential to have a scientifically established reference guideline. Limited information and criterion exist for evaluating common indoor contaminants including, but not limited to, bacteria, mold, pollen grains, insect bio-detritus, several other biogenic and a-biogenic entities, and physical factors such as humidity, temperature, water availability, light, etc. (Sahay and Wozniak, 2005; Spicer and Gangoff, 2005; Sahay et al., 2008). These constituents may influence our day-to-day life in terms of health and hygiene. To minimize risks associated with common indoor pollutants, one should accurately monitor and measure both biogenic and a-biogenic constituents and associated factors to determine healthy living conditions.

Some potential sources of indoor pollution are dampness, poor housekeeping, ventilation, nature, types of occupants, and other building characteristics (Heseltine and Rosen, 2009). When a definite source-cause is not established, identification, classification, and quantification of constituents are necessary in combating the issues associated with poor environmental quality in and around a closed, manmade structure. In this chapter, some important parameters are discussed in order to develop a numerical reference guideline as a standard for indoor air/environment quality for assessing pollution and pollutants.

6.2 COMMON INDOOR POLLUTANTS

The indoor environment retains a variety of pollutants. They are released from several macro and micro sources. Their presence in and around indoor environments depends upon the intermittence and diversity of their originating body. The main reason for pollutant accumulation within a closed environment is building conditions, their utilization, inhabitant's activities, adequacy of ventilation, appropriateness of comfort factors and other phenomena directly or indirectly impacting its surroundings.

6.2.1 *COMBUSTION*

The combustion of fossil fuels and other organic material in and around manmade structure are among important sources for emitting indoor pollutants in the solid, liquid and gaseous phases. Suspended particulate matter, carbon monoxide, nitrogen oxides, sulfur oxides, polynuclear aromatic hydrocarbons (PAH), other obnoxious gases and contaminants of various physiochemical properties are among the main products as a result. Some of these pollutants are persistent, bio-accumulative, and toxic (PBT).

6.2.2 *SMOKE*

Smoke is considered to be one of the most dangerous agents of indoor pollutants. It contains a cocktail of various pollutants. Soot from incomplete combustion, particulate matters, carbon monoxides, light hydrocarbons, volatile organic compounds (VOC), PAH, Polychlorinated biphenyls (PCB), and heavy metals (Pb, Hg, etc.) are identified as important ingredients in its makeup. Environmental tobacco smoke itself is considered the most toxic indoor pollutant. Tobacco burning itself emits over 4,000 chemicals both as vapors and particles. A comprehensive study on open burning, stove cooking, fireplace use in indoor environments, tobacco smoking, industrial smoke plumes and other likewise sources are essential for appropriately addressing it.

6.2.3 *VOLATILE OR MICROBIOLOGICAL VOLATILE ORGANIC COMPOUNDS*

VOC and MVO are groups of chemical compounds that originate from a variety of organic chemicals that are widely used as ingredients in household products or released by microorganisms. It is believed that the concentration of these compounds is 2 to 5 times higher inside homes than outside, irrespective of their location, rural or industrial. Groups of chemicals such as various alcohols, aldehydes, ketones, terrenes, esters, aromatic compounds, amines, and other sulfur containing substances may also occur as VOC/MVOC in indoor environments. Presence of these compounds in the indoor environment could lead in determining its toxicity. They can also be utilized as marker or fingerprint to determine the location of source.

6.2.4 RESPIRABLE PARTICULATES

Particles that are generally 10 microns or less are categorized as respirable particles. It represents a wide spectrum of both chemical and physical contaminants of indoor environments. These particles are suspended in the ambient environment for a longer duration of time and can be dispersed over a wide area/distance. The sizes of these particulates are vital in determining the health implications. When referring to solids and liquids that are 2.5–10 microns in size, the term coarse particles are used; anything under 2.5 microns are said to be fine particles. They mostly originate due to ambient pollution. Chemical reactions such as internal combustion of fossil fuels, forest burning, etc. and physical phenomena such as phase change (evaporation of saltwater, etc.) are believed to be primary sources of their production. Ventilation, infiltration, and occupant traffic are identified as main activities for the introduction of respirable particles from dust, construction activities, printing, photocopying, manufacturing processes, smoking, etc. To ensure good indoor environments, the source of these pollutants must be identified and controlled.

6.2.5 BIOAEROSOLS

Aerosols of biological origin or emitted/derived by living organisms are commonly known as "Bioaerosols." They may originate from many micro and macro creatures. Viruses, mycoplasma, bacteria, fungi/mold spores, pollen grains, etc. are some common biopollutants reported from indoor environments. Constituents originating from living sources have a variety of classifications, such as allergens (protein of various animal and plants), bacterial toxin (exo and endotoxins), fungal toxins (mycotoxins), and others are often found in indoor environments. An assessment of bioaerosols is indicative of a possible scenario of health and hygiene in and around indoor environments in most cases. Bioaerosols survive in both outdoor and indoor environments and are influenced by a number of factors including existing environmental conditions. Biological agents may enter the indoors from outside sources by people, pets/animal, insects, infiltration or propagate inside due to use of contaminated products. Places such as water intrusion, wet insulation, carpet, wooden flooring, drywall/ gypsum board, ceiling tile, wall covering, furniture, stagnant water in air conditioner, dehumidifiers, humidifiers, air handler unit coil, drip pans for water collection, cooling towers, etc. are vulnerable and likely to remain an important area for isolation and enumeration of bioaerosols and associated materials in indoor sites.

6.2.6 PLANT AND ANIMAL BORNE MATERIALS

Recent trends gained considerable interest in identifying materials that are not true bioaerosols, but originated from plants or animals. Cockroaches; dust mites; other insects; plant trichomes; hair and dander from humans, cats, dogs and others; cysts, droplets and spores of various animals and plants; and bits of plants, insects and animals have been identified from livable spaces. These materials may play a significant role as indoor biopollutants. Linking these entities as pollutants may provide a solution-orientated management for a variety of health and hygiene related problems of the indoor environment. Nuisance dusts, carpets, upholsteries, and furnishings are reservoirs of these important particles. They may persist and preserve themselves over a shortened or prolonged time.

6.2.7 ENVIRONMENTAL CONDITIONS

Surrounding and ambient environmental conditions act as indoor pollution. Global climate change is a disturbing weather pattern, which leads to designing tight buildings for various needs beside energy conservation. It has often been observed that additional thermal insulation and decreased ventilation leads to temperatures being too hot or too cool and a humidity level that is too high or low. Light, brightness, glare, and dampness are also significant contributors as indoor pollutants. Pressurization and/or a breach in building envelops are also an indicator of influential environmental conditions. Ventilation through air conveyance system in energy tight buildings often impact their environmental conditions.

6.2.8 NOISE AND VIBRATION

Noise and vibration are also identified as important indoor pollutants that can have an adverse impact on occupants. It has been observed that low frequency noises ranging from 20–100 hertz (Hz) is problematic in indoor environments. The Occupational Safety and Health Administration set a guideline at 90 decibels (dB) for industrial setups. Similarly, vibrations have a relationship with that of health. A causative link is observed with a resonance frequency of 1–20 Hz. A significant correlation may be notice between vibrations with irritability and dizziness specially in office workers.

6.2.9 ELECTROMAGNETIC RADIATION

This category of pollutants is a dangerous and silent killer. A number of equipment and technologies have become an integral part of both offices and residences that require high power charges. Computers, cell phones, microwaves, televisions, ultraviolet lights, and others contain radioactive materials that can be hazardous. They can release alpha, beta, and gamma radiation, which could potentially distribute into the surrounding environment. Some of these electromagnetic radiations are capable of ionization in materials and biological damage to human tissue.

6.2.10 OTHER CHEMICALS AND GASEOUS CONTAMINANTS

Asbestos, paints, plastics, pesticides, perfumes, fuels for cooking & heating, adhesive glue, lead, detergents, caustics, cleaners, acids, greenhouse gases, rotten fruits & vegetables, unpreserved foods, soil gas radon, carbon monoxides, sulfur oxides (SO_x), nitrous oxides (NO_x) and other inorganic and organic gases are identified as difficult-to-identify sources of indoor pollutants. Limited information is available regarding their nature and concentration for reasonably linking it with health and hygiene effects.

6.3 HEALTH AND HYGIENE

Indoor air pollutants may exert their effects on health and hygiene. Development and multiplication of microbes along with other physical, chemical and environmental factors are often identified as the main concern of public health. Considering the variety of microorganisms, and their possible synergistic effects with other factors, the most endangered populations are children, women, and the elderly (who spend a relatively substantial amount of time indoors). In absence of evidence-based assessments, the scope of proper management regarding a healthy indoor environment may be inadequate. Therefore, a potential connection and quality of evidence is extremely valuable. They may vary widely, but are considered helpful nonetheless, in ascertaining risk factors, exposure of pollutants, etc. in establishing a proper reason for explaining health implications arise due to such elements. It is essential to have a proper understanding of indoor contaminants to reduce the potential issues leading to health and hygiene related to the occupants. Some common human health effects due to indoor bio-contaminants are presented in Table 6.1.

This section describes a general understanding on type of sickness or other aliments associated with indoor pollutants.

6.3.1 ALLERGY AND ASTHMA

Allergy due to indoor pollution is referred to as a hypersensitivity of the immune system in response to conditions or substances in and around closed environments. Increasing evidence illustrates that some of the above-described indoor pollutants are associated with allergy and asthma. It has been observed that allergies and asthma due to indoor pollutants are increased worldwide over the latter part of 20th century (Asher et al., 2006;

TABLE 6.1 Summarizes the Major Indoor Pollutants, Health Effects and Sources

Origin	Spawn	Health Effects	Indoor Source
Algae	Organisms	Asthma Rhinitis	Outdoor air, Water
Bacteria	Organisms Spores Endotoxin Exotoxin	Diseases Infection Fever Septic Pneumonia	Stagnant water Damp surfaces HVAC condensations Decomposition Contaminated food or water
Chemicals	Heavy Metals Corrosives Combustion products Consumer items Pesticides Tobacco smoke Soil gas MVO'C VOC'S	Irritations Fatigue Rashes Rhinitis Infection Cancer Dermatitis Symptom complexes	Building materials Dust and debris Paints Cooking and Breaking Decomposition Infiltration Water/Liquids Effluents Soil under building
Fungi	Organisms Molds/Spores Mycotoxin MVOC'S	Allergy Asthma Diseases Dermatitis Infection Pneumonitis	Stagnant water Damp surfaces HVAC condensations Decomposition Contaminated food or water Outdoor air
Insect	Particulates Feces	Asthma Rhinitis	House dust
Mammals	Dander Saliva	Asthma Rhinitis	Pets
Plants	Pollen grains Trichomes	Allergy Asthma Rhinitis	Outdoor air Indoor plants
Protozoa	Organisms Antigen	Infection Pneumonitis	Stagnant water Contaminated food or water
Viruses	Organisms Virion	Infections Diseases	Humans

WHO, 2008). A number of pollutants may be allergenic in nature to those who are susceptible, especially young and old individuals.

Indoor contaminants may cause short and long-term hypersensitive reactions (allergies). Hypersensitive reactions are exaggerated immune responses resulting in tissue inflammation or damage. Such responses are categorized based on the timing of the reaction as well as the nature of the immune components involved. The most common allergenic responses caused by indoor pollutants include Type I, Type III, and Type IV hypersensitivities. Type I hypersensitivities involve an immediate, but localized response to allergens such as fungi, pollen, dust mites, or animal dander. Common symptoms of a Type I response include itchy or watery eyes, runny nose, sinusitis, coughing or sneezing, congestion, chest tightness, and shortness of breath. Type III hypersensitivities involve delayed responses (usually within hours or days) caused by the formation of insoluble antigen-antibody complexes. Symptoms of Type III hypersensitivities may include fatigue, muscle and joint pain, respiratory disorders, chest pressure, and general flu-like symptoms. Type IV hypersensitivity, as with the Type III, represents a 'delayed' reaction. Delayed hypersensitive reactions are wholly or partly responsible for extrinsic allergic alveolit is and contact dermatitis—a common skin disorder.

6.3.2 INFECTIONS

Infection is generally referred to as a compromised state when deleterious, microbial entities erupt and proliferate within a host. Amongst indoor constituents, various microbiota have been observed as a potential source of infection. Exposure (usually through inhalation and contact) of pathogenic organisms may be capable of eliciting infection in a host. Infectious agents are perpetually found in indoor environments. Viruses, mycoplasmas, bacteria, fungi, protozoa, etc. are important etiological agents of biological origin associated with infection. Strains of *Norovirus*, influenza virus, methicillin-resistant *Staphylococcus aureus* (MRSA), *Legionella, Aspergillus, Giardia* and others are identified as common causes of infection. Hepatitis, gastroenteritis (the dreaded stomach bug), influenza, MRSA, tuberculosis, legionnaires, pontiac fever, and giardiasis are consequences of infection caused by these biogenic agents.

6.3.3 DISEASE

A marked disorder with specific signs and symptoms resulting in impaired or aberrant behavior is defined as disease. Typical indoor pollutants, irrespective of their origin, may elicit disease in individuals or populations. There is a wide range of natural and manmade elements around us identified as disease causing agents. Epidemiological, clinical, and toxicological evidence suggests that these agents may be related to numerous diseases and health conditions. Depending on duration and nature of exposure, these constituents may produce specific or non-specific symptoms.

In 2000, indoor air pollution was responsible for more than 1.5 million deaths and 2.7% of the global burden of disease (WHO/SDE/PHE/07.01rev). It is often difficult to determine which pollutants are the causes of a particular disease or symptoms, even if indoor pollution is the problem. The disease due to indoor pollutants usually target respiratory, pulmonary, dermal, nervous, and circulatory system. Disease symptoms may appear soon after the exposure of indoor pollutants, but it may also be delayed and can take up to weeks, months, or even years to develop. Exposure to household pollution may cause pneumonia, especially amongst children, elderly, and those with compromised immune systems. Particulate matter inhaled from indoor air pollution as a result of household solid fuels burning (WHO, 2014) in households are listed as a significant disease-causing element. Chronic exposure to household air pollution caused by cooking with solid fuels leads to stroke that can be fatal. Ischemic heart disease can be attributed to the exposure of household air pollution. Exposure to household air pollution has been reported as a factor for chronic obstructive pulmonary disease. Lung and other cancers may also develop up on the exposure of indoor pollutants. Particulate matter and other pollutants of indoor environments may cause some chronic and communicable diseases impacting proper functioning of body organs, impairing immune response, and reducing the oxygen-carrying capacity of the blood.

6.3.4 OTHER SICKNESSES

Health effects due to indoor pollutants other than what has been described above collectively may be termed as a symptom complex. These sicknesses are often difficult to predict and may depend on several important variables such as the duration and frequency of exposure, concurrent exposures to other sources (e.g., outdoor), and the type of agents involved, the physiological condition of the agent besides the sensitivity of the exposed individual. Symptoms like mucosal irritation in eyes and upper airways, pulmonary issues, upshot nervous system, tiredness, fever and chills, pnuemonitis, coughing, lethargy, arthralgic and myalgia, lung infection, weight loss, etc., are some common complaints by occupants due to indoor pollutants. Cardiovascular concerns due to extraneous constituents of indoor environments are predicted as important risks to humans. Furthermore, exposures to antigens and irritants of indoor particulates such as proteins, organic dust, low molecular weight chemicals, fungal glucans, mycotoxins, and other secondary metabolites may have complex results with unknown etiological mechanisms.

Examples of suspected mold-related effects include cough, congestion, wheezing, chest tightness, runny nose, headaches, flu-like symptoms, muscle and joint pain, fatigue, dizziness, nosebleeds, eye irritations, confusion, memory loss, and anxiety. Non-biological pollutants such as nuisance dusts, ozone, oxides of carbon, nitrogen, sulfur, and a host of other chemicals have been reported as toxic substances from indoor environments and are capable of initiating health related issues in occupants. Cutaneous and respiratory manifestations are some common indicators of ambient particulate matter's detrimental abilities.

6.3.5 MULTIPLE CHEMICAL SENSITIVITY

Adverse medical conditions with a variety of non-specific symptoms as a result of possible exposure to chemical, biological, or physical agents is commonly known as "Multiple Chemical Sensitivity (MCS)." Headache, fatigue, dizziness, nausea, congestion, itching, sneezing, sore throat, chest pain, changes in heart rhythm, breathing problems, muscle pain or stiffness, skin rash, diarrhea, bloating, gas, confusion, trouble concentrating, memory problems, and mood changes are commonly reported symptoms of MCS. Scented products, pesticides, synthetic fabrics, smoke, petroleum products, paints, leads, metals, gases, and other abrasive materials have been suspected as possible causes of the symptoms. Some of these compounds may act via multiple mechanisms and may be responsible for more than one type of symptom. Additionally, inhalation of certain things as described above may produce symptoms of disease that mimic immunological syndromes, but are not immunologically mediated. Chemicals such as formaldehyde produce a pseudoallergic reaction that resembles immediate hypersensitivity, although a demonstrable antibody is not detectable. Irritation of mucosal surfaces may stimulate protective responses (e.g., sneezing, coughing, and tearing) that appear superficially to be immunological in nature, but are related to the stimulation of epithelial irritant receptors by chemicals. The mechanism of MCS is a complex phenomenon and believed to be a complex mixture of both medical and psychological signs. It may occur due to a short exposure to extremely high concentrations of suspected chemicals or a long exposure to relatively low levels of similar chemicals.

6.3.6 BUILDING DISORDERS

Sick Building Syndrome (SBS), Building Related Illness (BRI), Organic Dust Toxic Syndrome (ODTS), Dirty Sock Syndrome (DSS) and Mold Linked Illness (MLI) are listed as some important heterogeneous groups of disorders that may link to indoor pollutants. Non-specific symptoms such as eye, nose, throat irritation, headache, fatigue, or other discomfort that cannot be associated with an identifiable cause, but appear to be linked to time spent in a building are generally known as SBS. BRI refers to the diagnosable illness accompanied by documentable physical signs and laboratory findings that are associated with an exposure of indoor pollutants, e.g. infectious diseases, hypersensitivity diseases, and inhalation fevers. When symptoms are poorly characterized following the exposure of high organic dust levels such as humidifier fever, short-lived, febrile reaction, etc. are often categorized as ODTS. DSS often associated with HVAC. It is called as DSS due to its typical smell like dirty socks emanates from HVAC ducts. Although the exact cause for this condition is not yet established but it is highly anticipated that it occurs due to bacterial and other chemical infestation in HVAC. It is worth mentioning that this problem is unique to very hot and very humid conditions. Many illnesses are believed to be caused by mold without any objective evidence of disease and pathogenicity of the involved fungus/fungal product classified as MLI. This term is widely used for legal ramifications and has limited importance in environmental diagnostics.

6.4 ASSESSMENT OF INDOOR POLLUTANTS

Assessment of pollution and pollutants within indoor environments is a highly complex phenomenon; however, there are steps that may be easily initiated. These may include initial walkthroughs, background evaluations, field diagnostics, heating ventilation and air conditioning systems (HVAC), environmental sample laboratory evaluations, pollutant pathways, source-cause determinations, and action plans.

6.4.1 INITIAL WALKTHROUGH

A walkthrough is an important step for an initial investigation of indoor pollution and pollutants. A common sense approach includes utilizing looking, smelling, and hearing to distinguish normal vs. abnormal. The area inspected is evaluated for general cleanliness (or lack thereof). Inspection of a building can be comprised of the living area, utility, storage, etc. for proper ventilation, adequacy of light, nature of storage, signs of water intrusion, material used in the building, roofing, flooring (carpet, wood, solid, etc.), building utilization (residential/commercial), and other overall conditions. It is important to examine the location of fresh air intake and exhausts. A survey of the fresh air intake is vital in determining the potential sources of pollutants in the surrounding area. The building contour and outer landscape of the primary structure must be observed in order to determine the slope of the building. This helps determine the direction of water flow under natural conditions. It is important to take note on the building location, especially if it is located near a swampland, landfill, dumpster, etc. A building's functionality greatly depends on its ventilation system, whether it be mechanical or natural, and is essential in order to determine the prevailing pollutants within a building. All information should be taken into consideration on determining the overall building maintenance. It is a good idea to collect information on large renovation projects as their additions can have an impact on an existing indoor environment. Interviews are conducted with occupants in order to find potential help with determining a complaint versus a non-complaint area. This information must be documented and a record prepared for further evaluation (*Appendix I*).

6.4.2 BACKGROUND EVALUATION

Evaluating the existing conditions and functionalities of an occupiable space is an important and integral part to developing a hypothesis to discuss pollution/pollutant measurements. This important step enables an evaluator to understand aspects of indoor pollution and their impact on the surrounding environments. It is helpful in designing an overall critical path management (CPM) to address specifics on agents responsible for indoor pollution. A twofold approach is encouraged for a proper correlation between problems and solutions. Information on building architecture, materials, age, ventilation, function, uses, and surrounding environment are important for understanding the factors important for pollutants and pollution of indoor places. The second valuable element is the occupant habit, behaviors, and other practices that include physiochemical, biological, and environmental activities around them. An interpretation process for understanding a scenario can be initiated by observing the preexisting data as well as records obtained as a result of a walkthrough. Attempts should be made to emphasize and identify the causal factors responsible for influencing the overall health and hygiene conditions within surroundings. An environment impact assessment and energy audit is helpful in assessing the nature and extent of the pollution along with the pollutants. Table 6.2 can be cited as a good example for a background evaluation of indoor pollutants.

6.4.3 FIELD DIAGNOSTICS

Field diagnostics is a unique tool to scientifically validate the hypothesis that signifies the nature of pollution and pollutants. The main focus and idea of field diagnostics is to narrow down target and influential factors responsible for initiating pollution. It may involve an evidence-based

TABLE 6.2 Example Evaluating Buildings for Indoor Pollution and Pollutants

Parameter	Observation	Interpretation	Outcome	Action
Building Structure	–	–	–	–
Building Utilization	–	–	–	–
Comfort	–	–	–	–
Ecology	–	–	–	–
Energy	–	–	–	–
Health	–	–	–	–
Hygiene	–	–	–	–
Inhabitants	–	–	–	–
Water Supply	–	–	–	–

assessment for indoor pollution and its causal factors. Many times, the elimination of obvious approaches is adapted to narrow-down or identify the causal source to address the situation appropriately. Field diagnostics can be undertaken by studying real time data and collecting environmental samples for laboratory analysis for establishing quality of the components that may be responsible for indoor environmental pollution and its impacts. Some common approaches to initiate field diagnostics is to collect and record vital data/observation such as real time readings on temperature, humidity, water intrusion, flooding, lighting, sounds, pressurization, total particulate counts, volatile organic compounds, obnoxious gases, chemicals/compounds, flora and fauna, degradation, occupant activities, exposure, and other similar activities. This information helps an evaluator determine the type and portion of environmental samples required for laboratory analysis to appropriately respond to issues of concern.

A number of methods and techniques are available for collecting and isolating environmental samples for air, surface and liquid/water. Generally, grab and composite sampling methods are adapted to collect environmental samples. Grab samples are a discrete sample, which is collected at a specific location at a certain point of time; however, composite samples are made by thoroughly mixing several grab samples.

Each type of sample has its advantages and limitations. If the environmental medium varies spatially or temporally, then a single grab sample is not representative and more samples need to be collected. Composite samples may be used to reduce the analytical cost by reducing the number of samples. Some common and frequently used practices for collecting the above samples are listed in the following subsections.

6.4.3.1 A-Biogenic

A-biogenic samples are collected to understand the extent and types of physiochemical pollutants perpetuated in the ambient environment. Proper and adequate sample collection is the key element for meaningful analytical results. It is highly encouraged that sample collection must be undertaken as per the protocol or recommendation specified by a testing laboratory. Collected samples can be analyzed by utilizing a number of techniques such as spectrometry/spectroscopy, chromatography, flame ionization detector, other analytical procedures such as electrochemical, X-ray diffraction, gravimetric, microscopy, etc. depending on the requirements and needs.

6.4.3.1.1 Air

Air samples are an important module for determining the nature and extent of contaminants that may be responsible for indoor pollution. There are three common methods that can be used for collecting environmental air sample. A sample for ambient air in the gas phase is collected in a container (summa container, bags, etc.); actively passing air through a sorbent tube, filter or solution by using a sampling pump; and a passive sample by exposing a sorbent or other relevant media in the air by utilizing aseptic techniques.

6.4.3.1.2 Surface

Surface samples are vital in order to evaluate the content and deposition of indoor pollutants for monitoring indoor environments. Bulk, swab, wipe samples are collected by using aseptic technique from environments for testing various pollutants/surficial contaminants. The obtained result helps evaluators in understanding the nature and extent of abiological pollutants around specified sites from where samples were collected.

6.4.3.1.3 Liquid/Water

Collecting liquid/water samples from indoor environment is challenging. It really depends on the need of target analytes. Small or large volume of liquid/water samples are collected by using aseptic techniques. It is highly encourage to collect the water specimen in glass, stainless steel or Teflon coated containers/test tubes due to the inert nature of these materials. In indoor environments water samples may be collected from potable and no-potable sources. This includes ground water, precipitation, wastewater, flooding water, condensation, etc.

6.4.3.2 Biogenic

6.4.3.2.1 Air

Air samples are one of the important elements for studying the pollutants perpetuating in and around closed environments. The air sample for biological particulates is collected by utilizing active or passive mechanism. Impaction and impingements are the two active methods practice to collect air samples. Some popular mechanisms are described below for collecting biogenic samples from the ambient air.

Drum Trap (DT) – Airborne elements are collected on an adhesive tape mounted on a rotating disc powered by an electric motor in an air sealed drum with an orifice. The rotation of the disc is fixed with that of the exposure time. Hirst spore trap, Tilak air samplers, etc. are some common, commercially available samplers in this category. This is useful especially in collecting fungi/mold spores besides other particulates of biological significance.

Electrostatic Trap (ET) – Microbiological air samples (Fungal or mold spores/bacteria) are collected by drawing air with a constant flow rate and exposure time over media under the influence of an electrostatically charged environment. Charged particles are collected on their positively charged electrode. An Electrostatic Sampling Device (ESD), SASS® 3100, Portable Biohazard Sampler, etc. are good, commercially available samplers under this technique.

Filter Trap (FT) – Air samples are drawn on a filter mounted within a closed, airtight chamber by pulling the air through it with a constant airflow rate and exposure time. Micro-orifice uniform deposit impactor (MOUDI) filter made out of cellulose ester, polyvinyl chloride, and polycarbonate are widely used for mold/fungi sampling.

Impinger Trap (IP) – In this method, the sample is collected by dissipating the air into an airtight flask containing the media with a constant airflow rate and exposure time. Some common IP samplers include, but are not limited to, Greenberg-Smith impinger, AGI-30, etc.

Pore Trap (PT) – Air samples for microbiological (mold or fungal spores/bacteria) evaluations are collected by this sampler on media in an air-tight cylinder by collecting air through a perforated metal plate with a constant airflow rate and exposure time. Andersen, Burkard, Bio-culture, and Button Aerosol Samplers are routinely used based on this technique.

Rotorod Trap (RT) – The airborne fungal and other particulates are collected on a strip of sticky tape or surface mounted on a mechanical arm/surface attached to a spindle powered by an electric motor that can rotate with a specific number of rotations per minute for a determined exposure time. Rotorod samplers by Sampling Technology, Inc. are one of the most widely used samplers of this category.

Spore Trap (ST) – Air samples is collected on a gel-coated glass slip mounted inside an airtight chamber (cassette). A sample from air is pulled out with a constant airflow for a predetermined exposure time depending on the project goals. Flow rate is verified in the field utilizing an in-line flow meter. Air is passed over the coated slide causing airborne particles to adhere to the gel. Some commercially available devices of this category are Air-O-Cell, Micro 5, Allergenco-D, M2, Burkard volumetric samplers, etc.

Thermal Trap (TP) – The air samples are collected on a glass slip by placing it around a hot body into ambient air.

Gravity or Settle plates **(GP)** – In this method appropriate microbiological media (typically Malt Extract Agar for fungi and Typtic Soy Agar for bacteria) are opened and exposed for a given time for isolating the target microorganisms from ambient air. This is a passive mechanism for air sample collection.

Other than methods described above, modern technology such as laser or induce fluorescence is employed for real time detection and enumeration of microbial contaminants. The viable particles in air are isolated by a device equipped with this technology for immediate detection and enumeration of microbial contaminants. Commercially, the BioLaz® instrument from Particle Measuring Systems is available in market which is designed specifically for use in the pharmaceutical and medical products sectors. TSI's BioTrak® Real-Time Viable Particle Counter instrument uses similar Laser Induced Fluorescence (LSI) technology, but is also capable of simultaneous total and viable particle counts.

6.4.3.2.2 Surface

Environmental surface samples for evaluating biopollutants may be collected by bulk, surface imprint, swab, wipe, and HEPA vacuuming. These samples may be collected from a desired site by utilizing aseptic technique with proper protective equipments. Appropriate precautions must be taken to prevent cross-contamination. All the collected samples must be placed in an appropriate container before submitting to the laboratory. Except for a few exceptions, these samples can be transported to the laboratory in ambient conditions (avoid excess heat or cold). Collected samples should be transported to the laboratory as soon as possible. A portion of building materials such as carpeting, dust cakes on air filters, settled dust (e.g., rafter dusts), sheet rock, furniture, curtains, and other office equipment may be collected in a unused (preferably sterile) paper or visqueen bags as bulk sample. A tape imprint by using adhesive tape (Bio-Scan 400) can be collected to examine common bio-contaminants of the indoor surface. Surface samples are also collected by wiping or swabbing a selected surface area with a swab or wipe (dry or wet with moistened and absorptive medium) across a surface. Vacuum samples are taken by vacuuming selected areas by using HEPA vacuum cleaners. This method is often used for collecting surface samples from a relatively larger area.

6.4.3.2.3 Liquid/Water

Liquid/water samples may be collected from various sources located in and around indoor sites for verifying biopollutants. Points of use (faucets, shower heads, etc.), storage tanks, sources of condensation (HVAC, humidifiers, dehumidifiers, etc.), groundwater, precipitation (rain or snow), surface water (lakes, river, runoff, etc.), waste water (domestic, industrial process, runoff, etc.) are some good points of sample collection. Depending upon the project goals, an adequate volume of sample is collected by utilizing aseptic techniques. Liquid/water samples are collected by drawing the appropriate volume (10–1000 mL) in a sterile container. Pollutants are distributed in the aqueous phase and in the particles suspended in the water. Solids and liquids with densities less than water (such as oils and grease) tend to float on the surface, while those with a higher density sink to the bottom. The composition of stagnant water varies with the source, nature, and also with ambient temperatures. Therefore, samples should be collected by identifying the suspected site for recovery of potential bio-pollutants.

6.4.4 HEATING, VENTILATION AND AIR CONDITIONING SYSTEM (HAVC)

A hygiene assessment of the heating, venting and air-conditioning (HVAC) equipment is one of the key elements in field diagnostics. It is important for both energy conservation and indoor pollution, specifically in those cases where a facility is equipped with a mechanical air-conveyance system. It is believed that HVAC systems are responsible for 50 to 60% of building generated indoor air quality (IAQ) problems. At the same time, a proper maintenance and management is capable of resolving up to 80% of IAQ related issues.

6.4.4.1 Design

An appraisal of HVAC system designs is the first step for building health and hygiene evaluation. It has been observed often that a faulty and inappropriate system will not only contribute to add indoor pollutants, but also waste precious energy. It is highly encouraged that during the process of field diagnostics that close attention should be given to understanding the total heating and cooling load, conditions of ventilation and distribution systems, suitability of materials used (ductwork, coil, condenser, drain pans, etc.), filtration mechanisms, pressure relationships, accessibility of systems, and overall hygiene conditions such as visual observation for settle dusts, debris, bio-film, etc.

6.4.4.2 Operation

Information collection during the field diagnostics on the system operation is crucial. Data such as total time of equipment operation, temperature set points, airflow, and test and balance reports on system components & functionality are import to collect for a proper evaluation. A number of equipments are in service in HVAC operations. Although the basic technology is the same, the functioning of equipment may vary depending on design and uses. Also, there is a marked differentiation between residential and commercial/industrial units. The HVAC components like an air handler unit (AHU), fan, blower motor, air distribution, filtration, air diffusion, outside air supply, and condensation are examined for their proper function during heating or cooling cycle.

6.4.4.3 Maintenance

HVAC system maintenance plays a significant role not only in controlling indoor pollutants, but also in energy conservation. It is essential to understand the basic components of an HVAC system in order to observe the overall system maintenance. Typically, it includes outdoor air intake, mixed-air plenum and outdoor air control, heating and cooling coils, fan, blowing motor, air filter, and humidification and/or de-humidification equipment. An optimal performance of an HVAC is directly proportional to the maintenance of these components. Evaluators should collect the data on the maintenance as it provides great support and opportunity in indoor pollutant reduction and enhance air quality.

6.4.5 Environmental Sample Evaluation

There are a number of techniques and methods available for analyzing environmental samples No one technique fits in every scenario, but rather, it should be case specific. Collected samples can be examined and evaluated in various ways utilizing appropriate protocols and techniques to understand the nature and extent of indoor pollutants. Typically, collected samples for testing pollutants are processed by using non-culture or culture methods. Some important approaches to evaluate indoor pollutants of environments are described in Table 6.3.

6.4.6 POLLUTANT PATHWAYS

Understanding the source, release, dispersal, dissemination, and impaction of pollutants in indoor environments strengthens our ability to address proactive or reactive issues appropriately pertaining health and hygiene. These factors help to formalize a theory/hypothesis on the likelihood of contaminants in an occupiable space through accurate measurement and testing. The obtained data, in conjunction with an assessment of effects, not only forms the basis of risk characterization, but also provides critical information required to render decisions regarding regulatory initiatives, remediation, monitoring, and proper management of the indoor environment.

6.4.6.1 Source

Diversified ranges of manmade and natural sources around the indoor environments capable of emitting both a-biogenic and biogenic materials associated with indoor pollution. Building exterior, HVAC intake, heat

TABLE 6.3 Techniques for Analyzing Environmental Samples

Parameter	Matrix	Sample type	Analytical Technique
Allergens	Air and Surface	Spore trap, bulk, and surface	Microscopy, microbial culture
Bacteria	Air, Surface and Liquid	Culture plate impactor, bulk, surface and liquid	Microbial culture, biochemical, Immuno-chemical, molecular diagnostics
Fungi	Air, Surface and Liquid	Culture plate impactor, bulk, surface and liquid	Microscopic, microbial culture, biochemical, molecular diagnostics
House dust	Surface	Filtration, bulk and surface	Immunoassay
Humidity	Air, Surface	Air, Bulk and surface	Hygrometer, Infrared and Data logger
Metal Non-metals	Air, Surface and Liquid	Air trap, bulk, surface	X-ray diffraction, Fluorescence, GC-MS, ICP
MVOC'S	Air and Surface	Aerosols and bulk	Bioassay, GC-MS, HPLC
Particulate	Air	Aerosols	Laser Diode Particle Counter and weighing of filters
Suspended Particulate Matter	Air	Aerosols	Gravimetric analysis
Temperature	Air, Surface	—	Thermographs, thermometer or Data logger
VOC	Air	Dosimeter, Aerosols	GC- MS, HPLC

exchanger, supply air plenum, ductwork, supply air diffuser, plumbing system, carpet, interior building furnishing, fixture, and other synthetic materials are some common manmade sources either emanating or harboring pollutants. Lower life forms (phytoplankton, zooplanktons, etc.), flora, and fauna serve as a natural source for a number of pollutants. Inadequate building construction, maintenance, and housekeeping along with substandard ventilation may cause pollutants to rapidly grow within a built environment. Pollution causing agents may be collected from manmade activities or part of a natural cycle as a reservoir called "sink." The sorption and desorption characteristics of contaminants is of fundamental importance to explain the sink effect in indoor environments. It is essential to have the knowledge of sink-effect to identify the source of pollutants in indoor environments. The sink behavior is one of important scaling system to establish a potential source emitting pollutants in indoor environments.

6.4.6.2 Release

The release of pollutants from its source into the indoor environment is a complex phenomenon and not well understood. Although pollutants release mechanisms may vary depending on size, composition, source, etc., they are often considered good indicators of indoor environment quality. Activities such as anthropogenic, blowing, chemotaxis, decomposition, dusting, electrostatics, evaporation, hygroscopic, inertia, natural disaster, off-gassing, splash, trampling, and withering have been noticed as important releasing factors. Construction or remodeling of buildings, road construction, afforestation, smoking, and decomposition of inorganic and inorganic materials in and around built environments often releases particles that could pollute an indoor environment. Some commonly released particles due to the aforementioned conduct include VOC, carbon mono or dioxides, oxides of nitrogen and sulfur, metals, non-metals, and other hazardous chemicals along with microbial entities. The release of microbial and other biogenic particulates depends on existing flora and fauna including microflora of the ambient environment.

The two specific mechanisms for pollutants release are known as active and passive method. In active methods, contaminants are released from their source on the cost of their inherent energy, e.g., off-gassing, fungal spore libration upon maturity. In case of a passive mode, particulates are discharged from their place of origin by the action of external energy. Blowing away of dust and debris, shedding of spores under gravity, rain splash of chemicals or microbial entities commonly occurs as a result of passive mechanism.

6.4.6.3 Dispersal

The transport of pollutants from their source is a key stage as it determines whether a pollutant will accumulate or be diluted in the ambient environment. Dispersion is influenced by several factors including environmental conditions and physical parameters. Changes in pollutants dispersion behavior after the release from their source may influence overall indoor environment quality irrespective of release mechanisms.

There are mainly two types of dispersion:

Vertical dispersion, related to the vertical temperature and humidity gradient of the surface layer, the ambient air's layer influenced by the surface below it. The nature, buoyancy, and composition of particulates are also important in the dispersal of such particulates.

Horizontal dispersion, referred to as transport, is related to air circulation, direction, and growth/concentration of pollutants. Contaminants adaptation and composition are significant for its dispersion. For example, a high-pressure zone within the closed environment pushes the pollutants toward the low-pressure zone. Conversely, low-pressure situations are generally associated with a stronger presence of the pollutants. Furthermore, low temperature and moisture restrict the pollutant deposits around indoor environments. During dispersion, pollutants may be transformed by complex forms to secondary pollutants such as bio-particulates, gases, and certain VOC, etc. There is static layer of air generally referred as the laminar boundary layer varying in thickness from 10 cm to 1 meter from the ground. This layer is thicker in still conditions and pollutant dispersal is negligible or none. The turbulent layer extents above the laminar boundary and much activate for pollutant dispersal point of view.

6.4.6.4 Dissemination

Pollutants with both biological and non-biological origins are disseminated mainly due to anthropogenic, ventilation, and other activities by occupants in the indoor environment. Activities related with air movement, rain splash, sorption, desorption and refuse handling are noted as main phenomena for dissemination of contaminants. HVAC, water containing appliances (humidifiers, etc.), carpeting, stored organic materials, warm, moist and damp areas, and house dust are identified as reservoirs and common disseminating factors for indoor pollutants. Air circulation, water distribution systems, and inhabitant's activities have been identified as potential driving forces for pollution dissemination. The floating particulates in air cannot established community structure as seen on the ground. Nevertheless, they remain in the ambient air either floating individually or in a group of heterogeneous mixture in agglomerated or conglomerated form respectively. Hence, monitoring of pollutant dissemination provides vital clues in its management.

6.4.6.5 Impaction

Most indoor contaminants directly or indirectly impact health and hygiene. Indoor contaminants widely vary in their nature, origin, degree of risk, and mode of action on host or substratum. A perceptive impaction evaluation of existing indoor pollutants may provide information on risk factors associated with it. Depending on the bouncy, along with transport mechanisms, pollutants diffuse and settle in and around indoor sites. After inhabiting an ecological niche, these pollutants start impacting the host or substratum. The deposition gradients interact erratically on either habitat or its inhabitants. The health and hygiene implication due to such contaminants is a complex process of which biological, chemical, environmental, and physical factors play significant roles. Although limited knowledge in associating deposition gradients on health implications exist, risk assessments can still be performed by knowing the exposure and other characteristics of the contaminant. Allergies, infections, diseases, and other hygiene associated problems caused by pollutants are not solely dependent on their potency, but also depend on the conditions of the host or substrate. Method, concentration, and time of exposure for the aforesaid elements are preferably used in predicting associated risk factors. Three methods of pollutant exposure; inhalation, contact, and ingestion; are common amongst inhabitants. The susceptibility of subpopulations, such as children, elderly, and others with compromised immune systems may show an accelerated impact of environmental pollutants even in low dosages. Some pollutants could be markedly more concentrated indoors than outdoors. Indoor pollutants may have an important impact even at low concentrations over long or short exposure periods.

6.4.7 SOURCE-CAUSE DETERMINATION

Building assessments for indoor environmental concerns are challenging and require special skills for establishing a source-cause determination. There is no universal mechanism that institutes a theory for aforesaid relationship. However, multiple sampling approaches and epidemiological data would be helpful in obtaining a proper interpretation of complaints. The source-cause determination provides vital clues for understanding the extent of indoor pollutants and their mitigation. Pollutants relevant to health and hygiene originate from different sources, ranging from the natural atmosphere, flora, and fauna to artificial or manmade substances. Irrespective of source locations (outdoors or indoors), pollutants can spread through indoors depending on other variables. If the source and nature of pollutants are not identified and controlled, it gives rise to problems related with health and hygiene. In order to determine the cause of indoor pollution, a thorough observation for determining the source is an obvious choice. Proper identification of possible sources are helpful in hypothesizing the theory for explaining who, what, where, and how in terms of pollution causing factors. They also act as supportive factors for screening non-biological or biological pollutants.

Chances of getting chemical contaminants such as sulfates, mineral dusts, ash, SPM, gases, and other inorganic or organic compounds in closed environments is relatively higher in building located near industrial zones. Likewise, high humidity, limited ventilation, dampness, decomposition, microbial flora, and others are some diversified sources of indoor pollutants. Obviously, linking causes with that of source is considered a typical practice for indoor environment evaluation in terms of a good fit for the inhabitants. Table 6.4 provides information on source-cause relationships on indoor pollutants.

6.4.8 ACTION PLAN

In order to provide a healthy, productive, and comfortable inhabitable space in any building requires a job specific action plan (JSAP). No one-action plan fits in all. The goal of an action plan is to ensure an adequate

TABLE 6.4 Cause, Source, and Location of Indoor Pollutants

Cause	Source	Location
Fine particulates, carbon mono or dioxides, nitrogen oxides, sulfur oxides, arsenic, fluorine and other chemicals	Fossil fuel combustion (Coal/Kerosene/Diesels/Transport)	Outdoors/Indoors
Suspended Particulate Matters, Carbon mono-dioxide, Hydrocarbon, Organic compounds, Metals, Non-metallic mineral products, Bio-pollutants and other chemicals.	Emission from industry and manufacturing activities	Outdoor
Fertilizers, Pesticides, Oder and Other chemicals	House hold and Farming chemicals	Outdoors/Indoors
Particulates, Carbon mono & dioxides, Hydrocarbons, VOC'S and other Chemicals	Cooking (wood, coal, charcoal, crop residue, and dung)	Indoors
Microbial growth, Comfort Issues	Damp and humid conditions	Indoors
Microbial growth, Fiberglass, Amines, VOC, MVOC, Oder and Comfort issues	Ventilation, Insulation and Furnishing	Indoors
Radon, Microbial infestation and Comfort issue	Soil under building	Indoor
Fine particulates, Dust, Debris, Asbestos, Leads, Oder and Comfort	Construction or Remodeling	Outdoors/Indoors
Persistent Organic Pollution (eg. Polycyclic aromatic hydrocarbons etc.), Ozone, Oder, and Comfort issues.	Cables, computers, TV's, Textiles, Food and Fumes	Indoors
Microbes, Microbial toxins, Pollen grains, Pets hairs/dander, Plant Trichomes, Oder and Comfort issues	Inhabitants, Plants and Pets	Indoors

and timely response to address indoor pollution to prevent small complaints from becoming major health and hygiene problems. It is worth noting that the maintenance and proper management of a livable space significantly depends on the building functions, such as residential or commercial properties. Managing pollutants in a closed environment in order to lower health risks, enhance productivity, increase comfort, and reduce exposure to liability is a complicated task. However, environmental building diagnostics along with epidemiological evaluations is helpful in designing an effective action plan.

Establishing a baseline in absence of universally accepted guidelines for the indoor environment is the first step. This at least includes construction/design, location, function, operation, and other factors that could influence building conditions besides any previously known issues in this context. If any issues have been recorded in the past, all the existing records must be reviewed before taking further action. A building health check is often performed in cases of known or anticipated issues besides developing a baseline for normal conditions of a building. Attempts are made to pinpoint the problem as a result of building evaluation and laboratory findings. Indoor contaminants can be drawn in from outside or can originate within a building. If contaminant sources are not controlled, building health and hygiene problems can arise, even if the HVAC system is well-maintained and running properly. If sources are identified, an action plan should be executed for providing remedial measures or modifications to the environment in order to address the problem appropriately. Still, some problems may persist due to unidentified and uncontrolled pollutant sources. Biological growth is one such situation as making an action plan is difficult; however, by controlling nutrition, moisture and temperature sources, it can be minimized or altogether eliminated. Problems linked with ventilation, filtration, HVAC, or other inadequate maintenance and operation practices, can have a specific solution oriented plan of action. Building inhabitants and owners' can be educated on building functioning, maintenance, and issues raised due to pollutants by crafting a plan of action. A routine housekeeping schedule should be part of an action plan in order to reduce the risk of indoor pollution. Action plans for managing some of the activities identified as pollutant sources are beneficial for controlling indoor pollutants in building. Remodeling and renovation, painting, pest control, discharge of effluent, collection and recycling of solid and food waste, smoking, and pets often emit microbiological or chemical pollutants.

6.5 NUMERICAL REFERENCE POINTS FOR INDOOR POLLUTANTS

In absence of an inadequate and universally accepted guideline assessment to ensure a healthful indoor environment often noticed as challenging task. Changing specification in building codes, energy utilizations, public perceptions, cultural preferences, litigation treads, change in building materials, inhabitant behaviours and regulations make this task more interesting and call for evidence based assessment models. Interestingly, criteria used in establishing guideline or reference point for indoor environment not only depend on the toxicity of pollutants but also exposure on inhabitants along with their health conditions. This reference point is prepared to evaluate indoor environment for various contaminates that may be crucial for determining health and hygiene of a building.

We have examined and/or appraised data obtained from more than 248,500 environmental specimens prepared after processing 60,000 environmental samples, collected between June 1994 to April 2011 in and around building environments on a proactive or reactive basis by field technicians or individuals in and around the United States.

Environmental parameters such as temperature, relative humidity, moisture content and air-borne particulate counts were also evaluated. The temperature and relative humidity is recorded by data loggers, where as moisture content and air-borne particulate is determined by using moisture meters and Laser Diode Particle counters, respectively.

Air, surface, bulk, swab and liquid samples were collected from the indoor environment on a proactive or reactive basis by Pure Air Control Services (PACS), Inc. technicians or individuals by using standard method (Dillon et al., 2005). These samples were examined for constituents that are characterized as biological or a-biological in nature.

The collected specimens were analyzed or appraised for enumerating indoor pollutants that may responsible for influencing the quality of environment in and around buildings. For developing a numerical reference point pollutants identified from the indoor environment is divided into the following categories.

6.5.1 CULTURABLE BIOAEROSOLS

These specimens includes culturable bacteria and fungi isolated from various matrix of indoor environment

6.5.2 MICROSCOPIC CONTAMINANTS

All of the above air and surface-borne constituents are categorized into the following groups.

Opaque Particulates: These particles may originate from inorganic or organic sources in nature. They appear opaque when observed under light microscopy and have various shapes and sizes with regular or irregular dimensions. On average, they can be measured as less than 1 μm to greater than 50 μm, with some exceptions. These particles commonly include, but are not limited to, dust and debris, paint, combustions, emissions, ash, silica and likewise particulates.

Skin Cell Fragments: Fragments of dead skin cells are dispersed or deposited in and around indoor environments from human or other animal sources. The size range of skin cells varies greatly between less than 5 μm to greater than 50 μm.

Insect Biodetritius: These are either small insects or portions/parts of insects floating or deposited in and around indoor environments. They may vary in size from a few μm to > 1 millimeters.

Total Fibers: This includes fibers such as manmade fibers, fiberglass fibers, etc. Manmade fibers may come from natural raw materials, like cellulose, or from synthetic chemicals like rayon, nylon, etc. The size of these fibers varies from a few microns to a few millimeters; however, an average size range may be 1 μm to over 500 μm.

Plant trichomes: These are the hairy outgrowths from the aerial parts of plants of various shapes (elongated, globose, stellate, pendate, with or without septae, etc.) and sizes (few μm to over 1 mm). Plant trichomes are listed as other types of fiber under the "Total Fibers" category.

Fiberglass Fibers: These are materials made from extremely fine fibers of glass. They appear as a smooth-walled, elongated, tube-like structure under the microscope with varying size ranges (average range 1 μm to over 1000 μm). Due to its importance as an irritant, it is accounted for in a separate category.

Pollen Grains: These are microscopic particles of varying shapes (mostly globose, spheroidal to ellipsoidal without pore or with pore, colpi or combination of both) and sizes (5 μm to more than 200 μm). They are colorless or pigmented with various shade of yellow, brown, etc. and originate from angiospermic plants.

Fungal Elements/Spores: These are fungal structures of various shapes (globose, elongated, ellipsoidal and others with or without septation) and sizes (few μm to more than 100 μm). They are hyaline to dark in color.

Others: The following miscellaneous particles that are biogenic or a-biogenic in nature are reported in the "Others" category.

Algae: These are unicellular to multicellular structures of biogenic origin with pigmentation (mostly green, chlorophyll, etc.). They greatly vary in their shape (spherical or longitudinal, etc.) and size (25 μm to > 1 mm).

Black Particulates: These microscopic particles may originate from an organic source material. They greatly vary in their shape and size depending on their origin. However, an average size ranges between 1 μm to 5 μm with some exceptions and it may be regular or irregular in shape. Some important sources/causes of these particles in the indoor environment include, but are not limited to, combustion, burning of oil and candles, chimney soot, automobile exhaust, neoprene (rubber compound that is applied to the inside surface of fiberglass duct liner) and other organic materials emitted by copier machines, printers, abraded paints, etc.

Reddish-brown Particulates: These microscopic particles may originate from inorganic or organic source materials. These particles mainly come originate in indoor environments by rusting, coarse, weathering of materials, etc. These particles greatly vary in shape and size, measuring from 1 μm to over 100 μm.

Talc-like Particulates: These are thin, disk-like particles of variable size range (10 μm to 50 μm). They may be organic or inorganic in nature. Within an indoor environment, these particles mainly come from cornmeal, other grain flour, talcum powder, etc.

Myxomycetes: This is a group of fungus-like organisms, which exhibit characteristics of both protozoans (one-celled microorganisms) and fungi. They greatly vary in their shape and size (10 μm to 500 μm).

6.5.3 INDOOR ANIMAL ALLERGENS

The common animal allergens from the house dust sample are grouped into the following categories:

Dust mites: Mite allergens (common in mite fecal particles), Der p 1 (*Dermatophagoides pteronyssinus*) and Der f1 (*Dermatophagoides farina*).

Cat: Fed 1 cat allergen, which is common in cat fur, saliva, epithelial cells, sebaceous gland excretions and urine.

Cockroach: Common allergens evaluated are Bla g 1 and Bla g 2 (*Blattella*), which may originate from cockroach feces and saliva.

Dog: Can f 1 allergen is evaluated in dust samples. It comes from dog saliva or, in some cases, urine or feces.

6.5.4 RESPIRABLE-SIZE PARTICLE

Respirable-size particle counts are observed in and around indoor sites.

It includes observation on the thermal indoor environmental conditions, moisture and relative humidity.

6.5.5 CARBON DI-OXIDE

This parameter includes concentration of carbon di-oxide gas.

Using appropriate environmental culture or microscopic techniques 439 types of bacteria (Table 6.5), 353 forms of fungi (Table 6.6), 91 categories of pollen grains (Table 6.7) 36 miscellaneous biogenic or a-biogenic particulates (Table 6.8) (Barnett and Hunter, 2003; Bassett et al., 1978; Beneke and Roger, 1996; Domsch et al., 1993; Grant, 1990; Gregory, 1973; Hanlin, 1998; Holt et al., 2000; Koneman et al., 1997; Lewis, 1983; Murray et al., 1995) have been identified. Quantitatively, bacteria (50%) dominated over fungi (36%), followed by pollen grains (10%) and miscellaneous particulates (4%) (Figure 6.1A). Overall, bacteria collected from indoor environments by swab sample (51%) dominated over fungi collected by bulk method (22%) when analyzed by using culture method. Fungi (22%) dominated over bacteria (15%) when collected and analyzed utilizing bulk method with culturable analysis. However, bacteria (51%)

TABLE 6.5 Bacteria Reported From Indoor Environments by Culture Method

1	*Achromobacter xylosoxidans*	34	*Agrobacterium tumefaciens*
2	*Acidovorax avenae*	35	*Agrobacterium tumefaciens A*
3	*Acidovorax delafieldii*	36	*Agrobacterium vitis*
4	*Acidovorax* species	37	*Agrobacterium radiobacter*
5	*Acinetobacter anitratus*	38	*Agrobacterium* species
6	*Acinetobacter anitratus gs 13*	39	*Alcaligenes denitrificans*
7	*Acinetobacter anitratus gs 4*	40	*Alcaligenes faecalis*
8	*Acinetobacter calcoaceticus*	41	*Alcaligenes faecalis ss homari*
9	*Acinetobacter calcoaceticus gs 2*	42	*Alcaligenes latus*
10	*Acinetobacter calcoaceticus gs 3*	43	*Alcaligenes* species
11	*Acinetobacter genospecies 10*	44	*Alcaligenes xylosoxidans*
12	*Acinetobacter genospecies 15*	45	*Ancylobacter aquaticus*
13	*Acinetobacter johnsonii*	46	*Aquaspirillum dispar*
14	*Acinetobacter lwoffii*	47	*Aquaspirillum species*
15	*Acinetobacter radioresistens*	48	*Arthrobacter cumminsii*
16	*Acinetobacter radioresistens gs 12*	49	*Arthrobacter species*
17	*Acinetobacter* species	50	*Aureobacterium terregens*
18	*Actinobacillus* species	51	*Aureobacterium testaceum*
19	*Actinomyces hordeovulneris*	52	*Aureobacterium species*
20	*Actinomyces canis*	53	*Bacillus alcalophilus*
21	*Actinomycetes* species	54	*Bacillus amyloliquefaciens*
22	*Aerococcus viridans*	55	*Bacillus azotoformans*
23	*Aeromonas caviae*	56	*Bacillus badius*
24	*Aeromonas caviae DNA group 4*	57	*Bacillus brevis*
25	*Aeromonas hydrophilia DNA group 1*	58	*Bacillus cereu*
26	*Aeromonas media DNA group 5B*	59	*Bacillus circulans*
27	*Aeromonas media-like DNA group 5A*	60	*Bacillus coagulans*
28	*Aeromonas salmonicida*	61	*Bacillus fastidious*
29	*Aeromonas schubertii DNA group 12*	62	*Bacillus laevolacticus*
30	*Aeromonas* species	63	*Bacillus lentus*
31	*Aeromonas veronii/sobria DNA 8*	64	*Bacillus licheniformis*
32	*Agrobacterium rhizogenes*	65	*Bacillus megaterium*
33	*Agrobacterium rhizogenes A*	66	*Bacillus mycoides*

TABLE 6.5 (Continued)

67	*Bacillus pasteurii*	101	CDC Group A – 5
68	*Bacillus pumilus*	102	CDC Group B-1/B – 3
69	*Bacillus species (*not *B. anthracis)*	103	CDC Group DF – 3
70	*Bacillus sphaericus*	104	CDC Group E
71	*Bacillus subtilis*	105	CDC Group E, Subgroup A
72	*Bacillus subtilis var globigii*	106	CDC Group EF – 4
73	*Bacillus thuringiensis*	107	CDC Group EO-2 (Eugonic Oxidizer-2)
74	*Bacillus trematum*		
75	*Bergeyella zoohelcum*	108	CDC Group II – H
76	*Bordetella bronchiseptica*	109	CDC Group II – I
77	*Brevibacillus brevis*	110	CDC group II-E subgroup A
78	*Brevibacterium acetylicum*	111	CDC Group IVC – 2
79	*Brevibacterium epidermidis*	112	*Cellulomonas cartae*
80	*Brevibacterium linens*	113	*Cellulomonas flavigena*
81	*Brevibacterium liquefaciens*	114	*Cellulomonas hominis*
82	*Brevibacterium mcbrellneri*	115	*Cellulomonas* species
83	*Brevibacterium otitidis*	116	*Cellulosimicrobium cellulans*
84	*Brevibacterium species*	117	*Cellulosimicrobium* species
85	*Brevundimonas diminuta*	118	*Chryseobacterium indologenes*
86	*Brevundimonas vesicularis*	119	*Chryseobacterium indoltheticum*
87	*Brochothrix campestris*	120	*Chryseobacterium meningosepticum*
88	*Brochothrix species*	121	*Chryseobacterium scophthalmum*
89	*Brochothrix thermosphacta*	122	*Chryseobacterium* species
90	*Burkholderia andropogonis*	123	*Chryseomonas luteola*
91	*Burkholderia cepacia*	124	*Citrobacter amalonaticus*
92	*Burkholderia cocovenenans*	125	*Citrobacter freundii*
93	*Burkholderia gladioli*	126	*Citrobacter koseri (C. diversus)*
94	*Burkholderia glumae*	127	*Citrobacter* species
95	*Burkholderia phenazinium*	128	*Clavibacter agropyri*
96	*Burkholderia* species	129	*Clavibacter michiganense*
97	*Buttiauxella gaviniae*	130	*Clavibacter sepedonicum*
98	*Buttiauxella species*	131	*Comamonas acidovorans*
99	*Cardiobacterium hominis*	132	*Comamonas* species
100	*Carnobacterium* species	133	*Comamonas terrigena*

TABLE 6.5 (Continued)

134	*Comamonas testosteroni*	167	*Enterobacter amnigenus*
135	*Corynebacterium afermentans*	168	*Enterobacter asburiae*
136	*Corynebacterium ammoniagenes*	169	*Enterobacter cancerogenus*
137	*Corynebacterium amycolatum*	170	*Enterobacter cloacae*
138	*Corynebacterium aquaticum*	171	*Enterobacter gergoviae*
139	*Corynebacterium aquaticum A*	172	*Enterobacter intermedium*
140	*Corynebacterium aquaticum B*	173	*Enterobacter sakazakii*
141	*Corynebacterium auris*	174	*Enterobacter* species
142	*Corynebacterium jeikeium*	175	*Enterococcus casseliflavus*
143	*Corynebacterium jeikeium A*	176	*Enterococcus faecalis*
144	*Corynebacterium jeikeium B*	177	*Erwinia* species
145	*Corynebacterium minutissimum*	178	*Escherichia blattae*
146	*Corynebacterium nitrilophilus*	179	*Escherichia coli*
147	*Corynebacterium pseudodiphtheriticum*	180	*Escherichia* species
		181	*Escherichia vulneris*
148	*Corynebacterium* species	182	*Ewingella Americana*
149	*Corynebacterium urealyticum*	183	*Exiguobacterium* species
150	*Curtobacterium albidum*	184	*Flavimonas oryzihabitans*
151	*Curtobacterium citreum*	185	*Flavimonas* species
152	*Curtobacterium flaccumfaciens*	186	*Flavobacterium balustinum*
153	*Curtobacterium luteum*	187	*Flavobacterium breve*
154	*Curtobacterium pusillum*	188	*Flavobacterium gleum*
155	*Curtobacterium* species	189	*Flavobacterium indologenes*
156	*Cytophaga fermentans*	190	*Flavobacterium indoltheticum*
157	*Cytophaga johnsonae*	191	*Flavobacterium johnsoniae*
158	*Deinococcus* species	192	*Flavobacterium meningosepticum*
159	*Delftia acidovorans*	193	*Flavobacterium mizutaii*
160	*Dermabacter hominis*	194	*Flavobacterium* species
161	*Dermacoccus nishinomiyaensis*	195	*Geobacillus stearothermophilus*
162	*Empedobacter brevis*	196	*Gluconobacter oxydans ss suboxydans*
163	*Enterobacter aerogenes*		
164	*Enterobacter agglomerans*	197	*Gordonia bronchialis*
165	*Enterobacter agglomerans Biogp 2A*	198	*Gordonia rubropertinctus*
166	*Enterobacter agglomerans Biogp 3B*	199	*Gordonia* species

TABLE 6.5 (Continued)

200	*Gordonia sputi*
201	*Helicobacter* species
202	*Hydrogenophaga flava*
203	*Intrasporangium calvum*
204	*Janthinobacterium lividum*
205	*Jonesia denitrificans*
206	*Kingella kingae*
207	*Klebsiella oxytoca*
208	*Klebsiella ozaenae*
209	*Klebsiella pneumoniae*
210	*Klebsiella* species
211	*Kluyvera cryocrescens*
212	*Kluyvera* species
213	*Kocuria kristinae*
214	*Kocuria rosea*
215	*Kocuria varians*
216	*Kurthia gibsonii*
217	*Kurthia sibirica*
218	*Kurthia* species
219	*Kurthia zopfii*
220	*Kytococcus sedentarius*
221	*Lactococcus plantarum*
222	*Leclercia adecarboxylata*
223	*Leifsonia aquatica*
225	*Listeria grayi*
224	*Leuconostoc paramesenteroides*
226	*Macrococcus carouselicus*
227	*Macrococcus* species
277	*Photobacterium logei*
228	*Mannheimia haemolytica*
229	*Methylobacterium* species
230	*Microbacterium arborescens*
231	*Microbacterium flavescens*
232	*Microbacterium imperiale*
233	*Microbacterium laevaniformans*
234	*Microbacterium saperdae*
235	*Microbacterium* species
236	*Microbacterium species* (CDC Gp A 4)
237	*Microbacterium species* (CDC Gp A 5)
238	*Microbacterium terregens*
239	*Microbacterium testaceum*
240	*Micrococcus agilis*
241	*Micrococcus diversus*
242	*Micrococcus luteus*
243	*Micrococcus lylae*
244	*Micrococcus roseus*
245	*Micrococcus* species
246	*Micromonospora species*
247	*Moraxella* species
248	*Morganella morganii*
249	*Myroides* species
250	*Neisseria sicca*
251	*Nesterenkonia halobia*
252	*Nocardia asteroids*
253	*Nocardia brasiliensis*
254	*Nocardia otitidiscaviarum*
255	*Nocardia* species
256	*Ochrobactrum anthropi*
257	*Oerskovia (Cellulomonas) turbata*
258	*Oerskovia xanthineolytica*
259	*Paenibacillus azotofixans*
260	*Paenibacillus pabuli*
261	*Paenibacillus polymyxa*
262	*Paenibacillus* species
263	*Pandoraea* species
264	*Pantoea agglomerans*
265	*Pantoea agglomerans biogroup 3*

TABLE 6.5 (Continued)

266	*Pantoea agglomerans biogroup 4*	301	*Pseudomonas fulva*
267	*Pantoea dispersa*	302	*Pseudomonas maculicola*
268	*Pantoea* species	303	*Pseudomonas mendocina*
269	*Pantoea stewartii*	304	*Pseudomonas pseudoalcaligenes*
270	*Pasteurella anatipestifer*	305	*Pseudomonas putida*
271	*Pasteurella anatis*	306	*Pseudomonas putida biotype A*
272	*Pasteurella multocida*	307	*Pseudomonas putida biotype B*
273	*Pasteurella* species	308	*Pseudomonas* species
274	*Pasteurella volantium*	309	*Pseudomonas stutzeri*
275	*Pediococcus acidilactici*	310	*Pseudomonas syringae*
276	*Photobacterium damsela*	311	*Pseudomonas vesicularis*
278	*Photorhabdus luminescens*	312	*Pseudomonas viridilivida*
279	*Photorhabdus* species	313	*Psychrobacter denitrificans*
280	*Phyllobacterium* species	314	*Psychrobacter immobilis*
281	*Proteus mirabilis*	315	*Psychrobacter phenylpyruvicus*
282	*Proteus myxofaciens*	316	*Psychrobacter* species
283	*Proteus penneri*	317	*Rahnella aquatilis*
284	*Proteus* species	318	*Ralstonia paucula*
285	*Proteus vulgaris*	319	*Ralstonia pickettii*
286	*Providencia heimbachae*	320	*Ralstonia* species
287	*Providencia rettgeri*	321	*Raoultella planticola*
288	*Providencia* species	322	*Raoultella terrigena*
289	*Providencia stuartii*	323	*Rathayibacter tritici*
290	*Pseudomonas aeruginosa*	324	*Rhizobium radiobacter*
291	*Pseudomonas alcaligenes*	325	*Rhizobium rhizogenes*
292	*Pseudomonas alcaligenes biovar A*	326	*Rhizobium* species
293	*Pseudomonas alcaligenes biovar B*	327	*Rhodococcus australis*
294	*Pseudomonas andropogonis*	328	*Rhodococcus equi*
295	*Pseudomonas aurantiaca*	329	*Rhodococcus erythropolis*
296	*Pseudomonas boreopolis*	330	*Rhodococcus fascians*
297	*Pseudomonas corrugata*	331	*Rhodococcus rhodochrous*
298	*Pseudomonas diminuta*	332	*Rhodococcus* species
299	*Pseudomonas fluorescens*	333	*Roseomonas genomospecies 5*
300	*Pseudomonas fluorescens, type G*	334	*Roseomonas* species

TABLE 6.5 (Continued)

335	*Rothia mucilaginosa*
336	*Rothia* species
337	*Saccharomonospora viridis*
338	*Saccharopolyspora rectivirgula*
339	*Salmonella* species
340	*Sanguibacter inulinus*
341	*Sanguibacter keddieii*
342	*Sanguibacter* species
343	*Serratia ficaria*
344	*Serratia liquefaciens*
345	*Serratia marcescens*
346	*Serratia odorifera*
347	*Serratia plymuthica*
348	*Serratia rubidaea*
349	*Serratia* species
350	*Shewanella algae*
351	*Shewanella putrefaciens*
352	*Shewanella putrefaciens* A
353	*Shewanella putrefaciens* B
354	*Shewanella putrefaciens* C
355	*Shewanella putrefaciens* D
356	*Shigella* species
357	*Sphingobacterium multivorum*
358	*Sphingobacterium* species
359	*Sphingobacterium spiritovorum*
360	*Sphingobacterium thalpophilum*
361	*Sphingomonas paucimobilis*
362	*Sphingomonas paucimobilis* A
363	*Sphingomonas paucimobilis* B
364	*Sphingomonas sanguinis*
365	*Sphingomonas* species
366	*Sphingomonas yanoikuyae*
367	*Staphylococcus arlettae*
368	*Staphylococcus aureus*
369	*Staphylococcus auricularis*
370	*Staphylococcus capitis*
371	*Staphylococcus caprae*
372	*Staphylococcus carnosus*
373	*Staphylococcus caseolyticus*
374	*Staphylococcus cohnii*
375	*Staphylococcus cohnii ss cohnii*
376	*Staphylococcus cohnii ss urealyticus*
377	*Staphylococcus epidermidis*
378	*Staphylococcus felis*
379	*Staphylococcus gallinarum*
380	*Staphylococcus haemolyticus*
381	*Staphylococcus haemolyticus 1*
382	*Staphylococcus haemolyticus 2*
383	*Staphylococcus haemolyticus 3*
384	*Staphylococcus hominis*
385	*Staphylococcus hominis 1*
386	*Staphylococcus hominis 2*
387	*Staphylococcus hominis 3*
388	*Staphylococcus hyicus*
389	*Staphylococcus hyicus ss chromogenes*
390	*Staphylococcus hyicus ss hyicus*
391	*Staphylococcus intermedius*
392	*Staphylococcus kloosii*
393	*Staphylococcus kloosii* A
394	*Staphylococcus lentus*
395	*Staphylococcus lugdunensis*
396	*Staphylococcus saprophyticus*
397	*Staphylococcus schleiferi*
398	*Staphylococcus schleiferi ss coagulans*
399	*Staphylococcus schleiferi ss schleiferi*
400	*Staphylococcus sciuri*
401	*Staphylococcus sciuri ss lentus*

TABLE 6.5 (Continued)

426	*Vibrio harveyi*	421	*Variovorax paradoxus*
402	*Staphylococcus sciuri ss sciuri*	422	*Vibrio alginolyticus*
403	*Staphylococcus* species	423	*Vibrio campbellii*
404	*Staphylococcus warneri*	424	*Vibrio carchariae*
405	*Staphylococcus xylosus*	425	*Vibrio fluvialis*
406	*Staphylococcus xylosus 1*	427	*Vibrio metschnikovii*
407	*Staphylococcus xylosus 2*	428	*Vibrio pelagius 1*
408	*Stenotrophomonas maltophilia*	429	*Vibrio* species
409	*Streptomyces albus*	430	*Vibrio tubiashii*
410	*Streptomyces anulatus (S. griseus)*	431	*Vibrio vulnificus*
411	*Streptomyces coelicolor*	432	*Weeksella zoohelcum*
412	*Streptomyces lateritius*	433	*Xanthomonas campestris*
413	*Streptomyces somaliensis*	434	*Xanthomonas campestris pv vesicator*
414	*Streptomyces* species	435	*Xanthomonas oryzae*
415	*Suttonella indologenes*	436	*Xanthomonas oryzae pv oryzae* B
416	*Thermoactinomyces sacchari*	437	*Xanthomonas oryzae pv oryzae* E
417	*Thermoactinomyces thalpophilus*	438	*Xanthomonas* species
418	*Thermoactinomyces vulgaris*	439	*Yersinia* species
419	*Tsukamurella inchonensis*	440	*Iresin*
420	*Tsukamurella* species		

TABLE 6.6 Fungi Reported From Indoor Environments

Sl. No.	Name of Fungi	B	M	Sl. No.	Name of Fungi	B	M
1	*Absidia* species			9	*Acremonium murorum*		
2	*Absidia corymbifera*			10	*Acremonium strictum*		
3	*Absidia spinosa*			11	*Agrocybe* species		
4	*Acremonium* species			12	*Albugo* species		
5	*Acremonium chrysogenum*			13	*Alternaria* species		
				14	*Alternaria alternata*		
6	*Acremonium fusidioides*			15	*Alternaria brassicicola*		
				16	*Alternaria radicina*		
7	*Acremonium* like spores			17	*Alternaria tenuissima*		
8	*Acremonium kiliense*			18	*Apiospora montagnei*		

TABLE 6.6 (Continued)

Sl. No.	Name of Fungi	B	M
19	*Apiosporina species*	Green	Green
20	*Arthrinium species*	Green	Green
21	*Arthrobotrys species*	Green	Green
22	*Arthroderma species*	Green	Red
23	*Arthroderma cuniculi*	Green	Red
24	*Arthroderma insingulare*	Green	Red
25	*Arthroderma quadrifidum*	Green	Red
26	*Aspergillus species*	Green	Green
27	*Aspergillus alutaceus*	Green	Red
28	*Aspergillus candidus*	Green	Red
29	*Aspergillus clavatus*	Green	Red
30	*Aspergillus flavipes*	Green	Red
31	*Aspergillus flavus*	Green	Red
32	*Aspergillus fumigatus*	Green	Red
33	*Aspergillus glaucus*	Green	Red
34	*Aspergillus japonicus*	Green	Red
35	*Aspergillus nidulans*	Green	Green
36	*Aspergillus niger*	Green	Green
37	*Aspergillus niveus*	Green	Red
38	*Aspergillus oryzae*	Green	Red
39	*Aspergillus parasiticus*	Green	Red
40	*Aspergillus restrictus*	Green	Red
41	*Aspergillus sclerotiorum*	Green	Red
42	*Aspergillus sydowii*	Green	Red
43	*Aspergillus terreus*	Green	Green
44	*Aspergillus/Penicillium-Like Spores*	Red	Green
45	*Asperisporium species*	Red	Green
46	*Aspergillus terricola*	Red	Green
47	*Aspergillus ustus*	Green	Red
48	*Aspergillus versicolor*	Green	Red
49	*Aspergillus wentii*	Green	Red
50	*Aureobasidium pullulans*	Green	Red
51	*Beauveria species*	Green	Red
52	*Beauveria bassiana*	Green	Red
53	*Beltrania species*	Green	Green
54	*Beltrania querna*	Green	Red
55	*Beltraniella species*	Green	Red
56	*Bipolaris species*	Green	Green
57	*Bipolaris spicifera*	Green	Red
58	*Bispora species*	Green	Green
59	*Bispora betulina*	Green	Red
60	*Blastomyces species*	Green	Red
61	*Botryotrichum piluliferum*	Green	Red
62	*Botryotrichum species*	Green	Red
63	*Botrytis cinerea*	Green	Red
64	*Botrytis species*	Green	Red
65	*Brachysporium obovatum*	Green	Red
66	*Brachysporium species*	Green	Red
67	*Broomella acuta*	Green	Red
68	*Broomella species*	Green	Green
69	*Bulleromyces albus*	Green	Red
70	*Candida species*	Green	Red
71	*Candida albicans*	Green	Red
72	*Candida diversa*	Green	Red
73	*Candida edax*	Green	Red
74	*Candida guilliermondii*	Green	Red
75	*Candida krusei*	Green	Red
76	*Candida parapsilosis*	Green	Red
77	*Candida parapsilosis A*	Green	Red

TABLE 6.6 (Continued)

Sl. No.	Name of Fungi	B	M
78	*Candida parapsilosis B*	Green	Orange
79	*Candida pseudotropicalis*	Green	Orange
80	*Candida silvae*	Green	Orange
81	*Candida sorboxylosa*	Green	Orange
82	*Candida tropicalis*	Green	Orange
83	*Capronia species*	Green	Green
84	*Cercospora species*	Red	Green
85	*Chaetomium species*	Green	Green
86	*Chaetomium elatum*	Green	Orange
87	*Chaetomium globosum*	Green	Orange
88	*Chrysonilia species*	Green	Orange
89	*Chrysonilia sitophila*	Green	Orange
90	*Chrysosporium species*	Green	Orange
91	*Chrysosporium asperatum*	Green	Orange
92	*Chrysosporium merdarium*	Green	Orange
93	*Cladosporium species*	Green	Green
94	*Cladosporium cladosporioides*	Green	Orange
95	*Cladosporium herbarum*	Green	Orange
96	*Cladosporium macrocarpum*	Green	Orange
97	*Cladosporium sphaerospermum*	Green	Orange
98	*Collectotrichoum species*	Green	Green
99	*Conidiobolus species*	Green	Orange
100	*Conidiobolus coronatus*	Green	Orange
101	*Coprinus species*	Orange	Green
102	*Corynespora species*	Orange	Green
103	*Cryptococcus species*	Green	Orange
104	*Cryptococcus albidus*	Green	Orange
105	*Cryptococcus albidus var aerius*	Green	Orange
106	*Cryptococcus albidus var diffluens*	Green	Orange
107	*Cryptococcus laurentii*	Green	Orange
108	*Cryptococcus luteolus*	Green	Orange
109	*Cryptococcus terreus B*	Green	Orange
110	*Cunninghamella species*	Green	Orange
111	*Cunninghamella elegans*	Green	Orange
112	*Curvularia species*	Green	Green
113	*Curvularia geniculata*	Green	Green
114	*Curvularia lunata*	Green	Green
115	*Cylindrocarpon species*	Green	Orange
116	*Cylindrocarpon candidum*	Green	Orange
117	*Cylindrocarpon cylindroides*	Green	Orange
118	*Debaryomyces hansenii A*	Green	Orange
119	*Debaryomyces hansenii C*	Green	Orange
120	*Debaryomyces species*	Green	Orange
121	*Delitschia species*	Green	Green
122	*Dictyosporium species*	Orange	Green
123	*Dinemasporium species*	Green	Green
124	*Diplocladiella species*	Orange	Green
125	*Diplococcium species*	Green	Orange

TABLE 6.6 (Continued)

Sl. No.	Name of Fungi	B	M
126	*Diplococcium spicatum*	Green	Orange
127	*Drechslera species*	Green	Green
128	*Drechslera hawaiiensis*	Green	Orange
129	*Drechslera rostrata*	Green	Orange
130	*Emericella nidulans*	Green	Orange
131	*Emericella nivea*	Green	Orange
132	*Emericella rugulosa*	Green	Orange
133	*Endomycopsella vivi*	Green	Orange
134	*Epicoccum species*	Green	Green
135	*Epicoccum nigrum*	Green	Orange
136	*Epicoccum purpurascens*	Green	Orange
137	*Erysiphae (Powdery Mildews)*	Orange	Green
138	*Eupenicillium lapidosum*	Green	Orange
139	*Eupenicillium species*	Green	Orange
140	*Eurotium amstelodami*	Green	Orange
141	*Eurotium chevalieri*	Green	Orange
142	*Eurotium herbariorum*	Green	Orange
143	*Eurotium species*	Green	Green
144	*Exophiala jeanselmei*	Green	Orange
145	*Exophiala species*	Green	Orange
146	*Exosporium species*	Green	Green
147	*Exserohilum species*	Green	Green
148	*Fusarium species*	Green	Green
149	*Fusarium aquaeductuum*	Green	Orange
150	*Fusarium arthrosporioides*	Green	Orange
151	*Fusarium culmorum*	Green	Orange
152	*Fusarium moniliforme*	Green	Orange
153	*Fusarium oxysporum*	Green	Orange
154	*Fusarium roseum*	Green	Orange
155	*Fusarium solani*	Green	Orange
156	*Fusarium sporotrichioides*	Green	Orange
157	*Ganoderma species*	Orange	Green
158	*Geotrichum candidum*	Green	Orange
159	*Gliomastix species*	Orange	Green
160	*Gliocladium species*	Green	Orange
161	*Gliocladium viride*	Green	Orange
162	*Glomerella species*	Green	Orange
163	*Gonatobotryum apiculatum*	Green	Orange
164	*Gonatobotryum fuscum*	Green	Orange
165	*Gonatobotryum species*	Green	Orange
166	*Gonytrichum chlamydosporium*	Green	Orange
167	*Gonytrichum species*	Green	Orange
168	*Graphium species*	Green	Orange
169	*Helicomyces species*	Orange	Green
170	*Hormographiella species*	Green	Green
171	*Humicola species*	Green	Orange
172	*Humicola fuscoatra*	Green	Orange
173	*Humicola grisea*	Green	Orange
174	*Idriella lunata*	Green	Orange
175	*Idriella species*	Green	Green
176	*Lecythophora species*	Orange	Green
177	*Leptosphaeria species*	Orange	Green
178	*Leptosphaerulina species*	Orange	Green
179	*Lophiostoma species*	Orange	Green

TABLE 6.6 (Continued)

Sl. No.	Name of Fungi	B	M
180	*Massarina species*	Orange	Green
181	*Memnoniella species*	Green	Green
182	*Memnoniella echinata*	Green	Green
183	*Monodictys species*	Green	Green
184	*Microsporum species*	Green	Orange
185	*Microsporum gypseum*	Green	Orange
186	*Microsporum nanum*	Green	Orange
187	*Monilia species*	Green	Orange
188	*Monodictys species*	Green	Green
189	*Mortierella species*	Green	Orange
190	*Mucor-Rhizopus like Spores*	Orange	Green
191	*Mucor/Rhizopus species*	Orange	Green
192	*Mucor species*	Green	Orange
193	*Mucor circinelloides*	Green	Orange
194	*Mucor hiemalis*	Green	Orange
195	*Mucor hiemalis*	Green	Orange
196	*Mucor plumbeus*	Green	Orange
197	*Mucor racemosus*	Green	Orange
198	*Mycelia sterilia*	Green	Orange
199	*Mycogone species*	Green	Orange
200	*Myrothecium species*	Green	Orange
201	*Neurospora species*	Green	Orange
202	*Nigrospora species*	Green	Green
203	*Nigrospora sphaerica*	Green	Orange
204	*Oidiodendron species*	Green	Orange
205	*Oidiodendron griseum*	Green	Orange
206	*Oidiodendron tenuissimum*	Green	Orange
207	*Oidium species*	Orange	Green
208	*Oospora species*	Green	Orange
209	*Paecilomyces species*	Green	Green
210	*Paecilomyces carneus*	Green	Orange
211	*Paecilomyces farinosus*	Green	Orange
212	*Paecilomyces lilacinus*	Green	Orange
213	*Paecilomyces marquandii*	Green	Orange
214	*Paecilomyces variotii*	Green	Orange
215	*Papularia species*	Green	Green
216	*Papulaspora immersa*	Green	Orange
217	*Papulaspora species*	Green	Orange
218	*Penicillium species*	Green	Green
219	*Penicillium atrovenetum*	Green	Orange
220	*Penicillium brevicompactum*	Green	Orange
221	*Penicillium canescens*	Green	Orange
222	*Penicillium chrysogenum*	Green	Orange
223	*Penicillium citrinum*	Green	Orange
224	*Penicillium claviforme*	Green	Orange
225	*Penicillium corylophilum*	Green	Orange
226	*Penicillium daleae*	Green	Orange
227	*Penicillium decumbens*	Green	Orange
228	*Penicillium digitatum*	Green	Orange
229	*Penicillium expansum*	Green	Orange
230	*Penicillium herquei*	Green	Orange
231	*Penicillium implicatum*	Green	Orange
232	*Penicillium islandicum*	Green	Orange
233	*Penicillium italicum*	Green	Orange
234	*Penicillium janthinellum*	Green	Orange
235	*Penicillium jensenii*	Green	Orange
236	*Penicillium lanosum*	Green	Orange

TABLE 6.6 (Continued)

Sl. No.	Name of Fungi	B	M
237	*Penicillium lividum*		
238	*Penicillium nigricans*		
239	*Penicillium oxalicum*		
240	*Penicillium purpurogenum*		
241	*Penicillium restrictum*		
242	*Penicillium rubrum*		
243	*Penicillium rugulosum*		
244	*Penicillium sacculum*		
245	*Penicillium simplicissimum*		
246	*Penicillium solitum*		
247	*Penicillium spinulosum*		
248	*Penicillium steckii*		
249	*Penicillium stoloniferum*		
250	*Penicillium thomii*		
251	*Penicillium variabile*		
252	*Penicillium verrucosum*		
253	*Penicillium waksmanii*		
254	*Periconia species*		
255	*Peronospora species*		
256	*Pestalotia species*		
257	*Phialophora americana*		
258	*Phialophora richardsiae*		
259	*Phialophora species*		
260	*Phoma species*		
261	*Phoma eupyrena*		
262	*Phoma leveillei*		
263	*Pichia fluxum*		
264	*Pithomyces species*		
265	*Pithomyces chartarum*		
266	*Plectosphaerella cucumerina*		
267	*Pleiochaeta setosa*		
268	*Pleospora species*		
269	*Pleospora herbarum*		
270	*Pseudocercospora species*		
271	*Puccinia species*		
272	*Pythium species*		
273	*Rhinocladiella species*		
274	*Rhinocladiella anceps*		
275	*Rhizomucor miehei*		
276	*Rhizomucor pusillus*		
277	*Rhizopus oryzae*		
278	*Rhizopus species*		
279	*Rhizopus rhizopodiformis*		
280	*Rhizopus stolonifer*		
281	*Rhodotorula* species		
282	Rhodotorula glutinis		
283	Rhodotorula minuta		
284	Rust spores		
285	Schizosaccharomyces octosporus		
286	Scolecobasidium constrictum		
287	*Scolecobasidium* species		
288	Scolecobasidium tshawytschae		
289	*Scopulariopsis* species		

TABLE 6.6 (Continued)

Sl. No.	Name of Fungi	B	M
290	Scopulariopsis brevicaulis	Green	Orange
291	*Sepedonium* species	Green	Orange
292	*Spegazzinia* species	Green	Green
293	Spegazzinia tessarthra	Green	Orange
294	*Spondylocladiella* species	Green	Green
295	Sporidiobolus johnsonii B	Green	Orange
296	Sporangia of *Mucor-Rhizopus*	Orange	Green
297	*Sporidesmium* species	Orange	Green
298	*Sporormiella* species	Orange	Green
299	Sporothrix species	Green	Green
300	Sporothrix schenckii	Green	Orange
301	*Sporotrichum* species	Green	Orange
302	*Stachybotrys* species	Green	Green
303	*S. chartarum*	Green	Green
304	*S./Memnoniella*-Like Spores	Orange	Green
305	Staphylotrichum coccosporum	Green	Orange
306	*Stemphylium* species	Green	Green
307	Stemphylium sarciniforme	Green	Orange
308	Sterigmatomyces elviae	Green	Orange
309	Syncephalastrum species	Green	Orange
310	Syncephalastrum racemosum	Green	Orange
311	*Syncephalastrum* like spores	Orange	Green
312	*Talaromyces* species	Green	Orange
313	Talaromyces emersonii	Green	Orange
314	Talaromyces flavus	Green	Orange
315	Taeniolella species	Orange	Green
316	*Tetraploa* species	Green	Orange
317	*Torula* species	Green	Green
318	Torula herbarum	Green	Orange
319	Torulomyces lagena	Green	Orange
320	Torulopsis glabrata	Green	Orange
321	*Trichocladium* species	Green	Green
322	*Trichoderma* species	Green	Green
323	Trichoderma harzianum	Green	Orange
324	Trichoderma viride	Green	Orange
325	*Trichophyton* species	Green	Green
326	*Trichosporon* species	Green	Orange
327	Trichothecium roseum	Green	Orange
328	*Tritirachium* oryzae	Green	Orange
329	*Tritirachium* species	Green	Orange
330	*Ulocladium* species	Green	Green
331	*Ulocladium* spores	Orange	Green
332	Ulocladium botrytis	Green	Green
333	*Ustilago* species	Orange	Green
334	Ulocladium chartarum	Green	Orange
335	Venturia species	Orange	Green
336	*Verticillium* species	Green	Green
337	Verticillium alboatrum	Green	Orange
338	Wallemia sebi	Green	Orange
339	Wickerhamiella domercqiae	Green	Orange
340	*Xylaria* species	Orange	Green
341	*Yeast* species (unidentified)	Green	Green
342	*Zygophiala* species	Orange	Green

TABLE 6.6 (Continued)

Sl. No.	Name of Fungi	B	M
343	Zygorrhynchus species	Reported	Absent
344	Zygorrhynchus moelleri	Reported	Absent
345	*Zygosporium* species	Reported	Absent
346	Zygosporium gibbum	Reported	Absent
347	Zygosporium masonii	Reported	Absent
348	Ascospores (undifferentiated)	Absent	Reported
349	Basidiospores (undifferentiated)	Absent	Reported
350	Dark Fungal Hyphal Elements	Absent	Reported
351	*Dark Fungal Spore Elements*	Absent	Reported
352	*Fungal Hyphal Elements*	Absent	Reported
353	*Fungal Spore Elements*	Absent	Reported

Index:

B = Bioassay M = Microscopy

Absent (red)

Reported (green)

TABLE 6.7 Pollen Grain Type Identified From Indoor Environments

1	*Acalypha* species	16	*Carya* species
2	*Acer* species	17	*Casuarina* species
3	*Acoelorrhaphe* species	18	*Celtis* species
4	*Aesculus* species	19	*Chenopodiaceae* family
5	*Alnus* species	20	*Chenopodium* species
6	*Amaranthus* species	21	*Citrus* species
7	*Ambrosia* species	22	*Cocos* species
8	*Arecaceae* family	23	*Cornaceae* species
9	*Artemisia* species	24	*Corylus* species
10	*Asteraceae* family	25	*Cruciferae* species
11	*Baccharis* species	26	*Cupressaceae* family
12	*Betula* species	27	*Cupressus* species
13	*Betulaceae* family	28	*Cyperaceae* family
14	*Caprifoliaceae* family	29	*Daucus carota*
15	*Carex* species	30	*Empetraceae* family

TABLE 6.7 (Continued)

31	*Eschscholzia* californica	62	*Parietaria* species
32	*Eucalyptus* species	63	*Parthenocissus* species
33	*Eupatorium* species	64	*Phoenix* species
34	*Fagaceae* family	65	*Pinaceae* (Pine) family
35	*Fraxinus* species	66	*Platanus* species
36	*Ginkgo* species	67	*Poaceae* (Grass) family
37	*Hamamelidaceae* family	68	*Polygonaceae* family
38	*Hamamelis* species	69	*Populus* species
39	*Ilex* species	70	*Pseudophoenix* species
40	*Iresine* species	71	*Quercus* (Oak) species
41	*Iva* species	72	*Rhamnaceae* family
42	*Juglans* species	73	*Rhapidophyllum* species
43	*Juniperus* species	74	*Rosaceae* family
44	*Lauraceae* Family	75	*Roystonea* species
45	*Leitneria* species	76	*Rumex* species
46	*Ligustrum* species	77	*Rutaceae* (Citrus) family
47	*Liquidambar* species	78	*Sabal* (Palmetto) species
48	*Liriodendron* species	79	*Sequoia* species
49	*Lonicera* species	80	*Serenoa* species
50	*Maclura* species	81	*Taxodium* species
51	*Magnolia* species	82	*Taxus* species
52	*Melaleuca* family	83	*Thrinax* species
53	*Melilotus* species	84	*Tilia* species
54	*Mimosa* species	85	*Typha* species
55	*Moraceae* family	86	*Ulmaceae* family
56	*Morus* species	87	*Ulmus* (Elm) species
57	*Myricaceae* family	88	*Urtica* species
58	*Myrtaceae* family	89	*Viburnum* species
59	*Nyssa* species	90	*Vitaceae* (Grape) family
60	*Oleaceae* (Olive) family	91	*Xanthium* species
61	*Papaveraceae* family		

dominated over the fungi (1%) when the sample was collected by swab method with culture analysis. Airborne fungi dominated over airborne bacteria in the indoor environments based on spore trap (bio-aerosol) culture method. Bacteria (11%) dominated over the fungi (less than 1%) when water samples were collected from indoor environments and analyzed with standard microbiological culture method (Figure 6.1B). Spore trap analysis from indoor environments reveals the dominance of opaque particles (68%) over skin cell fragments (16%), others (13%), fungal elements (2%), fibers including plant trichomes (1%), insect biodetritus (less than 1%), pollen grains (less than 1%) and fiberglass fibers (less than 1%) (Figure 6.1C). Surficial evaluation for indoor entities also exhibited the prepotency of opaque particles (69%) over other particles (14%), skin cell fragments (13%), fibers including plant trichomes (3%), fungal elements (1%), fiberglass fibers (less than 1%), pollen grains (less than 1%) and insect biodetritus (less than 1%) (Figure 6.1D).

All of the samples collected from indoor environments exhibited the presence of opaque particles with a mean concentration of 33,336 counts per cubic meter (cts/m^3) and 3110 counts per centimeters squared (cts/cm^2) for air and surface, respectively (Table 6.9). Skin cell fragments (SCF) were tested positive in all the samples collected from the indoor environment; however; only 93% of the surface samples were positive for the same. The mean concentration of SCF is recorded as 7,553 cts/m^3 and 585 cts/cm^2 from air and surface, respectively. Approximately, 42% of the indoor air samples tested positive for insect biodetritus, whereas, in the case of surface samples, it is 20%. The mean concentration of insect biodetritus was 196 cts/m^3 for indoor air samples and 2 cts/cm^2 for indoor surface samples. The airborne fibers are frequently observed in spore trap samples (98%) collected from indoor air. The samples collected from the indoor surface tested positive for fibers in case of 92% samples. The mean concentration of fibers is shown in Table 6.6. We have reported that the majority of the air samples (82%) collected from indoor air tested negative for fiberglass fibers. But in the case of surface samples, 36% were found to be containing fiberglass fibers. The average concentration of these contaminants reported 5 cts/m^3 and 4 cts/cm^2, in the case of air and surface samples. Only 31% indoor air samples (spore trap method) taken from residential and commercial buildings tested positive for pollen grains with-

TABLE 6.8 Miscellaneous Particulates Identified From Indoor Environments by Light Microscopy

1	*Algae*	19	Dermatophagoides species
2	*Bird Feathers*	20	Intact Dust Mites
3	*Black Fibers*	21	Intact Insects
4	*Black Particles*	22	Magenta Fibers
5	*Blue Fibers*	23	Manmade Fibers
6	*Blue-Green Fibers*	24	Manmade Fibers, Not Pigmented
7	*Brown Fibers*	25	Myxomycetes
8	*Cysts*	26	Opaque Particles
9	*Fern Spores*	27	Orange Fibers
10	*Fiberglass Fibers*	28	Pink Fibers
11	*Gray Fibers*	29	Pink-Blue Fibers
12	*Green Fibers*	30	Plant Fibers (Trichomes)
13	*Green-Blue Fibers*	31	Purple Fibers
14	*Hair, Animal*	32	Red Fibers
15	*Hair, Human*	33	Reddish-Brown Particles
16	*Insect Biodetritus*	34	Talc-Like Particles
17	*Intact Dermatophagoides farinae*	35	Violet Fibers
18	*Dermatophagoides pteronyssinus*	36	Yellow Fibers

TABLE 6.9 Summary of Statistical Analysis

IEQ Parameter	Unit	Mean (Avg.)	Table Reference Number	
			Low	**High**
Microbiology				
Bioaerosol – Bacteria	CFU/m^3	153	175	350
Bioaerosol – Fung	CFU/m^3	322	350	700
Bulk – Bacteria	CFU/gm	49389	50,000	100,000
Bulk – Fungi	CFU/gm	73009	75,000	150,000
Swab – Bacteria	CFU	172109	170,000	340,000
Swab – Fungi	CFU	2998	3,000	6,000
Water – Bacteria	CFU/mL	37884	40,000	80,000
Water – Fungi	CFU/mL	29	30	60

TABLE 6.9 (Continued)

Spore Trap				
Opaque Particles	cts/m^3	33336	35,000	70,000
Skin Cell Fragments	cts/m^3	7553	7,500	15,000
Insect Biodetritus	cts/m^3	196	200	400
Fibers	cts/m^3	500	500	1000
Fiber Glass	cts/m^3	5	5	10
Pollen	cts/m^3	14	15	30
Fungal Elements/Spores	cts/m^3	979	1000	2,000
Other	cts/m^3	6125	6000	12000
Surface Microscopy				
Opaque Particles	cts/cm^2	3110	3000	6000
Skin Cell Fragments	cts/cm^2	585	600	1200
Insect Biodetritus	cts/cm^2	2	4	8
Fibers	cts/cm^2	120	120	240
Fiber glass	cts/cm^2	4	4	8
Pollen	cts/cm^2	3	4	8
Fungal Elements/Spores	cts/cm^2	50	50	100
Other	cts/cm^2	657	650	1300
Total Particles and Moisture				
Respirable Particles	P/l	17552	25000	50000
Moisture	%	10	0	100

out a distinct trend. Contrary to the air sample only 24% surface samples were tested positive for pollen grains without a set pattern. List of all the reported pollen grains from indoor environment is presented in Table 6.4. The mean concentration of pollen grains in indoor air samples is 14 cts/m^3 and 3 cts/cm^2 in indoor surface samples (Table 6.9). All of the indoor environmental samples tested positive for miscellaneous airborne particles. The mean concentration of these particles is given in Table 6.9.

Approximately 86% of the indoor air samples tested positive for bacteria, whereas, 89% of the samples showed the presence of fungi. However, 50% of the environmental bulk samples yielded bacterial growth and about 63% tested positive for fungi. The airborne bacterial flora in the indoor air was recurrently dominated by *Micrococcus luteus* (14%) over Gram-negative bacilli (13%), *Bacillus* species (12%), *Staphylococcus* species (12%), *Kytococcus sedentarius* (11%) and others. A list of airborne bacteria reported from the indoor environment is presented in Table 6.5. The most frequent mycroflora recovered from the indoor air was *Cladosporium cladosporioides* (30%), *Cladosporium* species (24%), *Penicillium* species (18%), Mycelia sterilia (14%) and *Penicillium brevicompactum* (13%) followed by other taxa. A complete list of fungi identified from the indoor air is given in Table 6.6. *Cladosporium* species (79%) was also recorded as the most repeatedly trapped fungi from indoor air by the spore trap method (using Air-O-cells) and examined by light microscopy (with a magnification up to 1000 times). Dematiaceous Fungal Hyphal Elements (DFH) (66%), *Aspergillus* – *Penicillium* like spores (Asp. & Pen. spores) (64%) and Ascospores (58%), followed by others were also generally reported. However, on indoor surfaces our study reveals the dominance of DFH (23%) over Dematiaceous Fungal Spore Element (DFS) (20%), Asp. & Pen. spores (12%), *Cladosporium* species (11%) and *Curvularia* species (7%), followed by others, when samples were evaluated with microscopic techniques (non-culture based). Table 6.3 shows the list of fungal taxa identified from indoor air/environment by microscopic method. It is our observation that only about 5% of the air samples were not containing any fungal structures; although, in the case of surface samples this number was observed to be about 32% when the samples were analyzed by non-cultured methods (microscopy). *Bacillus subtilis* (35%) was reported as the most common bacteria from the residential home, whereas the bacterial flora in surface samples from commercial buildings was dominated by Gram-negative bacilli (7%). The bacterial flora in commercial buildings is lower than that of the residential facilities. We have noticed that the *Cladosporium cladosporioides* dominated the surface mycroflora (culture method) both in residential as well as commercial facilities; although, they are common in occurrence in residential facilities (22%) in comparison to the commercial buildings (6%). Our observation picked out that the microbial (bacteria/fungi) flora in residential complexes is more frequent and diverse than those of commercial buildings.

Fifty-five percent of the indoor samples (dust) tested positive for dust mite (Der p 1 and Der f 1) allergens with an average concentration of 5 micrograms per gram (mg/g) of sample material. The Mite group 2 allergens have tested positive in about 55% of the samples collected from indoor environments. The mean concentration of Mite group 2 allergens were less than one μg/g. Cat allergens (Fel d 1) were recorded in 98% of the samples tested which were collected from indoor environments. The cockroach allergens were positive for Bla g 1 and Bla g 2 in 73% and 15% of the samples collected during this investigation. The mean concentration of these allergens was less than 1 units/gram.

The monitoring of temperature from indoor environments reveals that it varies between 64–86°F. Our findings suggest that approximately 97% of the indoor environments which were monitored for carbon dioxide have a level that is below 300 ppm. Only 5% of the test sites exceeded the concentration of carbon dioxide at 1,100 ppm. The overall respirable airborne particles that were reported as positive in both air and surface samples collected from indoor environments with an average concentration is 17,552 particles per liter (p/L). The moisture content of indoor environments was recorded up to 85%, with an average of 10%. However, the relative humidity varies between 28–79%.

The speciation of microorganisms (bacteria/fungi) by means of microscopy is often not possible, especially in distinguishing a proper genus and speciation in a mixed vegetation of fungal populations. This might be the reason why more appropriate fungal identification (genus and speciation) is possible by culture method and should be adapted in specific scenario where speciation of microorganism is a requirement.

Only a handful of pollen grains, biogenic and a-biogenic entities have been reported from indoor environments, which may have been influenced due to the seasonal period, habit of the dwellers or the filtration system in place within modern buildings. It is evident that using the swab method is superior than collecting a bulk sample for indoor environmental bacterial evaluation; however, the environmental bulk method is deemed more appropriate for the collection of fungal specimens rather than the swab method. This might validate that fungi is capable of growing and penetrating deep into building materials. The findings on environmental bacteria collected from indoor environmental water samples reveals that the colonization of bacteria is much faster than those of fungi under a flooding scenario. The dominance of the reported opaque particles and skin cells from air and surface samples of the indoor environment can be correlated with the hygiene of an indoor environment. Even though fibers including plant fibers, pollen grains, insect biodetritus, fiberglass fibers and other particles are often reported, both from air as well as surfaces in indoor environments, they should not be interpreted as the only parameter during the evaluation of an indoor environment. Rather, the finding of these particles may be helpful in understanding a source-causation relationship.

People spend a large part of their time each day indoors; in homes, offices, schools, healthcare facilities, or other private or public buildings. A good indoor environment is an important factor in health and hygiene; to establish this, it is essential to have information about what constitutes a good indoor environment. The management of a good indoor environment requires information on engineering design, mechanical systems, building materials, environmental conditions and other associated conditions. Building environments are complex ecosystems, with a wide variety of physiochemical, biological and environmental factors producing a complex scenario of biogenic or a-biogenic components. These components include common indoor contaminants, toxins, allergens and other living or non-living entities. Some of them are directly or indirectly associated with health and hygiene and may influence the dwellers and dwelling conditions. Monitoring of indoor environments is one of the essential mechanisms in understanding the ecology of building environments and in making recommendations for creating a healthy living. Some common building contaminants may pose a risk to health and hygiene. The indoor environment of any operating building is constructed with many building materials that are microbial nutrient sources, as well as with a myriad of potential niches artificially maintained (either by design or through building failure). During this study, it was noticed that bacteria, fungi (mold causal organisms), opaque particles, skin cell fragments, insect biodetritius, fibers, pollen grains and some other particulates of inorganic and organic nature were frequently reported as indoor contaminants both from air and surface samples. Dust collected from the indoor environment also tested positive for mite, cat, cockroach, and dog allergens.

Data generated during the study is stored in a proprietary database "Computer Assisted Air Management Program" (CAAMP). The resulting data was compiled using statistical methods to create a tiered ranking system of Low, Medium, and High concentrations to give a clear, concise measure of relative contamination in buildings for common air- and surface-borne contaminants. The data compiled for temperature, relative humidity and animal allergen concentration are adapted from other sources and were closely consistent with our findings (ANSI/ASHRAE Standard 55-2004; ANSI/ASHRAE Standard 62.1-2-2010; Platts-Mills and Deweck, 1989; Luczynska et al., 1990; Juniper et al., 1993; Custovic et al., 1997; Platts-Mills et al., 1997; Leung et al., 2003; Indoor Biotechnologies, Ltd. 2000) The average concentration of the above reported constituents is presented in Table 6.9. The data sets do not represent a systematically designed study; rather, they reflect the common contaminants of both healthy and sick buildings under prevailing environmental conditions. However, the outcome suggests that the mean (after taking the outlier top and bottom 2% or up to 10% in some cases) and the value at 67th percentile is often very similar to each other in most of the biogenic and a-biogenic factors. A consistent trend is also noticed between concentrations of reported particles with that of the percentile of samples studied. The mean value was taken as the "Low" guideline, while the "High" guideline was determined as two times the mean, or doubling of the mean. The value in between "Low" and "High" is considered as a tolerance level and referred to as "Medium." The Low, Medium and High scale, with a color scheme of GREEN, YELLOW and RED, respectively, was developed to easily interpret the severity of any issues in indoor environments for the general public Table 6.10 exhibits the reference guideline for indoor environment assessment.

These findings correlate and support a World Health Organization (WHO) report (1984), which has suggested that as many as 1/3rd of new or remodeled buildings worldwide may generate excessive complaints related to indoor air quality; in other words, this leaves 2/3rd without potential complaints. The findings of the study performed are also consistent with a US Environmental Protection Agency report (2001) that reveals that as many as 30–50% of building structures may encourage the growth of biological pollutants.

Statistical analysis on large sets of data compiled from real world samples collected in and around buildings provides a unique scaling system to determine the normal indoor environmental condition. A more detailed and systematic study is strongly suggested and recommended to further consolidate the above scaling system for investigating indoor air/environments. Nevertheless, the above listed (Table 6.10) data should be considered in order to monitor the indoor air/environment under prevailing conditions. These reference points could be helpful in evaluating the common contaminants of building both qualitatively and quantitatively. This guideline is not intended to evaluate inhabitant's health however; it is helpful for the correlation of health and exposure to individuals. These reference points should be used only as guidance. It is not recommended as a site-specific assessment tool nor is it a substitute for building diagnostic evaluation for understanding indoor air/environment quality. The indoor

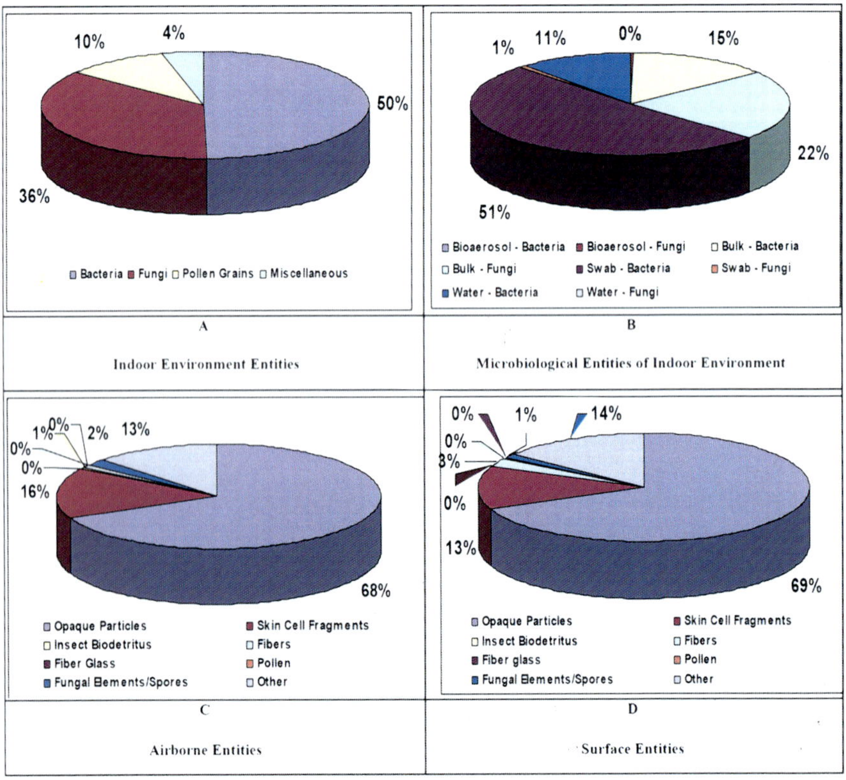

FIGURE 6.1 Comparison of Indoor Environment Entities

TABLE 6.10 IEQ Reference Points for Good Indoor Environments

	Guidelines				
Ieq Parameters	**Low**	**Moderate**	**High**	**Units**	**Source**
Comfort					
Temperature – Summer	73		> 79	°F	ANSI/ASHRAE Standard 55 (2004)
Temperature – Winter	68		>74	°F	
Relative Humidity	30-60			%	ANSI/ASHRAE Standard 62.1&2 (2010)
Carbon Dioxide	700 + Outside Air			ppm	
Microbiology					
Bioaerosol – Bacteria	175	176–349	350	CFU/m^3	EDLab COMPUTER ASSISTED AIR MANAGEMENT PROGRAM June 1994 to April 2011
Bioaerosol – Fungi	350	351–699	700	CFU/m^3	
Bulk – Bacteria	50000	50001–99999	100000	CFU/m^3	
Bulk – Fungi	75000	75001–149999	150000	CFU/m^3	
Swab – Bacteria	170000	170001–339999	340000	CFU/m^3	
Swab – Fungi	3000	3001–5999	6000	CFU/m^3	
Water – Bacteria	40000	40001–79999	80000	CFU/m^3	
Water – Fungi	30	31–59	60	CFU/m^3	
Spore Trap					
Opaque Particles	35000	35001–69999	70000	cts/m^3	
Skin Cell Fragments	7500	7501–14999	15000	cts/m^3	
Insect Biodetritus	200	201–599	400	cts/m^3	
Fibers	500	501–999	1000	cts/m^3	
Fibers – Fiberglass	5	6–9	10	cts/m^3	
Pollen	15	16–29	30	cts/m^3	
Fungal Elements	1000	1001–1999	2000	cts/m^3	
Other	6000	6001–11999	12000	cts/m^3	
Surface Microscopy					
Opaque Particles	3000	3001–5999	6000	cts/m^2	
Skin Cell Fragments	600	601–1199	1200	cts/m^2	
Insect Biodetritus	4	5–7	8	cts/m^2	
Fibers	120	121–239	240	cts/m^2	
Fibers – Fiberglass	4	5–11	12	cts/m^2	
Pollen	4	5–7	8	cts/m^2	
Fungal Elements	50	51–99	100	cts/m^2	
Other	650	651–1299	1300	cts/m^2	

TABLE 6.10 (Continued)

	Guidelines				
Ieq Parameters	**Low**	**Moderate**	**High**	**Units**	**Source**
Animal Allergens					
Dust Mites Group 1 (Der p1 + Der f1)	2	3–9	10	μg/g	Platts-Mills & Deweck (1989); Luczynska et al. (1990); Juniper et al. (1993); Leung et al. (2003)
Dust Mites Group 2	0.2	0.3–0 .9	1.0	μg/g	Custovic et al. (1997)
Cat (Fel d 1)	0.2	0.3–0 .9	1.0	μg/g	Luczynska et al. (1990); Juniper et al. (1993); Custovic et al. (1997); Leung et al. (2003)
Dog (Can f 1)	0.2	0.3–0 .9	1.0	μg/g	Luczynska et al. (1990); Juniper et al. (1993); Custovic et al. (1997); Leung et al. (2003)
Cockroach (Bla g 1)	1	1.1–7.9	8	Units/g	Custovic et al. (1997); Leung et al. (2003)
Cockroach (Bla g 2)	0.2	0.3–0.9	1	Units/g	Platts-Mills et al. (1997); Leung et al. (2003)
Particulates and Moisture					
Total Respirable Particulates	25000	25001–49999	50000	p/l	
Moisture Content	0-35	36-50	51–100	%	Tramex, USA

environment varies greatly depending upon the building engineering, geographical location, use of building and other physical and environmental conditions. Therefore, it is highly recommended that these guidelines should be carefully used in the likewise scenarios. These numbers should not be correlated directly with occupants health. These reference points provide information on many biogenic and a-biogenic agents of a closed environment. The reference guideline assists the general public, industrial hygienists, health authorities and others to identify acceptable and unacceptable levels of indoor contaminants. It is also helpful in monitoring the remedial activities. These reference points are indicative of the hygiene of indoor air/environments in terms of common building pollutants.

ACKNOWLEDGMENTS

The authors are grateful to Pure Air Control Services, Inc. for providing the company's resources to complete this chapter. We are thankful to Ms. Cyndy Bailey, Operation Manager of Pure Air Control Services for administrative support and encouragement. The authors appreciate the effort and time devoted by Mr. Francisco Aguirre, Director Building Science's division PACS for his critical knowledge sharing. We gracefully acknowledge the effort made by Mr. Rony I Iraq, EDLab's Quality Assurance Manager for reviewing manuscript and valuable contribution towards preparation of this document. We extend are thanks to Mr. Mark Weimer, Computer Programmer for assisting us in managing our Computer Assisted Air Management Program (CAAMP) and by helping in analyzing the data. We deeply appreciate all of our technicians and analysts who have helped us in data collection and laboratory evaluation of collected samples. We gratefully acknowledge all of our customers and anyone who has helped us directly or indirectly during this endeavor.

KEYWORDS

- **allergens**
- **building assessment**
- **environmental diagnostics**
- **health and hygiene**
- **indoor environments**
- **pollutant**
- **reference points and guideline**

REFERENCES

American Society of Heating, Refrigerating and Air-Conditioning Engineers, Inc. (2004). *ASHRAE STANDARD Thermal Environmental Conditions for Human Occupancy.* ANSI/ASHRAE Standard 55, 2004.

American Society of Heating, Refrigerating and Air-Conditioning Engineers, Inc. (2010). *ASHRAE STANDARD Ventilation for Acceptable Indoor Air Quality.* ANSI/ASHRAE Standard 62.1 and 62.2, 2010.

Analytical Profile Index. *API 5th Edition.* France: BIOMERIEUX S.A., 1999.

Asher, M. I., Montefort, S., Bjorksten, B., Lai CKW, Strachan, D. P., Weiland, S. K., et al. Worldwide time trends in the prevalence of symptoms of asthma, allergic rhinoconjunctivitis, and eczema in childhood; ISAAC phase one and three repeat multicountry cross-section surveys. *Lancet* 2006, 368(9537), 733–743.

Baker, D. B. Social and Organizational Factors in Office Building-Associated Illness. In, J., E. Cone and, M., J. Hodgson (Eds.), *Problem Buildings: Building-Associated Illness and the Sick Building Syndrome* Philidelphia, PA: Hanley & Belfus, Inc. 1989, pp. 607–624.

Barnett, H. L., Hunter, B. B. *Illustrated Genera of Imperfect Fungi.* St. Paul, MN: APS Press. 2003.

Bassett, I. J., Crompton, C. W., Parmelee, J. A. *An Atlas of Airborne Pollen Grains and Fungal Spores of Canada.* Ottawa, Ontario: Biosystematics Research Institute, 1978.

Beneke, E. S., Rogers, A. L. *Medical Mycology and Human Mycoses.* Belmont, CA: Star Publishing Company. Biolog, Inc. 1998, *Biolog MicrologTM Microbial Identification System 4.01C.* Hayward, CA: Biolog, Inc., 1996.

Burge, H. Health Effect of Biological Contaminants. In: B. A. Berven, R. B. Gammage (Eds.), *Indoor Air and Human Health* (pp. 171–178). Boca Raton, FL: CRS Press, 1996.

Custovic, A., Green, R., Fletcher, A., Smith, A., Pickering, C. A.C., Chapman, M. D., Woodcock, A. Aerodynamic Properties of the Major Dog Allergen Can f 1: Distribution in Homes, Concentration, and Particle Size of Allergens in the Air. *American Journal of Respiratory and Critical Care Medicine*, 1997, 155(1), 94–98.

Dillon, H. K., Heinsohn, P. A., Miller, J. D. *Field Guide for the Determination of Biological Contaminants in Environmental Samples, Second Edition.* VA: American Industrial Hygiene Association (AIHA), 2005.

Domsch, K. H., Games, W., Anderson, T. H. *Compendium of soil fungi.* Eching, Germany: IHW-Verlag, 1993.

Flannigan, B., Samson, R. A., Miller, J. D. *Microorganisms In Home and Indoor Work Environments: Diversity, Health Impacts, Investigation and Control.* Boca Raton, FL: CRC Press, 2001.

Grant Smith, E. G. *Sampling and Identifying Allergenic Pollen and Molds.* San Antonio, TX: Blewstone Press, 1990.

Gregory, P. H. *The Microbiology of the Atmosphere 2nd ed.* NY: John Wiley & Sons. 1973.

Hanlin, R. T. *Illustrated Genera of Ascomycetes Vol. I, II and III.* St. Paul, MN: APS Press, 1998.

Heseltine, E., Rosen, J., (Eds.) *WHO Guidelines for Indoor Air Quality: Dampness and Mould.* Germany: World Health Organization, Europe, 2009.

Holt, J. G., Krieg, N. R., Sneath, P. H. A., Staley, J. T., Williams, S. T. (Eds.) *Bergey's Manual of Determinative Bacteriology, 9th ed.* Philadelphia, PA: Lippincott Williams & Wilkins, 2000.

Indoor Biotechnologies, Ltd. *Rapid Test for Dust Mites*. Charlottesville, VA: INDOOR Biotechnologies, Inc., 2000.

Juniper, E. F., Guyatt, G. H., Ferrie, P. J., Griffith, L. E. Measuring Quality of Life in Asthma. *American Review of Respiratory Disease*, 1993, 147(4), 832–838.

Koneman, E. W., Allen, S. D., Janda, W. M., Schreckenberger, P. C., Winn, Jr., W. C. *Color Atlas and Text Book of Diagnostic Microbiology, 5th ed.* Philadelphia, PA: Lippincott-Raven Publishers, 1997.

Leung, D. Y.M., Sampson, H. A., Geha, R. S., Szefler, S. J. *Pediatric Allergy: Principles and Practice*. St. Louis, MO: Saunders Elsevier, 2003.

Lewis, W. H., Vinay, P., Zenger, V. E. *Airborne Allergenic Pollen of North America*. Baltimore, MD: The John Hopkins University Press, 1983.

Luczynska, C. M., Li, Y., Chapman, M. D., Platts-Mills, T. A. E. Airborne Concentrations and Particle Size Distribution of Allergen Derived from Domestic Cats (Felis domesticus). *American Review of Respiratory Disease*, 1990, 141(2), 361–367.

Macher, J., Ammann, H. A., Milton, D. K., Burge, H. A., Morey, P. R. *Bioaerosols: Assessment and Control*. Cincinnati, OH: ACGIH, 1999.

Mandrioli, P., Comtois, P., Levizzani, V. *Method in Aerobiology*. Bologna, Italy: Pitagora Editrice. Martinez, K. 2004, Biologically derived airborne contaminants in 2004 TLVs and BEIs. *American Conference of Governmental Industrial Hygienists*, 1998, 1–25.

Murray, P. R., Baron, E. J., Pfaller, M. A., Tenover, F. C., Yolken, R. H. (Eds.). *Manual of Clinical Microbiology, 7th Ed.* Washington, D.C.: ASM Press, 1995.

National Institute for Occupational Safety and Health. *NIOSH Safety and Health Topic: Indoor Environmental Quality*, 2005.

Platts-Mills, T. A. E., Deweck, A. L. Dust Mite Allergens and Asthma – A Worldwide Problem. *Journal of Allergy and Clinical Immunology*, 1989, 83(2), 416–427.

Platts-Mills, T., Vervloet, D., Thomas, W., Aalberse, R., Chapman, M. Indoor allergens and asthma: report of the Third International Workshop. *The Journal of Allergy and Clinical Immunology*, 1997, 100(6 Pt 1), S2–S24.

Sahay, R. R., Wozniak, A. L. Air Quality Guidelines Established for Microbiological Assessment of Residential and Commercial Buildings. *Mold*, June 2005, 2–5.

Sahay, R. R., Parvataneni, S. R., Barnes, R. A., Aguirre, F., Wozniak, A. L., Gasana, J., Singh, A. B. Assessment of Surficial Mold in Indoor Environments. *Indian Journal of Aerobiology*, 2008, 21(1), 13–23.

Samson, R. A., Huekstra, E. S., Frisvad, J. C. (Eds.). *Introduction to Food and Airborne Fungi, 7th ed.* Wageningen, The Netherlands: CBS, 2004.

Spicer, R., Gangoff, H. Establishing Site Specific Reference Levels for Fungi in Outdoor Air for Building Evaluation. *Journal of Occupational and Environmental Hygiene* 2005, 2(5), 257–266.

Triamex Limited. *Triamex MEP Moisture Encounter Plus*. Littleton, CO: Triamex Ltd.

US Environmental Protection Agency (EPA). *Mold Remediation in Schools and Commercial Buildings*. Washington, D.C., 2001.

World Health Organization, 2007. Indoor Air Pollution: National Burden of Disease Estimates, WHO/SDE/PHE/07.01 rev.

APPENDIX I

Record for IEQ Evaluation

Appointment:	
Date:	
Time:	

Administrative Information/Location

Company:
Contact:
Position:
Address:
City: ST: Zip:
Phone:
Cell:
Fax:
Email:
Web:

Project Location (1)

Name:
Address:
City: ST: Zip:
Contact:

Project Location (2)

Name:
Address:
City: ST: Zip:
Contact:

IEQ Related Questions

1) What are the occupant IEQ symptoms?
- ☐ Headaches ☐ Eye Irritation ☐ Lethargy
- ☐ Coughing ☐ Sneezing ☐ Fatigue
- ☐ Dizziness ☐ Tight Chest
- ☐ Flu-Like ☐ Respiratory Irritation
- ☐ Other:

2) Occupant / Illness:
- # of occupants in home / building:
- # of occupant complaints:

3) Do symptoms clear up within 2 hours after leaving bldg?
☐ Yes ☐ No

4) If no, which symptom(s) persist throughout week?

5) Is temperature and humidity under control?
☐ Yes ☐ No

Average Temp: Average Humidity:

6) Has there been a history of water or moisture intrusion?
☐ Roof ☐ Windows ☐ Plumbing ☐ Cracks

7) What have you done to date to fix IAQ concerns?

8) What is your perception of concern?

9) Is this a legal case? ☐ Yes ☐ No
Atty. Represented:

10) Has an attorney been retained?
☐ Yes ☐ No

Building Attributes

Yr. of Construction/Bldg Age	
# of Floors?	
Square Footage?	
Building Use?	☐ Office ☐ School ☐ Hospital ☐ Other
Basement?	
Operable Windows?	
Filtration Type?	
HVAC Equipment Type?	
Air Handler Type / # of units	
Ductwork Type?	
Cooling Tower?	
Special Features?	☐ Computer Room ☐ Lab ☐ Kitchen ☐ Loading Dock
Other:	
Recent Construction Renovation?	☐ Yes ☐ No
What Type?	

Comments:

Evaluation parameters

- ☐ Symptom patterns, if any
- ☐ Nature and complaints
- ☐ Design or construction issues
- ☐ Sample collection
- ☐ Type of environmental test
- ☐ Laboratory and field analysis
- ☐ Further action
- ☐ Remedial action, if any

IEQ management	Description of Source
☐ Proactive	
☐ Reactive	
☐ Sample collection	
☐ Environmental Diagnostics	
☐ Source identifie issued	
☐ Remediation requied	
☐ Post remediation verification	
☐ Legal issue	
☐ Health and Hygiene issue	
☐ Microbial proliferation	
☐ Epidemic	
☐ IEQ consultation	

PART III

POLLEN ALLERGY IN TROPICS AND TEMPERATE REGIONS

CHAPTER 7

POLLEN ALLERGY IN IRAN

MOHAMMAD-ALI ASSAREHZADEGAN

Immunology Research Center, Iran University of Medical Sciences (IUMS), Tehran, Iran

Immunology Department, School of Medicine, Iran University of Medical Sciences (IUMS), Tehran, Iran, Tel: +98-(21)-86703264, Fax: +98-21-88622652, E-mail: assarehma@gmail.com, assareh.ma@iums.ac.ir

CONTENTS

7.1 INTRODUCTION

Respiratory allergies, particularly allergic rhinitis, are the most common allergies within Iranian populations and the incidence is expected to increase (Khazaei et al., 2003; Mirsaid-Ghazi et al., 2003; Mohammadzadeh et al., 2013; Shakurnia et al., 2010). Recent studies showed that the prevalence of allergic rhinitis in Iranian children is high, and more attention must be given to the control of allergic rhinitis in Iran (Assarehzadegan et al., 2013a; Assarehzadegan et al., 2013b; Fereidouni et al., 2009;

Khazaei et al., 2003; Mohammadzadeh et al., 2013). Based on limited reports, the prevalence of respiratory allergy has been determined to be between 10 and 30% in various studies (Entezari et al., 2009; Khazaei et al., 2003; Mohammadzadeh et al., 2008; Shakurnia et al., 2010; Mohammadzadeh et al., 2013).

Aeroallergens play an important role in the pathogenesis of respiratory allergic diseases. Pollens, mites, and molds are the main sources of allergens (Assarehzadegan et al., 2013a; Assarehzadegan et al., 2013b; Entezari et al., 2009; Farhoudi et al., 2005; Fereidouni et al., 2009; Kashef et al., 2003; Khazaei et al., 2003; Mohammadzadeh et al., 2013; Mohammadzadeh et al., 2008; Shakurnia et al., 2010; Singh, 2014; Singh and Dahiya, 2002). Geographical variation in the pattern of sensitization to common aeroallergens is usually observed across different regions within a country which could be related to the type of allergens existing in those regions, and variations in the local airspora profile (Assarehzadegan et al., 2013a; Bartra et al., 2007; Beggs, 2004; Singh and Kumar, 2004; Singh and Kumar, 2003). Several studies have reported on the aeroallergen sensitivity of Iranian patients with respiratory allergies (Assarehzadegan et al., 2013a; Farrokhi et al., 2015; Fereidouni et al., 2009; Kashef et al., 2003; Teifoori et al., 2014) indicating significant variation in sensitization sources depending on the report. In spite of the different geographical localization of these studies, all results showed that pollen allergy is the most prevalent, and members of the Amaranthaceae family are important allergenic sources.

Recently, dusty storms have been occurring in the south and southwestern provinces of Iran particularly Khuzestan and Bushehr, with semitropical climates (Assarehzadegan et al., 2013a; Gheybi et al., 2014; Shahsavani et al., 2012). The major sources of these dust storms, called the Middle Eastern dust storms, are believed to be the Arabian Peninsula, Kuwait, Iraq, and parts of Iran (Gheybi et al., 2014; Shahsavani et al., 2012). Previous studies showed that the prevalence of allergic diseases was increasing in southern parts of Iran, which are closely located near the mentioned sources of the Middle Eastern dust storms in this region (Assarehzadegan et al., 2013a; Assarehzadegan et al., 2013b; Gheybi et al., 2014; Shakurnia et al., 2010). It is suggested that exposure to the chemical and biological composition of particulate matter during the Middle Eastern dust storms could be a cause of the increase in the prevalence of allergic diseases in the population living in the southern parts of Iran.

Generally, there are limited studies regarding the prevalence of sensitization to aeroallergens in different regions in Iran. Moreover, further studies are required to investigate the effect of the dust storm on hospital visits, admission frequency, respiratory allergic diseases onset and mortality in local residents.

7.2 GEOGRAPHY AND FLORA OF IRAN

7.2.1 *LOCATION*

Geographically, Iran with an area of about 1,648,000 km^2 is located in the southwest of Asia and lies approximately between 25N and 40N in latitude and between 44E and 64E in longitude. It borders the Caspian Sea, Persian Gulf, and the Gulf of Oman. Its mountains have helped to shape both the political and the economic history of the country for several centuries. The mountains enclose several broad basins, or plateaus, on which major agricultural and urban settlements are located (Aghaei et al., 2013; Heshmati, 2007).

7.2.2 *CLIMATE*

There are different climatic districts in Iran (Figure 7.1). The country's climate is mainly arid or semi-arid, except the northern coastal areas and parts of western Iran. The climate is extremely continental with hot and dry summers and very cold winters, particularly in inland areas. Apart from the coastal areas, the temperature in Iran is characterized by the relatively large annual range of about 22°C to 26°C. The rainy period in most of the country is from November to May, followed by a dry period between May and October with precipitation being rare. The average annual rainfall of the country is about 240 mm with maximum amounts in the Caspian Sea plains, Alborz and Zagros slopes with more than 1,800 and 480 mm, respectively (Heshmati, 2007).

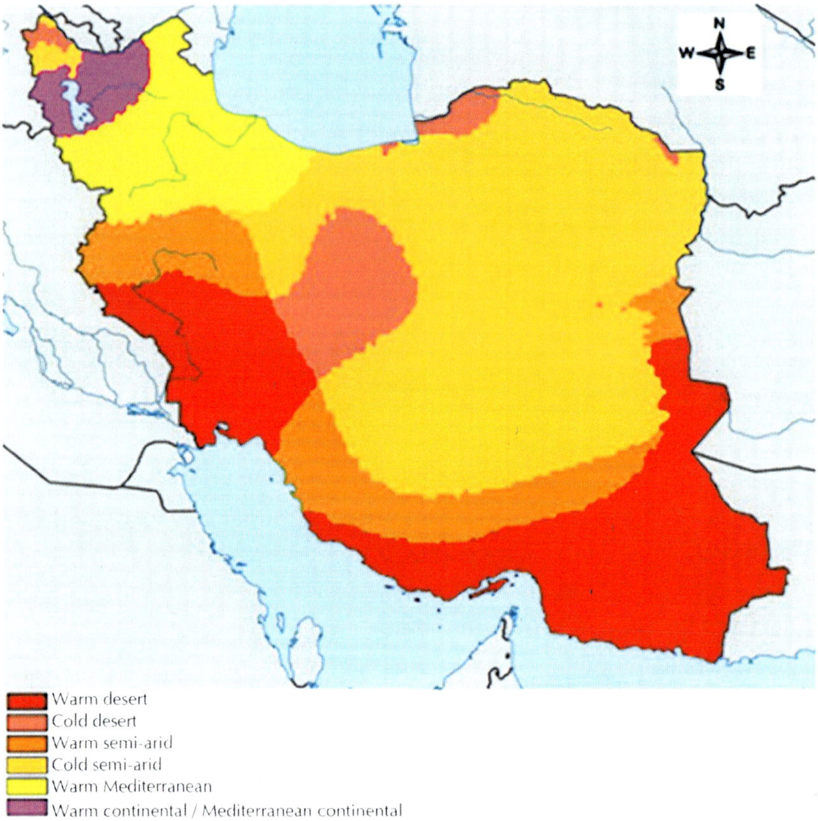

FIGURE 7.1 Climate map of Iran.

7.2.3 FLORA OF IRAN

Due to the diversity of climate, topography, and edaphic conditions, limited areas of vegetation in Iran are very different and heterogeneous (Figure 7.2). Iran hosts of 167 families of vascular plants, 1215 genera, some of them only exhibiting one species and some of them exhibiting about 800 species (Aghaei et al., 2013; Heshmati, 2007). Total taxa in Iran are about 8000 which include about 6417 species, 611 subspecies, 465 varieties, and 83 hybrids. Of these, about 1810 are endemic to Iran. With approximately six thousand recorded species of ferns and flowering plants, Iran harbors one of the richest floras of the Near Eastern countries,

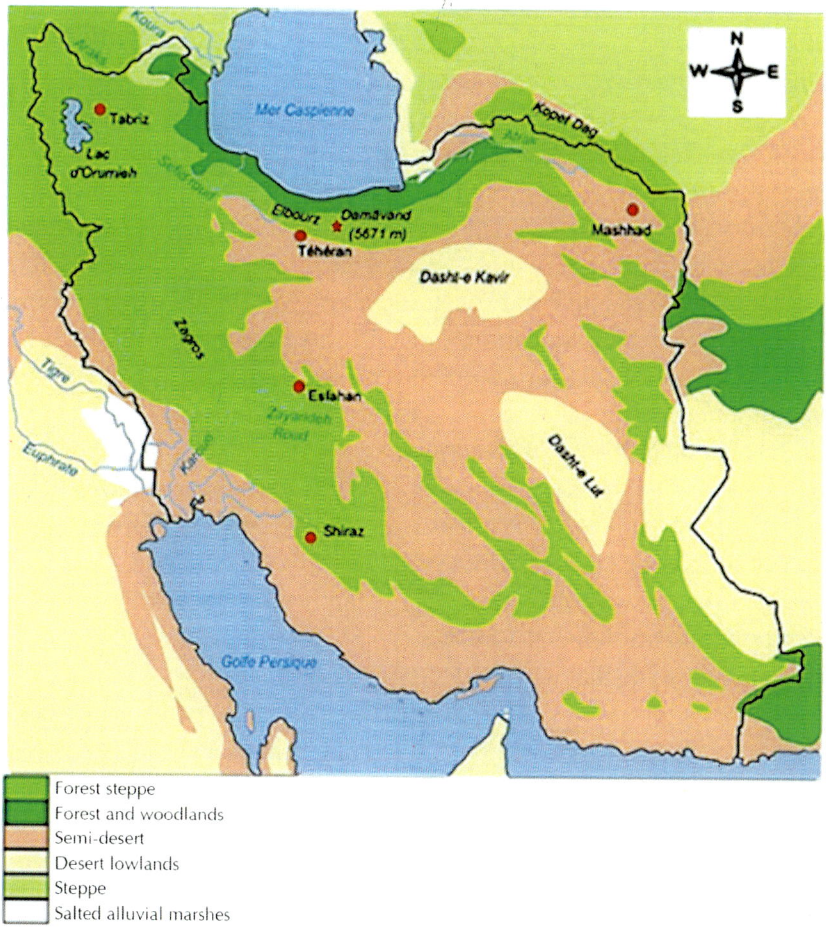

FIGURE 7.2 Biotope map of Iran.

ranging from subtropical forests to dry-adapted woodlands, dwarf shrubs and thorn cushion formations, and semi-desert shrublands (Aghaei et al., 2013; Akhani, 2003; Heshmati, 2007).

7.3 PREVALENCE OF POLLEN ALLERGY IN IRAN

There were limited systematic reviews regarding the prevalence of allergic rhinitis in Iran, but in a systematic review, the prevalence of asthma symptoms in Iran was reported to be about 13.4% (ranged from 2.7% to 35.4%) (Entezari et al., 2009). Moreover, in another systematic review and descriptive meta-analysis, the overall prevalence of allergic rhinitis in children 6–7 years of age was 11.9% and in children aged 13–14 was 21.2% (Mohammadzadeh et al., 2013). Based on these studies the prevalence of asthma and allergic rhinitis in Iran is high and the incidence of respiratory allergies has been increasing in the last few decades in keeping with the rising incidence of atopy worldwide.

In one cross-sectional study in Bushehr city, in the southwestern region of Iran, located along the coastal region on the Persian Gulf with a hot and humid climate, the results of skin prick tests (SPT) for indoor and outdoor aeroallergens among 743 patients with asthma and allergic rhinitis, showed that 73.3% of weed pollens, 73.3% for trees and 67.9% for grasses were SPT positive. The sensitivity to *Chenopodium album* and *Salsola kali* (*Russian thistle*) pollens were significantly associated with the severity of allergic rhinitis. Moreover, sensitivity to Bermuda grass and *Chenopodium album* pollens were significantly associated with the severity of asthma (Farrokhi et al., 2015).

In another study that was conducted to evaluate the prevalence of positive skin tests for various aeroallergens among allergic patients in Ahvaz, southwest Iran, 299 participants with allergic rhinitis (seasonal or perennial) were tested (Assarehzadegan et al., 2013a). Ahvaz, the largest and the capital of Khuzestan province, is located in the southwest of Iran with an approximate population of 1.4 million (census 2006). Ahvaz has a desert climate with long, extremely hot summers and mild, short winters. It is consistently one of the hottest cities in Iran, with summer temperatures regularly reaching 45°C, sometimes exceeding 50°C, with many sandstorms and dust storms common during the summer period while in winters the minimum temperature could fall to approximately +5°C. Ahvaz is also an industrial city that has petrochemical, silk textile, and sugar production and steel companies. Recently, dust storms over southwestern of Iran, particularly Ahvaz, have added an anthropogenic source of air pollution to this city. Skin prick tests using 23 common allergen extracts were performed on all patients in the above-mentioned study. Skin reaction to *Salsola kali* was the most common among the allergens (72.9%). Other prevalent weeds were *Amaranthus retroflexus* (70.9%), *Chenopo-*

dium album (67.9%), and *Kochia scoparia* (66.6%). Ninety-five percent of patients with a positive skin prick test for outdoor allergens were also sensitized to at least to one of the allergens belonging to the Amaranthaceae and Chenopodiaceae families. Among grasses pollen, the most prevalent allergens were *Poa pratensis* (54.8%) and *Cynodon dactylon* (52.5%). Moreover, among pollen of trees, the common prevalent allergens were *Prosopis juliflora* and *Fraxinus americana* (Ash) pollen with 65.9% and 52.5%, respectively.

Surprisingly, in spite of a very limited presence of Ash tree in Ahvaz or Bushehr cities, southwest Iran, the Ash pollen was a common type of sensitizing tree pollen in these studies (Assarehzadegan et al., 2013a; Farrokhi et al., 2015). This may be due to confirmed cross-reactivity between pollens of ash and olive (Guerra et al., 1995; Hemmer et al., 2000; Niederberger et al., 2002), a tree with a close taxonomical relationship tree, which is cultivated in orchards and sometimes in parks and gardens throughout the area. It is also possible that the high rate of sensitization to ash pollen is due to cross-reactivity among pollens of ash and grasses and weeds, as has been previously reported (Assarehzadegan et al., 2013a; Guerra et al., 1995; Hemmer et al., 2000; Niederberger et al., 2002).

Moreover, Forouzan et al. (2014) reported one of the biggest thunderstorm asthma epidemics in the world from Iran. This thunderstorm asthma occurred on the evening of November 2, 2013, in Ahvaz city. After the thunderstorm, the emergency departments of hospitals in Ahvaz encountered a sudden rise in the number of patients presenting with acute bronchospasm attacks. Of a total of 2000 patients who were interviewed initially, almost all patients complained of shortness of breath and had wheezing in lung auscultation. Although the mechanism of this relationship is not clear yet, different climate changes, that is, temperature drop, higher humidity, thunder and lightning, and increased wind can raise the concentration of allergen particulates, whose inhalation, particularly during seasons with high levels of allergens, intensifies asthma attacks (Forouzan et al., 2014; Girgis et al., 2000). Since not all types of storms cause asthma, meteorological and aeroallergens seem to be simultaneously involved in the development of the condition.

In order to determine the prevalence of type 1 allergy in patients with allergic disorders in Sistan-Blouchestan province, in the southeast of Iran with hot desert climate, 1286 patients during a 7-year period were studied (Khazaei et al., 2003). Although dust mites and fungal species are the predominant sensitizing allergens, pollens of grasses (43.4%), weeds (35.5%), and trees (41.3%) are major sources of allergens in the southeast of Iran. The association of these allergens with atopy suggests a role in the pathogenesis of allergic diseases in this area. The major allergenic pollens are derived from wind-pollinated plants rather than from insect-pollinated plants and the clinically important pollens vary according to location (Khazaei et al., 2003; Mothes and Valenta, 2004).

The results of a study in Mashhad city, the second largest city in Iran, located in the Northeast with a semiarid climate, hot summers, and cold winters, showed that the importance of pollen and, in particular, weed pollen as a trigger of allergic symptoms in the northeast Iran. In this study, the rate of sensitization to weeds, grasses, and trees pollen were 96%, 75% and 66%, respectively. All the four most common aeroallergens in this study were weeds (*A. retroflexus, S. kali, C. album, K. scoparia*) from the Amaranthaceae family, which are botanically close and have a high degree of cross-reactivity, possibly because of the presence of common allergenic determinants. These weeds are found throughout the world and they are highly adaptable and drought-tolerant and found on saline soils, deserts, and coasts (Fereidouni et al., 2009).

The prevalence of skin reactivity to different aeroallergens in patients with allergic rhinitis in Shiraz city, South of Iran with hot semi-arid climate, showed that pollens are the major aeroallergens responsible for allergic rhinitis in Shiraz (92.4%) (Kashef et al., 2003). Among pollens, the highest positive rate belonged to weeds (75.4% of pollens). *A. retroflexus* was positive in 62.1% of all allergic rhinitis patients in this region. The second common pollen was grass (63.9% of pollens), among which timothy grass and extract of mixed grasses were responsible for higher positive tests. The third common pollen was from allergenic trees (55.7% of pollens).

In one study in Tehran city, the capital of Iran, located north of Iran and with a semi-arid climate, 202 adult asthmatic patients were tested for specific IgE to allergens using the ImmunoCAP specific IgE assay (Teifoori et al., 2014). The results showed that pollen from allergenic plants was one of the most relevant allergen sources in the asthmatic population. The *Salsola kali* major allergen (Sal k 1) was the main cause for sensitization in the atopic patients suffering asthma. The prevalence of pollen sensitization found in this work was 37% of the total asthmatic population and 82% of the allergen-sensitized population.

Sensitization to aeroallergens among 226 allergic patients in Karaj city, located north of Iran and with cold semi-arid climate, were studied. The results showed that the most common aeroallergens were sycamore (57%), Chenopodium (53%), grasses (43%), ash (40%) and cedar (27%) (Farhoudi et al., 2005).

Several studies have reported on the aeroallergen sensitivity of Iranian patients with asthma or rhinitis (Assarehzadegan et al., 2013a; Behmanesh et al., 2010; Bemanian et al., 2012; Farhoudi et al., 2005), and they found different prevalence rates among atopic subjects and different percentages of allergen sensitization. However, all of these studies agree that pollen sensitization is the most prevalent and that Amaranthaceae, Poaceae and Fabaceae families are the most important allergenic sources.

Recent studies have shown that high incidence of respiratory allergy is related to the global increase of CO_2 and other greenhouse gasses, which leads to an increase in the production of pollens by plants, the allergenicity of pollens, increase in production period and distribution of pollens, and changes in plant pattern in areas (Clot, 2003; Damialis et al., 2007; Singh and Mathur, 2012). There is no doubt that environmental factors, especially air pollution, play an important role in increasing allergies worldwide. Nowadays, due to severe geographical and climate change, the dust storm becomes a common phenomenon in Iran (Keramat et al., 2011; Miri et al., 2007; Waness et al., 2011). To this date, there is no data available to report the effects of Middle East storms on public health particularly allergic diseases in this area. However, recently increasing evidence has been accumulated that indicated that exposure to particulate matters which contains various aeroallergens such as pollens and fungal spores, during dust storms could increase respiratory allergic diseases (Cakmak et al., 2012; Lei et al., 2004; Mari et al., 2003; Waness et al., 2011; Watanabe et al., 2011).

7.4 ALLERGENIC PLANTS IN IRAN

The geographical distribution of plants, climate, and air pollution has an important influence on their allergenic impact. Grasses, such as Bermuda grass and Kentucky bluegrass and weeds, such as Mugwort, can be found anywhere in Iran and, indeed, all over the world which is why they are very important in terms of pollen allergy. Some plants are only found in specific regions: Mesquite found mainly in the warm climate in arid and semi-arid regions of Iran; ragweed grows predominantly in Northern Iran; olive trees are found mainly in the Mediterranean climate. Consequently, allergies to the pollen of certain plants may be restricted to specific regions whereas allergies to common pollens (such as grasses) will be encountered throughout the world.

7.4.1 WEEDS

Pigweed and Russian thistle pollens are the most important sources of allergenic proteins in different parts of Iran. Although these allergenic weed pollination begins in summer and extends to late autumn, its pollinating season varies depending on the geographical location. The common allergenic weeds in Iran are listed in Table 7.1.

7.4.2 GRASSES

Grass pollen represents a major component of the airborne allergen load during the spring and summer months in most parts of the world. They are

TABLE 7.1 Common Allergenic Weeds in Iran

Family	Botanic name	Common name
Amaranthaceae	*Amaranthus retroflexus*	Pigweed
	Salsola kali	Russian thistle
	Chenopodium album	Lamb's quarters
	Kochia scoparia	Nettle
	Atriplex leucoclada	Orache
Asteraceae	*Xanthium spinosum*	Cocklebur
	Artemisia vulgaris	Mugwort
Plantaginaceae	*Plantago lancelota*	Plantain
Polygonaceae	*Rumex acetosella*	Sheep sorrel

responsible for the symptoms in the majority of allergic rhinitis patients and can also trigger asthma.

The grasses belong to the family Poaceae that is the fourth largest family of flowering plants, with more than 600 genera and 10,000 species (Esch et al., 2001; Lockey et al., 2014). There are 116 genera and 328 species of this family in different regions of Iran (Jafarpour and Manohar, 2014). The most allergenic grasses are Bermuda grass and Kentucky blue grass, which belong to the two subfamilies Chloridoideae and Pooideae, respectively (Assarehzadegan et al., 2013a; Assarehzadegan et al., 2013b; Fereidouni et al., 2009). The common allergenic grasses in Iran are listed in Table 7.2.

7.4.3 TREES

Besides weeds and grass pollens, trees are other important sources for pollen allergy. Wind-pollinated trees with heavy pollen production are the major sources of respiratory allergens (Lockey et al., 2004). The common allergenic plants in Iran are listed in Table 7.3. The most allergenic plants are Mesquite, Acacia spp. belonging to the Fabaceae family, white Ash belonging to the Oleaceae family, Sycamore belonging to the Platanaceae family and White poplar belonging to the Salicaceae family (Assarehzadegan et al., 2013a; Assarehzadegan et al., 2013b; Fereidouni et al., 2009).

TABLE 7.2 Common Allergenic Grasses in Iran

Family	Botanic name	Common name
Poaceae	*Cynodon dactylon*	Bermuda grass
	Sorghum halepense	Sorghum
	Phleum pratense	Timothy grass
	Poa pratensis	Kentucky blue grass
	Lolium perenne	Raygrass
	Dactylis glomerata	Orchard grass

TABLE 7.3 Common Allergenic Trees in Iran

Family	Botanic name	Common name
Fabaceae	*Prosopis juliflora*	Mesquite
	Acacia farnesiana	Acacia
	Albizia lebbeck	
Platanaceae	*Platanus orientalis*	Sycamore
Oleaceae	*Fraxinus excelsior*	Ash
	Olea europaea	Olive tree
Salicaceae	*Populus alba*	White poplar
Aceraceae	*Acer cappadocicum*	Maple tree
Simaroubaceae	*Ailanthus altissima*	Tree of heaven
Cupressaceae	*Cupressus sempervirens*	Cypress
Myrtaceae	*Eucalyptus camaldulensis*	Eucalyptus
Pinaceae	Pinus eldarica	Pine
Cupressaceae	*Juniperus communis*	Juniper

KEYWORDS

- **aeroallergen**
- **allergen**
- **allergy**
- **Iran**
- **pollen**
- **prevalence**

REFERENCES

Aghaei, R., Alvaninejad, S., Zolfaghari, R., Gharehlar, M. R. M., Esfahani, M. N., Shafagh, N., Rastegar, M. F., Malekiyan, R., Poria, M., Nouri, F., Flora, Life Form and Geographical Distribution of Plants in West-South Forests of Iran (Case Study: Vezg, Yasouj). *Flora,* 2013, 2–23.

Akhani, H., Notes on the flora of Iran: 3. Two new records and synopsis of the new data on Iranian Cruciferae since Flora Iranica. *Candollea,* 2003, 58(2), 369–385.

Assarehzadegan, M.-A., Shakurnia, A., Amini, A., The most common aeroallergens in a tropical region in Southwestern Iran. *World Allergy Organ J,* 2013a, 6, 7.

Assarehzadegan, M.-A., Shakurnia, A. H., Amini, A., Sensitization to common aeroallergens among asthmatic patients in a tropical region affected by dust storm. *J Med Sci,* 2013b, 13(7), 592–597.

Bartra, J., Mullol, J., Del Cuvillo, A., Davila, I., Ferrer, M., Jauregui, I., Montoro, J., Sastre, J., Valero, A., Air pollution and allergens. *J Investig Allergol Clin Immunol,* 2007, 17 Suppl 2, 3–8.

Beggs, P. J., Impacts of climate change on aeroallergens: past and future. *Clin Exp Allergy,* 2004, 34(10), 1507–1513.

Behmanesh, F., Shoja, M., Khajedaluee, M., Prevalence of aeroallergens in childhood asthma in Mashhad. *Maced J Med Sci,* 2010, 3(3), 295–298.

Bemanian, M. H., Alizadeh Korkinejad, N., Shirkhoda, S., Nabavi, M., Pourpak, Z., Assessment of sensitization to insect aeroallergens among patients with allergic rhinitis in Yazd City, Iran. *Iran J Allergy Asthma Immunol,* 2012, 11(3), 253–258.

Cakmak, S., Dales, R. E., Coates, F., Does air pollution increase the effect of aeroallergens on hospitalization for asthma? *J Allergy Clin Immunol,* 2012, 129(1), 228–231.

Clot, B. (2003), Trends in airborne pollen: An overview of 21 years of data in Neuchâtel (Switzerland). *Aerobiologia,* 19(3–4), 227–234.

Damialis, A., Halley, J., Gioulekas, D., Vokou, D., Long-term trends in atmospheric pollen levels in the city of Thessaloniki, Greece. *Atmospheric Environment,* 2007, 41(33), 7011–7021.

Entezari, A., Mehrabi, Y., Varesvazirian, M., Pourpak, Z., Moin, M., A systematic review of recent asthma symptom surveys in Iranian children. *Chron Respir Dis,* 2009, 6(2), 109–114.

Esch, R. E., Hartsell, C. J., Crenshaw, R., Jacobson, R. S., Common allergenic pollens, fungi, animals, and arthropods. *Clin Rev Allergy Immunol,* 2001, 21(2–3), 261–292.

Farhoudi, A., Razavi, A., Chavoshzadeh, Z., Heidarzadeh, M., Bemanian, M. H., Nabavi, M., Descriptive study of 226 patients with allergic rhinitis and asthma in Karaj city. *Iran J Allergy Asthma Immunol,* 2005, 4(2), 99–101.

Farrokhi, S., Gheybi, M. K., Movahed, A., Tahmasebi, R., Iranpour, D., Fatemi, A., Etemadan, R., Gooya, M., Zandi, S., Ashourinejad, H., et al., Common Aeroallergens in Patients with Asthma and Allergic Rhinitis Living in Southwestern Part of Iran: based on Skin Prick Test Reactivity. *Iran J Allergy Asthma Immunol,* 2015, 14(2), 133–138.

Fereidouni, M., Hossini, R. F., Azad, F. J., Assarehzadegan, M.-A., Varasteh, A., Skin prick test reactivity to common aeroallergens among allergic rhinitis patients in Iran. *Allergol et Immunopathol (Madr),* 2009, 37(2), 73–79.

Forouzan, A., Masoumi, K., Haddadzadeh Shoushtari, M., Idani, E., Tirandaz, F., Feli, M., Assarehzadegan, M. A., Asgari Darian, A., An overview of thunderstorm-associated asthma outbreak in southwest of Iran. *J Environ Public Health,* 2014, 504017.

Gheybi, M. K., Movahed, A. M., Dehdari, R., Amiri, S., Khazaei, H. A., Gooya, M., Dehbashi, F., Fatemi, A., Sovid, N., Hajiani, G., Tahmasebi, R., Dobaraderan, S., Assadi, M., Farrokhi, S., Dusty Air Pollution is Associated with an Increased Risk of Allergic

Diseases in Southwestern Part of Iran. *Iran J Allergy Asthma Immunol,* 2014, 13(6), 396–403.
Girgis, S. T., Marks, G. B., Downs, S. H., Kolbe, A., Car, G. N., Paton, R., Thunderstorm-associated asthma in an inland town in south-eastern Australia. Who is at risk? *Eur Respir J,* 2000, 16(1), 3–8.
Guerra, F., Galan Carmen, C., Daza, J., Miguel, R., Moreno, C., Gonzalez, J., Dominguez, E., Study of sensitivity to the pollen of *Fraxinus* spp. (Oleaceae) in Cordoba, Spain. *J Investig Allergol Clin Immunol,* 1995, 5(3), 166–170.
Hemmer, W., Focke, M., Wantke, F., Gotz, M., Jarisch, R., Ash (Fraxinus excelsior)-pollen allergy in central Europe: specific role of pollen panallergens and the major allergen of ash pollen, Fra e 1. *Allergy,* 2000, 55, 923–930.
Heshmati, G. A., Vegetation characteristics of four ecological zones of Iran. *Int J Plant Prod,* 2007, 2, 215–224.
Jafarpour, M., Manohar, M., Distribution of Poaceae, Chenopodiceae, Papaveraceae and Fumariaceae Plant Families in Fars, Iran. *Life Sci J,* 2014, 11(6), 182–193.
Kashef, S., Kashef, M. A., Eghtedari, F., prevalence of Aeroallergens in allergic Rhinitis in shiraz. *Iran J Allergy Asthma Immunol,* 2003, 2(4), 185–188.
Keramat, A., Marivani, B., Samsami, M., Climatic Change, Drought and Dust Crisis in Iran. *WASET,* 2011, 57, 10–13.
Khazaei, H. A., Hashemi, S. R., Aghamohammadi, A., Farhoudi, F., Rezaei, N., The study of type 1 allergy prevalence among people of South-East of Iran by skin prick test using common allergens. *Iran J Allergy Asthma Immunol,* 2003, 2(3), 165–168.
Lei, Y. C., Chan, C. C., Wang, P. Y., Lee, C. T., Cheng, T. J., Effects of Asian dust event particles on inflammation markers in peripheral blood and bronchoalveolar lavage in pulmonary hypertensive rats. *Environ Res,* 2004, 95(1), 71–76.
Lockey, R. F., Bukantz, S. C., Bousquet, J. *Allergens and allergen imunotherapy*, Marcel Dekker, Inc., 2004.
Lockey, R. F., Bukantz, S. C., Bousquet, J., Allegen and allergen immunotherapy. In: ESCH, R. E. (Ed.) *Grass pollen allergens.* Second ed., Marcel Dekker, Inc., 2014.
Mari, A., Schneider, P., Wally, V., Breitenbach, M., Simon-Nobbe, B., Sensitization to fungi: epidemiology, comparative skin tests, and IgE reactivity of fungal extracts. *Clin Exp Allergy,* 2003, 33(10), 1429–1438.
Miri, A., Ahmadi, H., Ghanbari, A., Moghaddamnia, A., Dust Storms Impacts on Air Pollution and Public Health under Hot and Dry Climate. *IJEE,* 2007, 1(2), 101–105.
Mirsaid-Ghazi, B., Imamzadehgan, R., Aghamohammadi, A., Darakhshan-Davari, R., Rezaei, N. (2003), Frequency of Allergic Rhinitis in School-age Children (7–18 Years) in Tehran. *Iran J Allergy Asthma Immunol,* 2(4), 181–184.
Mohammadzadeh, I., Barari-Savadkoohi, R. R. A.-N., The prevalence of allergic rhinitis in Iranian children: A systematic review and descriptive meta-analysis. *J Pediatr Rev,* 2013, 1(2), 19–24.
Mohammadzadeh, I., Ghafari, J., Savadkoohi, R. B., Tamaddoni, A., Dooki, M. R. E., Navaei, R. A., The Prevalence of asthma, allergic rhinitis and eczema in North of Iran. *Iran J Pediatr,* 2008, 18(2), 117–122.
Mothes, N., Valenta, R., Biology of tree pollen allergens. *Curr Allergy Asthma Rep,* 2004, 4(5), 384–390.

Niederberger, V., Purohit, A., Oster, J. P., Spitzauer, S., Valenta, R., Pauli, G., The allergen profile of ash (*Fraxinus excelsior*) pollen: cross-reactivity with allergens from various plant species. *Clin Exp Allergy,* 2002, 32(6), 933–941.

Shahsavani, A., Naddafi, K., Jaafarzadeh Haghighifard, N., Mesdaghinia, A., Yunesian, M., Nabizadeh, R., Arhami, M., Yarahmadi, M., Sowlat, M. H., Ghani, M., Jonidi Jafari, A., Alimohamadi, M., Motevalian, S. A., Soleimani, Z., Characterization of ionic composition of TSP and PM10 during the Middle Eastern Dust (MED) storms in Ahvaz, Iran. *Environ Monit Assess,* 2012, 184(11), 6683–6692.

Shakurnia, A. H., Assar, S., Afra, M., Latifi, M., Prevalence of asthma among schoolchildren in Ahvaz, Islamic Republic of Iran. *East Mediterr Health J,* 2010, 16(6), 651–656.

Singh, A. B., Pollen and Fungal Aeroallergens Associated with Allergy and Asthma in India. *Glob J Immunol Allerg Dis,* 2014, 2(1), 19–28.

Singh, A. B., Dahiya, P., Antigenic and allergenic properties of Amaranthus Spinosus pollen—a commonly growing weed in India. *Ann Agric Environ Med,* 2002, 9(2), 147–151.

Singh, A. B., Kumar, P., Aeroallergens in clinical practice of allergy in India—An overview. *Ann Agric Environ Med,* 2003, 10(2), 131–136.

Singh, A. B., Kumar, P., Aerial pollen diversity in India and their clinical significance in allergic diseases. *Indian J Clin Biochem,* 2004, 19(2), 190–201.

Singh, A. B., Mathur, C., An aerobiological perspective in allergy and asthma. *Asia Pac Allergy,* 2012, 2(3), 210.

Teifoori, F., Shams-Ghahfarokhi, M., Postigo, I., Razzaghi-Abyaneh, M., Eslamifar, A., Gutierrez, A., Sunen, E., Martinez, J., Identification of the main allergen sensitizers in an Iran asthmatic population by molecular diagnosis. *Allergy Asthma Clin Immunol,* 2014, 10(1), 41.

Waness, A., Abu El-Sameed, Y., Mahboub, B., Noshi, M., Al-Jahdali, H., Vats, M., Mehta, A., Respiratory disorders in the Middle East: A review. *Respiratory,* 2011, 16(5), 755–766.

Watanabe, M., Igishi, T., Burioka, N., Yamasaki, A., Kurai, J., Takeuchi, H., Sako, T., Yoshida, A., Yoneda, K., Fukuoka, Y., Nakamoto, M., Hasegawa, Y., Chikumi, H., Matsumoto, S., Minato, S., Horasaki, K., Shimizu, E., Pollen augments the influence of desert dust on symptoms of adult asthma patients. *Allergol Int,* 2011, 60(4), 517–524.

CHAPTER 8

ALLERGY: AN EMERGING EPIDEMIC IN SRI LANKA

ANURA WEERASINGHE

Fellowship of the Ceylon College of Physicians, Member of the Indian Association for Allergy Asthma and Applied Immunology, Professor of Medicine and Immunology Dr. Neville Fernando Teaching Hospital of South Asian Institute of Technology and Medicine, Sri Lanka, Professor on Assignment, Rajarata University of Sri Lanka

CONTENTS

ABSTRACT

Sri Lanka faces the dual burden of both communicable and non-communicable diseases as we see a declining trend in communicable diseases while non-communicable disease, especially allergic diseases are rising in epidemic proportions. In a hospital-based study, 8.8% of the patients reported to the outpatient department with an allergic disease, and the figure was 44% in the case of a field-based rural clinic. Airway allergic diseases, namely rhinitis and wheezing constituted a major proportion in both settings, with more rhinitis than wheezing in rural settings. The common sensitization pattern for both adults and adolescents was to house dust mite, blomia and cockroaches. Preliminary data on plant allergens shows sensitization to number plants of found in India suggesting the possibility of using allergens of Indian origin for skin prick testing. Another study looking at the possibility of hygiene hypothesis as the reason for increasing trend in allergies gave equivocal results, suggesting the need for evaluating other environmental factors. In a separate group of studies focusing on urticaria, treatable associated factors were noted in 39 % of patients. They included hypothyroidism, filaria, toxocariasis and fungal infections. A study comparing the quality of life of patients with urticaria from Australia and Sri Lanka revealed that Sri Lankan populations were more affected by wheals, and by interference on activities, mood and food choices, but were less affected by tiredness due to sleep disturbances, demonstrating environmental and cultural differences in the clinical manifestations of allergies. In conclusion, allergic diseases are rising in Sri Lanka. The commonest manifestation involves the respiratory tract and the sensitization pattern and certain clinical manifestations differ from temperate and developed countries.

8.1 INTRODUCTION

Allergy is a clinical state resulting from deranged immune mechanisms. In that situation, the immune system responds to substances in a harmful manner. Those substances – pollen, mold, animal dander, dust and dust mites, insect stings and certain foods – are known as allergens. The people who are prone to develop this kind of reactions are recognized as atopic individuals.

8.2 MECHANISM OF ALLERGY

The immune system responds to a challenge by producing antibodies in the group of IgG. However, in atopic individuals IgE is generated instead of IgG upon exposure to an allergen. IgE gets bound to mast cell, which is known as sensitization. Subsequent exposure to a similar allergen results in release of chemicals (e.g., Histamine) causing clinical manifestation (Figure 8.1).

8.3 CLINICAL MANIFESTATIONS OF ALLERGY

Wide spectrum of allergic manifestations occurs mainly due to histamine release. They could be mild to fatal ranging from running nose, abdominal pain, wheezing, hives and anaphylactic shock (Figure 8.2). Although the key chemical responsible for this is histamine, other biological products of mast cells such as derivatives of prostaglandins (e.g., leukotrine) and cytokines (e.g., interleukins four and five) contribute to the genesis of clinical signs and symptoms.

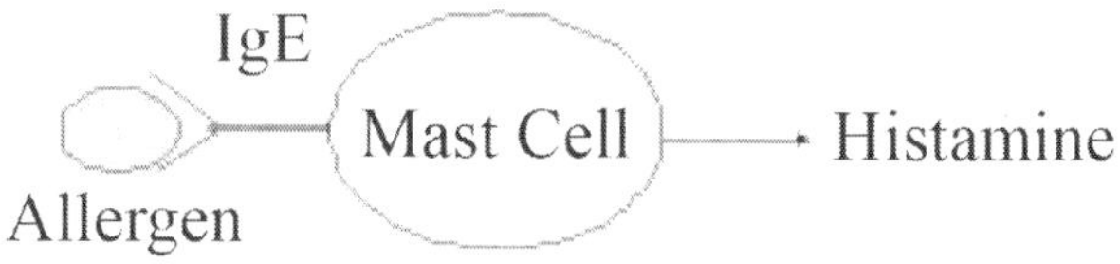

FIGURE 8.1 Release of histamine from a sensitized mast cell on encountering an allergen.

Nose → Running nose (Rhinitis)

Bronchi → Wheezing (Asthma)

Gut → Abdominal pain

Skin → Hives (Urticaria)

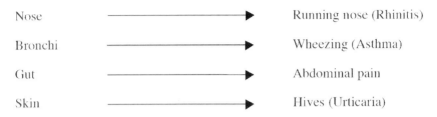

FIGURE 8.2 Clinical effects of Histamine.

8.4 GRAVITY OF THE PROBLEM

Twenty to thirty percent of the population in developed countries suffers from allergic diseases and allergy is the sixth leading cause of chronic diseases in the United States. We did descriptive cross-sectional study to find out the pattern of allergy among six thousand and eighty five patients attending the out patients department at the teaching hospital, Ragama (Weerasinghe et al., 2007). Five hundred and thirty seven of them (8.8%) were diagnosed as having an allergic disease. The majority of them (66%) were between 12 to 60 year age group and 22% were under 12 years and 12% were above 60 years. This corresponds with the normal demographic data of Sri Lanka (Figure 8.3) (Annual Health Bulletin 2003). Sixty five percent of them were female which could possibly be due to higher health seeking behavior of females.

Wheezing and rhinitis constituted the major allergic manifestations (Figure 8.4). Wheezing was the commonest allergic manifestation in all three age groups while urticaria, rhinitis and contact dermatitis were second common manifestation in less than 12 year, 12 to 60 years and over 60 year age groups. We did not find any life threatening events such as acute severe asthma and anaphylaxis as they were directly admitted to the emergency treatment unit.

Only 25% attributed the disease to an allergic reaction. Twenty five percent were found to be atopic which is comparable with the data from the developed countries. Thirty six percent has a positive family history, which was mainly maternal.

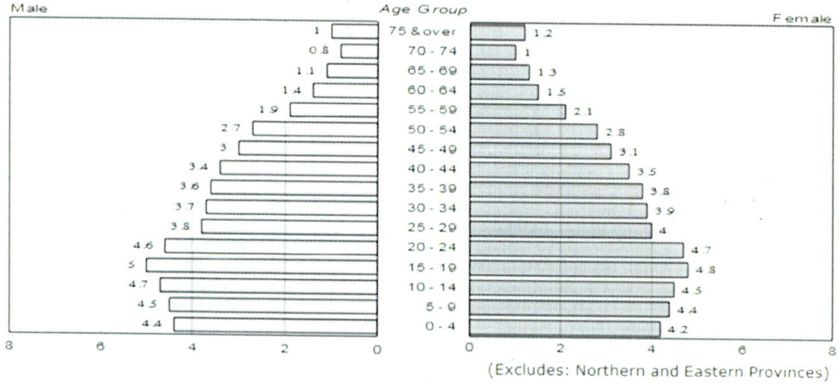

FIGURE 8.3 Normal Population distribution of Sri Lanka.
(Source: Annual Health Bulletin of Sri Lanka 2014.)

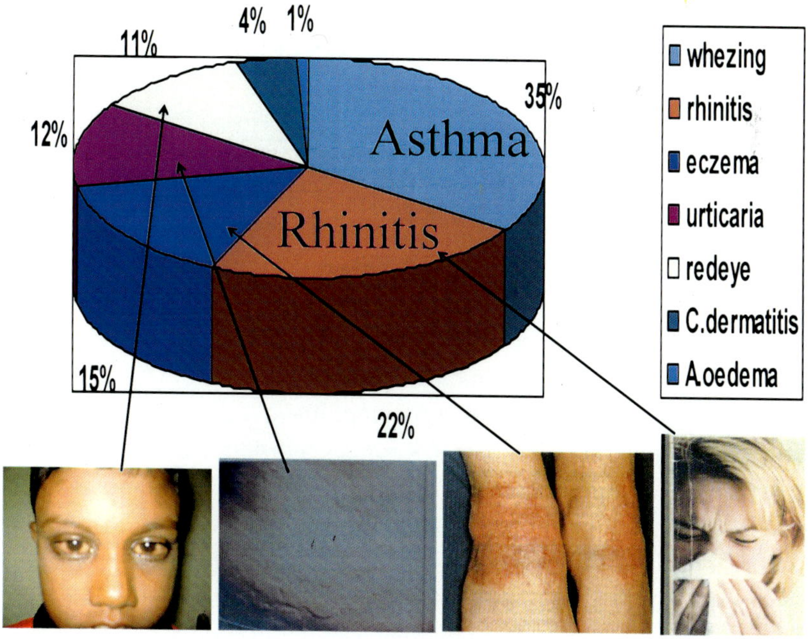

FIGURE 8.4 The prevalence of each allergic manifestation.

8.5 THE PREVALENCE OF ALLERGIC DISEASES IN RURAL SETTINGS

A descriptive cross sectional study was carried out among 588 subjects with mean age of 41±21 attending the free medical clinic at Kithulgoda in Kalutara district. Gender distribution was 60% females and 40% males. The prevalence of allergic diseases was 44.6% (n = 262). The prevalence of Bronchial Asthma/ Wheezing was 16.2% while the prevalence of Rhinitis was 22%. Other common allergies were Allergic Conjunctivitis 10.1%, Eczema 7.6%, Contact Dermatitis 3.7%, Angioedema 0.7% and anaphylaxis 0.2%.

The data from the rural setting portrait the correct picture of allergies indicating that rhinitis is the commonest allergic manifestation and they do not seek treatment at tertiary care centers. However, when they go into the stage of obstructive airway diseases, they come for treatment at hospital settings.

8.6 UNUSUAL CAUSE FOR A COMMON PRESENTATION

Myocardial infarction occurring during the course of type I hypersensitivity constitutes Kounis syndrome. We reported a case of a 38-year-old man who presented with anterior ST elevation myocardial infarction and peripheral blood eosinophilia. He had rhinitis and malaise for several days prior to presentation. There was no urticarial rash or pruritus to suggest hypersensitivity. Coronary angiogram revealed only mild plaque disease. Blood investigations revealed moderate eosinophilia and elevated IgE levels. CT of the thorax revealed fluid extravasation at multiple sites. Screening for a possible secondary cause of eosinophilia revealed hypersensitivity to multiple antigens. A diagnosis of Kounis syndrome was made. Within days of starting steroids and antihistamines, the patient's eosinophil count returned to normal with improvement of clinical picture. This case differs from classical Kounis syndrome as there was no acute allergic reaction (except atopic rhinitis). Fluid extravasation at multiple sites has not been described in previous cases (Gunawardena et al., 2015).

8.7 THE PATTERN OF ALLERGENS

The allergen which is responsible for inducing an attack of allergy differs from one person to another and from one geographical location to another. They fall into several categories such as food allergens and environmental allergens. We studied the pattern of allergen among asthmatics in Sri Lanka by skin prick test method (Weerasinghe et al., 2007).

A panel of 12 allergens extracts (Stellergen), a positive and a negative control were used. A drop of each allergen was placed over the anterior aspect of the forearm and a prick was made using a lancet. The diameter of the wheal was measure after 15 minutes. A diameter of 3 mm more than the negative control was regarded as positive (Figure 8.5).

Sixteen physician diagnosed asthmatics and sixteen non-asthmatics (control) were recruited to the study. The ethical approval was taken from the ethical review committee of the Faculty of Medicine, University of Kelaniya. The mean age of asthmatics was 39.5±15.5 years and 56% were females. The mean age of the control population was 32.4±12 years and 56% were females.

About 93% of the asthmatic group gave a positive reaction to at least one allergen while it was 75% in the non-asthmatic group. Mites (house dust mites and Blomia) and cockroaches were the main allergen responsible for bronchial asthma in Sri Lanka. It was interesting to note that cat fur dog hair and pollen were least responsible allergen in our population (Table 8.1).

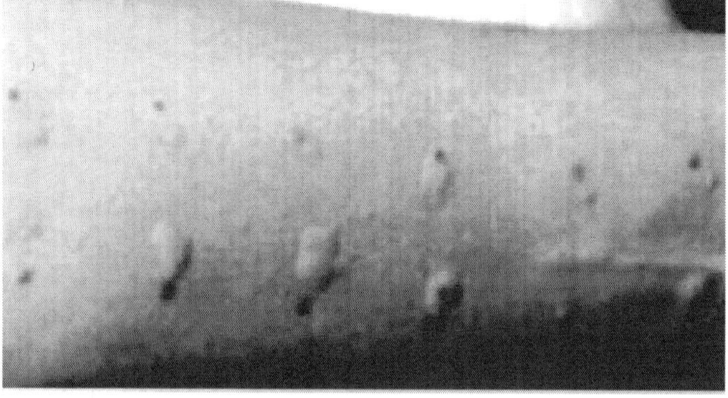

FIGURE 8.5 Skin wheal following skin prick test.

TABLE 8.1 Percentage of Skin Prick Sensitization of Asthmatics and Healthy Individuals

Asthmatics		Healthy individuals	
1.	Blomia	90%	42%
2.	House dust mite	90%	71%
3.	Cockroach	70%	57%
4.	Storage mites	60%	42%
5.	Latex	40%	28%
6.	Aspergillus	20%	71%
7.	Grass pollen	10%	42%
8.	Dog hair	10%	28%
9.	Cat fur	10%	28%
10.	Cow's milk	10%	42%
11.	Egg white	0	28%
12.	Cereals	0	14%

TABLE 8.2 The Pattern of Sensitization in a Farming Population

Allergen	%
Plant	100
Mosqitoes	83
HDM	66
Cockroches	66

TABLE 8.3 The Pattern of Plant Sensitization in a Farming Population

Scientific	Common	%
Cynodondactylon	Bermuda grass	66
Partheniumhysterophorous	White-top weed	58
Cassia siamea	Kassod tree	58
Xanthium strumarium	Cocklebur	41
Haloptelliaintergrifollia	Indian elm	41
Eucalyptus teriticonis	Forest red gum	41
Azadirachtaindica	Neem	16
Cassia fistula	Golden shower tree	8

In another study done in farmers with a mean age of 41 years at Medirigiriya Base Hospital in the north central province of Sri Lanka with the allergen produced in India provided by Dr. A. B. Singh revealed that all of them were sensitized to plant allergens (Table 8.2) and the breakdown of the plants is given in Table 8.3.

8.8 THE TREND IN ALLERGIC DISEASES

Epidemiological data shows that there is a steady rise in the incidence of allergic and autoimmune diseases with concomitant decrease in the incidence of many infectious diseases in the developed countries (Figure 8.6). In the United States the prevalence of food allergy has gone up by three fold between 1989 and 1994 and it is attributed mainly to peanuts. In Sri Lanka we face a double burden of having both communicable and non-communicable diseases. Based on the statistics from the ministry of health, asthma ranks number one according to the hospital admissions to the public sector (Annual Health Bulletin, 2003).

This rising trend of allergic diseases in more cleanly societies led the researches to think in terms of an inverse relationship between allergic diseases and improved hygienic status – the hygiene hypothesis.

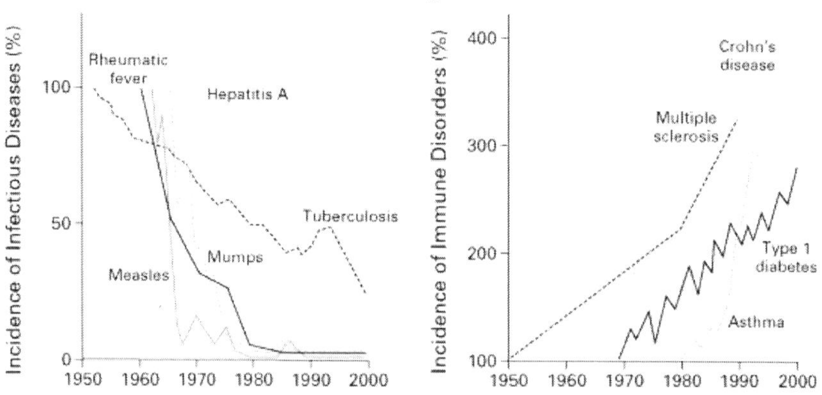

FIGURE 8.6 Inverse relation between the incidence of prototypical infectious diseases (Panel A) and the incidence of immune disorders (Panel B) from 1950 to 2000.

8.9 HYGIENE HYPOTHESIS

The increase in prevalence of allergic disorders in industrialized countries has been attributed to changes in lifestyle and the environment. Such changes have led, among others, to a lower exposure to microbes/microbial products. The hygiene hypothesis proposes that less frequent exchange of microbes may alter the immune system in such a way that upon encounter of an innocuous antigen, such as an aeroallergen, T-helper cell type (Th2) responses are readily induced, which lead to allergic disease. The hygiene hypothesis has remained controversial due to disagreement between epidemiological studies where exposure to microorganisms is not always associated with lower prevalence of allergies (Yazdandakhsh et al., 2005).

Observations in the 1970s and 1980s indicated that asthma and other allergic disorders were on the increase in industrialized countries (Nianan et al., 1992). This increase has continued, and it is estimated that about 40% of the developed countries' population are atopic (Crimi et al., 2001). The hypothesis that pollution can explain the increasing prevalence of allergic disorders was not supported by studies carried out in East and West Germany. Prevalence of allergies in East Germany, with a greater degree of pollution, was considerably lower than in West Germany (Von Mutius et al., 2005). Although there is some evidence that exposure to carbon particles might be involved in exacerbation of diseases such as asthma (Ohtani et al., 1994), it does not seem to be the only factor that has caused the recent rise in allergic diseases.

It is clear that allergen exposure and increased immunoglobin E (IgE) production is needed for the development of allergic disorders. However, whether the so-called allergic march can be explained solely by increasing exposure to allergens is questionable. In several of the studies which reported a lower prevalence of allergies in farming families (Braun-Fahrlander et al., 2002) or rural areas in developing countries (Scrivener et al., 2001). Exposure to allergens did not seem to explain the differences recorded in allergic disorders.

Another important factor that influences allergic disorders is food intake. For example, it is thought that breastfeeding (Oddy et al., 2004) and intake of 3-omega-fatty acids (Prescott et al., 2004) as well as intake of probiotics (Kalliomaki et al., 2001) might influence the expression of allergic disorders. However, there are as yet no large-scale studies of food consumption patterns that link detailed dietary intake to the prevalence of allergic disorders.

Epidemiological investigations on the increase in allergic disorders have shown that increase was not uniform across the general population with, for example, fewer allergies observed in farming communities as compared to urban environment (Riedler et al., 2001), and a considerably lower prevalence of allergic disorders is recorded in developing countries as compared to industrialized countries (ISAAC et al., 1998).

8.10 DOES HYGIENE HYPOTHESIS EXPLAIN THE RISING TREND OF ASTHMA IN SRI LANKA?

We investigated whether the rising incidence of asthma in Sri Lanka is attributed to the hygiene hypothesis (Weerasinghe et al., 2004). A house-to-house survey to detect individuals with wheezing in two remote farming villages (Galtammandiya & Siyabalagune, 2015) in Wallawaya was carried out. Five percent of the population (n = 1100) in Galtammandiya and 8% of the population (n = 355) gave a history of wheezing. This suggests that the hygiene hypothesis alone does not explain the rising incidence of asthma in Sri Lanka.

Therefore we studied the housing conditions of those villages in view of environmental factors for high prevalence of asthma in those two villages and found that the majority of them did not have good housing conditions suggesting the possibility of poor housing conditions as a predisposing factor for asthma in Sri Lanka (Table 8.4).

Sampling from the western province of Sri Lanka (Amarasekara et al., 2007). We further evaluated their total IgE levels to find out the usefulness in doing total IgE in the diagnosis of allergy in a setting of geohelminth infection (Table 8.5).

Prevalence of geohelminth infection in the study group was 15.5% and the prevalence of *Trichuristrichiura, Ascarislumbricoides,* Hookworm and Mixed infections was 14.3%, 4.2%, 0.2% and 20.3%, respectively. About 17%, 21% and 5% of the population had asthma, rhinitis and eczema, respectively.

TABLE 8.4 Housing conditions at Siyabalagune and Galthammandiya

Type of roof	Tiles	48%	Leaves (e.g., Iluk)	52%
Type of floor	Cement	22%	Clay	78%
Type of wall	Bricks	36%	Clay	64%
House area	>15x10 (sq. ft.)	25%	<15x10 (sq. ft.)	75%
Availability of separate kitchen	Yes	31%	No	63%

TABLE 8.5 Geometric Mean for total IgE in Different Groups

	Total IgE level (kU/L)
Geohelminth infected group	1039.4
Non-infected group	575*
Allergic group	933
Non-allergic group	639*p = 0.004.

8.11 ASSOCIATION OF GEOHELMINTH INFECTIONS WITH ALLERGY IN SRI LANKA

It is known that geohelminth infection is associated with allergy (Hagel et al., 1993). We investigated the prevalence of geohelminth infection and allergies in a group of 640 school children between the ages 9–11 years selected by stratified random.

It is concluded that serum total IgE concentration is strongly associated with the presence of geohelminth infection in children. Therefore, Serum total IgE level may not be a useful marker for the diagnosis of allergic diseases in children living in areas endemic to geohelminth infection.

8.12 TREATABLE ASSOCIATIONS OF URTICARIAL

We examined 113 patients with chronic urticaria presented for consultation at the Faculty of Medicine, Ragama and the private sector Institutions for a period of one year (Bandara et al., 2007). Ages ranged from 12 to 69 years (mean 38±13). 63% (n = 71) were females. Treatable association was found in 43(39%). Increased serum TSH in the range of 8–26 mU/L (11±4) was detected in 15(13%). Filarial antibodies in 10(9%), Toxocara antibodies in 14(12%) and clinical evidence of fungal infection in 3(3.5%) were found. None of them had evidence of angio-oedema or vasculitis. This study highlights the importance of investigating patients with chronic urticaria in view of treatable associations.

8.13 IMPACT OF URTICARIA ON THE QUALITY OF LIFE IN AUSTRALIAN AND SRI LANKAN POPULATION

Over a period of 6 months, patients attending Immunology clinic at Campbel Town Hospital in Sydney, Australia and at the faculty of Medicine University of Kelaniya, Sri Lanka were asked to fill out the modified chronic urticaria quality of life questionnaire (Jun et al., 2011). We obtained data from 125 patients (43 Australian vs 82 Sri Lankan). The study revealed that Sri Lankan populations were more affected by wheal, and by interference on activities, mood and food choices, but were less affected by tiredness due to sleep disturbances, demonstrating environmental and cultural differences in the clinical manifestations of allergies.

8.14 MANAGEMENT OF ALLERGY

Education, pharmacological management and immunotherapy constitute the main forms of management in allergy. Education is focused on alertness for the possibility of an allergic disease, identification of the trigger or the allergen and the avoidance of the allergen. Allergic manifestation could be an early manifestation of some internal diseases such as thyroid dysfunction, worm infestation, cancers and autoimmune diseases (Rumbyrt et al., 1995). Therefore, it is mandatory that such patients are properly investigated.

Pharmacological management includes the use of antihistamines, mast cell stabilizers and anti-inflammatory drugs The attending physician should make an attempt to use the minimum number of drugs at the lowest dosage to prevent undue side effects. Newer immunotherapeutic methods by administering allergens are aiming at curing allergy by inducing protective antibodies (IgG) and down regulating harmful immune responses.

8.15 POINTS TO NOTE

- Allergic diseases are on the rise.
- Respiratory allergic diseases constitute a major proportion of allergies.
- House dust mites and cockroaches play an important role.
- Plant allergens play an important role in farming population.
- Acquired allergy warrants investigation for a treatable underlying association.
- Allergic coronary angitis is to be considered as a cause of myocardial infarction.

KEYWORDS

- **allergic coronary angitis**
- **allergic diseases**
- **antihistamines**
- **respiratory allergic diseases**

REFERENCES

Amarasekera, N., Gunawardena, N., de Silva, N., Douglass, J., O'Hehir, R., Weerasinghe, A., Association between serum total IgE, allergic diseases and geohelminth infections in Sri Lankan Children. World Allergy Congress, 2007.

Amarasekera, N. D. D. M., Gunewardena, N. K., de Silva, N. R., Weerasinghe, A., Prevalence of childhood atopic diseases in the western province of Sri Lanka. *CMJ* 2010, 5, 5–8.

Bandara, D., Sanjeewa, B., Rathnayake, C., Weerasinghe, A., Treatable associations of urticaria. 41st Annual Academic Sessions of the Ceylon College of Physicians 2008.

Braun-Fahrlander, C., Riedler, J., Herz, U., Eder, W., Waser, M., Grize, L., Maisch, S., Carr, D., Gerlach, F., Bufe, A., Lauener, R. P., Schierl, R., Renz, H., Nowak, D., von Mutius, E., Allergy and Endotoxin Study Team. Environmental exposure to endotoxin and its relation to asthma in school-age children. *N Engl J Med* 2002, 347, 869–787.

Crimi, P., Minale, P., Tazzer, C., Zanardi, S., Ciprandi, G., Asthma and rhinitis in schoolchildren. The impact of allergic sensitization to aeroallergens. *J Invest Allergo Clin Immunol.* 2001, 11, 103–106.

Gunawardena, M. D. V. M., Weerasinghe, A., Herath, J., Amarasena, N., Myocardial infarction associated with eosinophilia and plasma extravasation at multiple sites. A variant of Kounis syndrome. *British Medical Journal* 2015, 10, 1136–1142.

Hagel, I., Lynch, N. R., Perez, M., Di Prisco, M. C., Lopez, R., Rojas, E., Modulation of the allergic reactivity of slum children by helminthic infection. *Parasite Immunolo* 1993, 15(6), 311–315.

Jun, J., Katelaris, C. H., Weerasinghe, A., Bandara, D. A., Impact of Chronic Urticaria on the quality of life in Australian and Sri Lankan populations. *Asia Pac Allergy.* 2011 Apr, 1(1), 25–29.

Kalliomaki, M., Salminen, S., Arvilommi, H., Kero, P., Koskinen, P., Isolauri, E., Probiotics in primary prevention of atopic disease, A randomized placebo-controlled trial. *Lancet.* 2001, 357, 1076–1079.

Ministry of Health Sri Lanka. Annual Health Bulletin, 2003.

Nianan, T. K., Russell, G., Respiratory symptoms and atopy in Aberdeen school-children, Evidence from two surveys 25 years apart. *BMJ.* 1992, 304, 873–875.

Oddy, W. H., Review of the effects of breastfeeding on respiratory infections, atopy and childhood asthma. *J Asthma.* 2004, 41, 605–621.

Ohtani, T., Nakagawa, S., Kurosawa, M., Mizuashi, M., Ozawa, M., Aiba, S., Cellular basis of the role of diesel exhaust particles in inducing Th2-dominant response. *J Immunol* 1994, 174, 2412–2419.

Prescott, S. L., Calder, P. C., N-3 polyunsaturated fatty acids and allergic disease. *Curr Opin Clin Nutr Metab Care.* 2004, 7, 123–129.

Riedler, J., Braun-Fahrlander, C., Eder, W., Schreuer, M., Waser, M., Maisch, S., Carr, D., Schierl, R., Nowak, D., von Mutius E ALEX Study Team. Exposure to farming in early life and development of asthma and allergy, A cross-sectional survey. *Lancet.* 2001, 358, 1129–1133.

Rumbyrt, J. S., Katz, J. L., Schocket, S. L. Resolution of chronic urticaria in thyroid autoimmunity. *J Allergy Clin Immunol* 1995, 96, 901–905.

Scrivener, S., Yamaneberhan, H., Zebenigus, M., Tilahun, D., GirmaS, Ali, S., McElroy, P., Custovic, A., Woodcock, A., Pritchard, D., Venn, A., Britton, J., Independent effects of intestinal parasite infection and domestic allergen exposure on risk of wheeze in Ethiopia, A nested case-control study. *Lancet.* 2001, 358, 1493–1499.

The International Study of Asthma and Allergies in Childhood Steering Committee. Worldwide variation in prevalence of symptoms of asthma, allergic rhinoconjunctivitis, and atopic eczema, ISAAC. *Lancet.* 1998, 351, 1225–1232.

Von Mutius, E., Martinez, F., Fritzsch, C., Nicolai, T., Roell, G., Thiemann, H. H., Prevalence of asthma and atopy in two areas of West and East Germany. *Am J Rspir Crit Care Med* 2005, 174, 358–364.

CHAPTER 9

ALLERGENIC POLLEN AND POLLEN ALLERGY IN EUROPE

GENNARO D'AMATO,[1,2] CAROLINA VITALE,[4] ALESSANDRO SANDUZZI,[2,5] ANTONIO MOLINO,[4] ALESSANDRO VATRELLA,[6] and MARIA D'AMATO[4]

[1]*Division of Respiratory and Allergic Diseases, Department of Chest Diseases, High Speciality A. Cardarelli Hospital, Napoli Italy*

[2]*University "Federico II," Medical School, Naples, Italy, E-mail: gdamatomail@gmail.com*

[3]*Division of Allergy, Department of Pediatrics Nippon Medical School, Tokyo, Japan*

[4]*First Division of Pneumology, High Speciality Hospital "V. Monaldi" and University "Federico II" Medical School Naples, Italy*

[5]*Second Division of Pneumology, High Speciality Hospital "V. Monaldi" and University "Federico II" Medical School Naples, Italy*

[6]*Department of Medicine and Surgery, University of Salerno, Via Giovanni Paolo II, 132, 84084 Fisciano SA, Italy*

CONTENTS

ABSTRACT

Aerobiological and allergological studies show that the pollen map of Europe is changing also as a result of cultural factors (e.g., importation of plants such as birch and cypress for urban parklands), greater international travel (e.g., colonization by ragweed in France, northern Italy, Austria, Hungary, etc.) and climate change. In this regard, the higher frequency of weather extremes, like thunderstorms, and increasing episodes of long-range transport of allergenic pollen represent new challenges for researchers. Furthermore, in the last few years the pathogenetic role of pollen and the interaction between pollen and air pollutants, gave new insights into the mechanisms of respiratory allergic diseases.

9.1 INTRODUCTION

Pollen allergy has a remarkable clinical impact all over Europe, and there is a body of evidence suggesting that the prevalence of respiratory allergic reactions induced by pollens in Europe has been on the increase in the past decades (D'Amato et al., 2015; D'Amato, Dal Bo et al., 1992; D'Amato et al., 1998; Burney et al., 1997; Asher et al., 2006).

The prevalence of pollen allergy is presently estimated to be up 40% and due to its associated costs is now a public health problem. Exposure to allergens represents a key factor among the environmental determinants of asthma, which include air pollution (D'Amato, Bergmann et al., 2014; D'Amato, Cecchi et al., 2014).

Since airborne-induced respiratory allergy does not recognize national frontiers, the study of pollinosis cannot be limited to national boundaries, as obviously happens with most diseases that can be prevented by avoiding exposure to the causative agent. In Europe, the main pollination period covers about half the year, from spring to autumn, and the distribution of airborne pollen taxa of allergological interest is related to five vegetational areas.

9.2 UPDATE ON ALLERGENIC POLLEN IN EUROPE

9.2.1 GRAMINEAE

Grass pollen is the major cause of pollinosis in many parts of the world (Eder et al., 2006; Friehoff, 1986). Although its frequency differs regionally, grass-induced pollinosis is the most common pollen allergy also in Europe. Upto 95% of patients allergic to grass pollen possess IgE specific for group 1 allergens and 80% for group 5 allergens, the two groups that constitute the major grass-pollen allergens (Valenta et al., 1993).

The antigens of grass pollen, like those of the other allergenic pollen grains, are rapidly released when allergen-carrying pollen comes into contact with the oral, nasal, or eye mucosa, there by inducing the appearance of hay-fever symptoms in sensitized patients. As a consequence, the concentration of airborne grass pollen influences the degree of symptoms in pollinosis patients. In London (UK), the lowest atmospheric concentration of grass pollen able to induce the appearance of hay-fever symptoms was shown to be 10–50 grains/m^3 (Davies et al., 1973). In Cardiff (Wales), 10% of pollinosis patients experienced symptoms in the presence of 10 grass-pollen grains/m^3, and again in London a concentration of more than 50 grains/m^3 induced symptoms in all pollinosis patients (Hyde 1972). In Bilbao (Spain), 100% of pollinosis patients experienced symptoms when the pollen count was above 37 grass-pollen grains/m^3 (Antepara et al., 1995). In Turku (Finland), a count of less than 30 grass-pollen grains/m^3 was significantly correlated with nasal symptoms at the start of the grass-pollen season (Rantio-Lehtimaki et al., 1991). The grass family (Gramineae) comprises more than 600 genera and over 10 000 species, of which more than 400 herbaceous, wind-pollinated plants are found in Europe (D'Amato et al., 1991). The most abundant airborne grass pollen originates from tall meadow grasses such as timothy (*Phleum pratense*), orchard grass (*Dactylis glomerata*), or meadow foxtail (*Alopecurus pratensis*). Cultivated rye (*Secale cereale*), which has remarkably high pollen production, is another potent source of allergens (Laffer et al., 1992). However, with very few exceptions, all grass-pollen types show a very high degree of cross reactivity (Martin et al., 1987; Aalberse et al.,

1992). In northern, central and eastern Europe the main grass flowering period starts at the beginning of May and finishes at the end of July. In the Mediterranean area, flowering usually starts and ends 1 month earlier (D'Amato, 1991). Pollination occurs about 2–3 weeks earlier at sea level than in mountainous regions. As mentioned above, pollen season tends to vary from year to year because of fluctuations in climatic factors, but maximum atmospheric concentration of grass pollen usually occurs 1–2 months after the start of the main flowering season. On the whole, in Europe, grass flowering notoriously peaks in June. Notwithstanding a decreased annual total grass-pollen count, probably because changes in agricultural practices and land use have led to a reduction in grasslands, the frequency of allergic sensitization to grass pollen does not seem to be decreasing (Emberlin et al., 1997). Recently Buters et al. (2015) studied the variation of the group 5 grass pollen allergen content of airborne pollen in relation to geographic location and time in season. It was observed that across Europe, the same amount of pollen released substantially different amounts of group 5 grass pollen allergen. This variation in allergen release is in addition to variations in pollen counts. Molecular aerobiology (i.e., determining allergen in ambient air) might be a valuable addition to pollen counting.

Grass allergens induce mostly nasal and conjunctival symptoms. Djukanovic et al. (1996) provided evidence that natural exposure to grass pollen may exacerbate asthma, and so, induce an inflammatory response involving T cells, mast cells and eosinophils.

9.2.2 TREES

The most allergenic tree pollen is produced by birch (Betula) in north, central, and eastern Europe, and by Olive (*Olea europaea*) as also cypress (Cupressus) in the Mediterranean regions.

9.2.2.1 Fagales

As in the grass family, there are high levels of allergenic cross-reactivity between the representative plants of the genera of the order Fagales (Ebner et al., 1995). This order comprises three families: Betulaceae, including the genera Betula (birch) and Alnus (alder); Corylaceae, including the genera Corylus (hazel), Carpinus (hornbeam), and Ostrya (hopbeam); Fagaceae, including the genera Quercus (oak), Fagus (beech), and Castanea (sweet chestnut). Birch is the major pollen-allergen-producing tree in northern Europe (Eriksson et al., 1996). In western Europe, the main flowering period usually starts at the end of March, and in central and eastern Europe, from the beginning to mid-April. Going northward, the flowering season starts, depending on the latitude, from late April to late May (northern Europe) (D'Amato, 1991; Spieksma, 1991). Pollen values peak 1–3 weeks after the start of the season. The duration of the main season is remarkably dependent on temperature and thus varies from 2 to as much as 8 weeks. Far shorter or longer periods, with yearly alternating low and high pollen production, has been observed in various European regions (Spieksma et al., 1995). The Corylaceae trees, hazel and alder, are the first (December–April) to shed pollen in the outdoor air in Europe, followed by birch, hornbeam and hop hornbeam.

As a consequence of this early pollination and of allergenic cross-reactivity, hazel and alder can act as primers of allergic sensitization to betulaceae pollen allergens, so that clinical symptoms become more marked during the birch-pollen season. Similarly, the onset of the oak season in spring, shortly before the beech-pollen season, which is usually quite mild, can prolong the birch season in western, central, and eastern Europe. Sweet-chestnut pollen appear in June and July in western and central Europe in the mountainous areas of southern Europe. In the central Alpine regions, the highest concentrations of Alnus viridis pollen are found at the end of May and in early June (D'Amato, 1991; Spieksma, 1991). Birch, followed by alder and hazel, has the greatest allergenic potency in this group of allergenic trees. In Europe, the percentage of subjects with a positivity skin prick test to birch allergens range from 5% in The Netherlands to 54% in Zurich (Switzerland) (Table 9.5). In recent years, the popularity of Betula as ornamental plant loved by architects, particularly in northern Italy, has caused a significant increase in allergic sensitization to this allergen (Spieksma et al., 1991; Ortolani et al., 1991; Troise et al., 1996; Prandini et al., 1991). In a large study of cross sensitization between allergenic plants in adult patients with asthma or rhinitis, Eriksson and Holmen

(1996) found that sensitization to birch pollen allergens was frequently associated with other allergens, that it induced mostly nasal symptoms, and that respiratory symptoms started at about 30 years of age. The Eriksson and Holmen study did not confirm the report by Bjorksten et al. (1980) of a correlation between the birth during the months of Betula flowering and the subsequent development of respiratory allergy to the same pollen.

9.2.2.2 Oleaceae

Olive (*Olea europaea*) pollen is considered as one of the most important causes of respiratory allergic disease in the Mediterranean region. In Spain, southern Italy, Greece and Turkey, olive pollen is an important cause of pollinosis (Florido et al., 1999; D'Amato et al., 1989; Gioulekas et al., 2004; Kirmaz et al., 2005; Liccardi et al., 1996). The main pollen season is from April to June. The frequency of olive-induced pollinosis is increasing as a consequence of improved diagnostic procedures and as a result of changes in farming practices (Liccardi et al., 1996). It is of interest that ecoenvironment and crop management are factors able to induce allergological changes, in different varieties or cultivars of olive tree (Conde et al., 2002).

The lowest prevalence among pollinosis patients in Europe of sensitization to O. europaea, as estimated by the skin prick test, is 1.1% in Sweden, and the highest is 53.9% in Switzerland. *Olea europaea* pollinosis is critically characterized by rhinoconjunctival symptomatology than bronchial asthma. Moreover, polysensitization to olive pollen is more frequent than monosensitization (Liccardi et al., 1996; Guerra et al., 1992). In sourthern Italy, the frequency of positivity to Olea pollen allergens among all skin prick test-positive patients is 13.49% in adults and 8.33% in children (D'Amato & Spieksma, 1990). In pollinosis patients of the Naples area, monosensitization to olive was identified in only 1.33% of children and in 2.28% in adults; in all the remaining patients, sensitization to olive pollen was associated with other allergens, mainly derived from pollen grains (Liccardi et al., 1996). Interestingly, children and adults with monosensitization to olive and living in the Naples area are frequently affected by year-long symptoms that usually do not increase during the olive-pollen season. A similar finding has recently described in Spanish (Bjorksten et al., 1980) and Turkish patients (Kirmaz et al., 2005). Pollen from other species of the Oleaceae family, e.g., Fraxinus excelsior and Ligustrum vulgare rarely induce allergic respiratory symptoms (Hemmer et al., 2000, Carinanos et al., 2002).

9.2.2.3 Cupressaceae

The genus Cupressus is widely spread in Mediterranean area, where the most common species are *C. sempervirens*, *C. arizonica*, *C. macrocarpa* and *C. lusitanica*. Cypress releases an enormous amount of anemophilous pollen and it has been recognized to be responsible for a large part of total annual amount of airborne pollen in several Mediterranean areas. In the city of Cordoba, southern Spain, Cupressaceae pollen represents at least 30% of the total pollen count during the winter season (Carinanos et al., 2002), whereas in Italy and Albania it reaches 20–40% of annual pollen rain (Ruiz et al., 1988; Mandrioli et al., 2000; Priftanji et al., 2000). In last decades, Cupressaceae pollen has been identified as source of increasing pollinosis in Mediterranean countries such as France (Charpin et al., 2000; Calleja et al., 2003), Israel (Geller-Bernstein et al., 2000), Spain (Subiza et al., 1995) and Italy (Italian Association of Aerobiology, 2002; Papa et al., 2001). It is also responsible for winter pollinosis in a period of the year when no other allergenic plants are flowering (Caramiello et al., 1991; D'Amato et al., 1992). The period of cypress pollination may last more than 1 month, because of the gradual mechanism of microsporophyllous maturation (from the bottom to the top of the flower) and furthermore because pollination shows a high variability from year to year, depending on meteorological factors (Hidalgo et al., 2003). Calleja and Farrera (2003) showed that the dates of maximum pollination differed by up to 29 days and precocity in pollination seems to run parallel to ongoing global warming. This phenological characteristic make cypress allergy tricky to treat, due to difficulties in identifying start and duration of pollen season. These observations prompted new studies addressed to set up phenological models able to forecast time and severity of cypress pollen seasons (Torriggiani et al., 2007). It should be noted that a high cross-reactivity exists within cupressacace family (Cupressus, Juniperus and Cryptomeria) and between cupressacae and Taxacee (Mari et al., 1996; Barletta et al., 1996; Caballero et al., 1996; Pharm et al., 1994), which have quite different pollination seasons, overlapping or preceding the cypress pollination period. This observation is of clinical importance, where cross-reacting and earlier flowering plants (*C. arizonica* is one of the most spread in several European areas) are well represented. The sensitization rate to Cupressaceae pollen antigens is highly variable depending on the population under study and on the exposure level. While in the general population it goes from 2.4 to 9.6%, the rate is much higher in pollinosis patients, being over 30% in some areas (Charpin, 2005). The increasing epidemiological impact of pollinosis induced by Cupressaceae plants is probable related to several factors: an increasing use of *C. arizonica* extracts (easier to prepare and chemically more stable specially in solution than *C. sempervirens* extracts (Ariano et al., 2001) and a better awareness to this allergy, that could be mistaken for viral infections due to its late winter occurrence.

A large French study showed that cypress allergy is characterized by higher prevalence of dry cough and a lower prevalence of conjunctivitis compared with grass pollen allergy (Charpin et al., 2003). However, asthma prevalence in sensitized patients seems to be very low (Agea et al., 2002). The latest clinical trials on efficacy of immunotherapy in cypress allergy, using standardized extracts, have led to significant improvements, using both the subcutaneous and the sublingual routes. However, the effects of specific immunotherapy should be further exploited (Charpin, 2005).

9.2.3 WEED URTICACEAE

Parietaria is the main allergenic genus of the Urticaceae (nettle) family. The most important species are *Parietaria judaica* and *Parietaria officinalis*. The major allergens of both species are small glycoproteins with molecular weights ranging between 10 and 14 kDa, with high cross-reactivity (Colombo et al., 2003). Recent findings showed that *P. judaica* pollen contains an aminopeptidase, which is able to disrupt epithelium barrier, enhancing the delivery of allergenic protein to dendritic cells (Cortes et al., 2006) *Parietaria judaica* grows mainly in coastal Mediterranean areas, but has also been found in the UK (Holgate et al., 1988). Parietaria pollen varies greatly according to the geographic area. Pollinosis caused by Parietaria is less frequent before the age of 10 years (D'Amato et al., 1983; Liccardi et al., 1992; Liccardi et al., 1996). The highest frequency of pollinosis caused by Parietaria occurs in subjects aged 10–30 years and is more frequent in population of coastal towns than in those living in rural, noncoastal areas. In Europe (Cvitanovic et al., 1986; D'Amato, Ruffili et al., 1991) and the USA (Kaufman, 1990), there is a greater frequency of reactivity to Parietaria. The extraordinarily long persistence in the atmosphere of Parietaria pollen in the Mediterranean area is responsible for a multi-seasonal symptomatology (Colombo et al., 1998). In some areas, like southern Italy, some patients have year-long symptoms.

In a retrospective cohort study, sensitization to *Parietaria judaica* markedly increased the risk of developing asthma, while no associations were shown for sensitization to house dust mite and other pollens (Polosa et al., 2005). Bronchial asthma or its equivalents, such as cough (severe in some cases) associated with rhinoconjunctivitis, is present in 52% of the monosensitized Parietaria patients in central and southern Italy, reaching a peak of 60% in Naples and Rome (D'Amato, Ruffili et al., 1992). Although the correlation was not significant, a higher number of Parietaria-monosensitized subjects living in the Naples area were born during the Parietaria pollen season and underwent an early exposure to the allergens released by this pollen (Liccardi, Visone et al., 1996). The frequency of positivity skin prick test to various types of pollen grains (particularly those of *Parietaria* spp.) implicated in pollinosis symptoms in atopic subjects has increased in the Naples area during the last 15 years (D'Amato, Ruffili et al., 1992). Severe oral allergy syndrome after the ingestion of pistachio nuts was described in two patients with monosensitization to Parietaria and a slight degree of cross-reactivity between Parietaria allergens and the pistachio nut was detected in both cases (Liccardi et al., 1999). The treatment of Parietaria hay fever is often a frustrating experience for both patients and clinicians because of the prolonged persistance of this pollen in the atmosphere. However, an increasing body of evidence supports use of sublingual specific immunotherapy for subjects with symptoms due to Parietaria pollen (Polosa et al., 2004; Pajno et al., 2004). The identification of a hypoallergenic fragment of Par j 2, able to upregulate natural immunity receptors (Toll-like receptors) and increase INFc might disclose new perspectives for immunotherapy (Pace et al., 2006).

9.2.3.1 Compositae

The Compositae (Asteraceae), is one of the largest plant families with almost 20,000 species. Ragweed (Ambrosia) and mugwort (Artemisia) are the most involved in pollenosis. The most common species of Artemisia are A. vulgaris (mugwort), which grows throughout Europe, *A. Annua* and *A. verlotorum*, which grow mainly in southern Europe. Mugwort is present in both urban and suburban areas. It flowers from late July to the end of August in northwest Europe. The genus Ambrosia (A.), which includes both A. artemisiifolia (short or common ragweed) and A. trifida (giant ragweed) has long been recognized as a significant cause of allergic rhinitis. A large random skin test survey demonstrated that 10% of the US population was ragweed sensitive (Gergen et al., 1987). More recently, Ambrosia pollen levels were significantly related to asthma and rhinitis in a study based on a symptoms diary and peak expiratory flow rates (Newhouse et al., 2004). The pollen of *A.artemisiifolia* is produced in enormous amounts and one single plant alone may produce millions of pollen grains. Since the pollen grains are small (18–22 lm) they are often involved in episodes of long distance transport (Mandrioli et al., 1998) The most representative species, *A.artemisiifolia*, was first signaled in Europe in 1860 (Touraine et al., 1966) and ragweed pollen is increasingly important from an allergological point of view in parts of Central and Eastern Europe. Its distribution covers the area at medium latitude characterized by continental climate and it started its expansion from Hungary, the most ragweed-polluted country (Makra et al., 2004), Croatia (Peternel et al., 2006), certain areas of France (Laiidi et al., 2003) and Italy (Ridolo et al., 2006). Furthermore, ragweed has been also detected in Bulgaria (Yankova et al., 2000), Austria (Jager et al., 2000), Switzerland (Taramarcaz et al., 2005), Czech Republic (Rybncek et al., 2001), Slovak Republic (Bartkova et al., 2003), Sweden, (Dahl et al., 1999) and Poland (Piotrowska et al., 2006). Ragweed and mugwort have nearly identical flowering seasonal periods and high degree of cross-reactivity. In a recent study was shown that patients with both ragweed and mugwort IgE reactivity on RAST and/or skin prick tests are actually co-sensitized. This observation is of clinical relevance especially in patients for whom specific immunotherapy is indicated (Asero et al., 2006). A large cross-reactivity between short and giant ragweed is also well known. However, recent data suggest the two plants are not allergenically equivalent. Due to this, in subjects sensitized to ragweed, diagnosis and eventually immunotherapy should be performed according to type of pollen species present in that specific area (Asero et al., 2005).

9.2.4 EMERGING POLLENS

In the last decades, the increased use of ornamental plants in parks and gardens, public and work places and houses provided new sources of aeroallergens. The first report of weeping fig (*Ficus benjamina*) allergy in plants keepers was published about 25 years ago (Axelsson et al., 1987). Since then, several cases were also reported among general population and non-atopic subjects (Schmid et al., 1993; Axelsson, 1995) and in a series of 2662 patients with a positive skin test to any aeroallergens the 2.5% reacted with *Ficus benjamina* (Hemmer et al., 2004). Findings showed the source of allergen to be in sap. (Kortekangas-Savolainen et al., 2006). A Ficus-fruit (i.e., fig and other tropical fruits) syndrome was identified in which *Ficus benjamina* latex is the cross-reacting allergen (Chen et al., 2000). In a population of 59 subjects with persistent rhinitis and exposed to indoor decorative plants in the domestic environment 78% were sensitized to at least one ornamental plant (weeping fig, yucca, ivy, palm tree and geranium) (Mahillon et al., 2006). Authors suggest indoor plants have to be considered as potential allergens causing perennial rhinitis and they should be included into the standard skin prick test panel in exposed patients. Recently different studies observed emerging pollen allergy (Rodriguez et al., 2007; Villalba et al., 2014; Velasco-Jiménez et al., 2014).

The Amaranthaceae, common weeds, have become increasingly relevant as triggers of allergy in the last few years, as they are able to rapidly colonize salty and arid soils in extensive desert areas. The genera Chenopodium, Salsola, and Amaranthus are the major sources of pollinosis from the Amaranthaceae family in southern Europe, western United States, and semidesert areas of Saudi Arabia, Kuwait, and Iran. In Spain, Salsola kali is one of the most relevant causes of pollinosis, together with olive and grasses. To date, 9 Amaranthaceaepollen allergens from Chenopodium album, Salsola kali, and Amaranthus retroflexus have been described and are listed in the International Union of Immunological Societies allergen nomenclature database. The major allergens of Amaranthaceae pollenbelong to the pectin methylesterase, Ole e 1-like, and profilin panallergen families, whereas the minor allergens belong to the cobalamin-independent methionine synthase and polcalcin panallergen families (Villalba et al., 2014).

Pistacia species grow in temperate regions, and are widespread in the Mediterranean area. Airborne pollen from Pistacia species, recorded in some Spanish provinces, is regarded by some authors as potentially allergenic, and therefore should be of particular interest, given that these species are actually being introduced as ornamentals in parks and gardens. A recent study analyzed daily and seasonal Pistacia airborne pollen counts in Córdoba city, in parallel with field flowering phenology data. Pistacia pollen counts in Córdoba were low, but sufficient to identify seasonal and daily patterns. The number of trees introduced as ornamentals should be carefully controlled, since widespread planting could increase airborne pollen levels (Velasco-Jiménez et al., 2014).

9.3 CONCLUDING REMARKS

The allergenic content of the atmosphere varies according to climate, geography and vegetation. Data on the presence and prevalence of allergenic airborne pollens, obtained from both aerobiological studies and allergological investigations, make it possible to design pollen calendars with the approximate flowering period of the plants in the sampling area. In this way, even though pollen production and dispersal from year to year depend on the patterns of preseason weather and on the conditions prevailing at the time of anthesis, it is usually possible to forecast the chances of encountering high atmospheric allergenic pollen concentrations in different areas. Aerobiological and allergological studies show that the pollen map of Europe is changing also as a result of cultural factors (e.g., importation of plants such as birch and cypress for urban parklands), greater international travel (e.g., colonization by ragweed in France, northern Italy, Austria, Hungary, etc.) and climate change.

KEYWORDS

- **Gramineae**
- **pollen allergy**
- **trees**
- **weed**

REFERENCES

Aalberse, R. C., Clinically significant cross-reactivities among allergens. *Int Arch Allergy Immuno* 1992, 99, 261–264.

Agea, E., Bistoni, O., Russano, A., Corazzi, L., Minelli, L., Bassotti, G., et al., The biology of cypress allergy. *Allergy*, 2002, 959–960.

Antepara, I., Fernandez, J. C., Gamboa, P., Jaurefui, I., Miguel, F., Pollen allergy in the Bilbao area (European Atlantic seaboard climate): pollination forecasting methods. *Clin Exp Allergy* 1995, 25, 133–140.

Ariano, R., Spadolini, I., Panzani, R. C., Efficacy of sublingual specific immunotherapy in Cupressaceae allergy using an extract of *Cupressus arizonica. A Double Blind Study Allergol Immunopathol (Madr)* 2001, 29, 238–244.

Asero, R., Weber, B., Mistrello, G., Amato, S., Madonini, E., Cromwell, O., Giant ragweed specific immunotherapy is not effective in a proportion of patients sensitized to short ragweed: Analysis of the allergenic differences between short and giant ragweed. *J Allergy Clin Immunol* 2005, 116, 1036–1041.

Asero, R., Wopfner, N., Gruber, P., Gadermeier, G., Ferreira, F., Artemisia and Ambrosia hypersensitivity: co-sensitization or co-recognition? *Clin Exp Allergy* 2006, 36, 658–665.

Asher, M. I., Montefort, S., BjorkstenB, Lai CKW, Strachan, D. P., Weiland SK et al. Worldwide time trends in the prevalence of symptoms of asthma, allergic rhinoconjunctivitis, and eczema in childhood: ISAAC Phases One and Three repeat multicountry cross-sectional surveys. *Lancet* 2006, 368, 733–743.

Axelsson, I. G., Allergy to *Ficus benjamina* in nonatopic subjects. *Allergy* 1995, 50, 284–285.

Axelsson, I. G., Johansson, S. G., Zetterstrom, O., Occupational allergy to weeping fig in plant keepers. *Allergy* 1987, 42, 161–167.

Barletta, B., Afferni, C., Tinghino, R., et al. Cross reactivity between *Cupressus arizonica* and *Cupressus sempervirens* pollen extracts. *J Allergy Clin Immunol* 1996, 98, 797–804.

Bartkova -Scevkova, J., The influence of temperature, relative humidity and rainfall on the occurence of pollen allergens (Betula, Poaceae, Ambrosia artemisiifolia) in the atmosphere of Bratislava (Slovakia). *Int J Biometeorol* 2003, 48, 1–5.

Bjorksten, F., Suoniemi, I., Koski, V., Neonatal birch pollen contact and subsequent allergy to birch pollen. *Clin Allergy* 1980, 10, 585–591.

Burney PGJ, Malmberg, E., Chinn, S., Jarvis, D., Luczynska, C., Lai, E., The distribution of total and specific serum IgE in the European community respiratory health survey. *J Allergy Clin Immunol* 1997, 99, 314–322.

Buters, J., Prank, M., Sofiev, M., et al. Variation of the group 5 grass pollen allergen content of airborne pollen in relation to geographic location and time in season *J Allergy Clin Immunol* 2015 Jul, 136(1), 87-95.e6. doi: 10.1016/ j.jaci.2015.01.049. Epub 2015 May 617, 18

Caballero, T., Romualdo, L., Crespo, J. F., Pascual, C., Munoz-Pereira, M., MartinEsteban, M., Cupressaceae pollinosis in the Madrid area. *Clin Exp Allergy* 1996, 26, 197–201.

Calleja, M., Farrera, I., Cypress: a new plague for the Rhone-Alpes region? Allerg Immunol (Paris), 2003, 35, 92–96. 13 Caramiello, R., Gallesio, M. T., Siniscalco, C., Leone, F., Aerobiological data and clinical incidence in urban and extra urban environments. *Grana* 1991, 30, 109–112.

Carinanos, P., Alcazar, P., Galan, C., Dominguez E Privet pollen (*Ligustrum* sp.) as potential cause of pollinosis in the city of Cordoba, south-west Spain. *Allergy* 2002, 57, 92–97.

Charpin, D., Allergy to cypress pollen. *Allergy* 2005, 60, 293–301.

Charpin, D., Boutin-Forzano, S., Gouitaa, M., Cypress pollinosis: atopy or allergy? *Allergy*, 2003, 58, 383–384.

Charpin, D., Epidemiology of cypress allergy. *Allerg Immunol (Paris)* 2000, 32, 83–85.

Chen, Z., Duser, M., Flagge, A., Maryska, S., Sander, I., Raulf-Heimsoth, M., et al. Identification and characterization of cross-reactive natural rubber latex and *Ficus benjamina* allergens. *Int Arch Allergy Immunol* 2000, 123, 291–298.

Colombo, P., Bonura, A., Costa, M. A., Izzo, V., Passantino, R., Locorotondo, G., et al. The allergens of Parietaria. *Int Arch Allergy Immunol* 2003, 130, 173–179.

Colombo, P., Duro, G., Costa, M. A., Izzo, V., Mirisola, M., Locorotondo, G., et al. An update on allergens. Parietaria pollen allergens. *Allergy* 1998, 53, 917–921.

Conde Hernandez, J., Conde Hernandez, P., Gonzalez Quevedo Tejerýna, M. T., et al. Antigenic and allergenic differences between 16 different cultivars of *Olea europaea*. *Allergy* 2002, 71, 60–65.

Cortes, L., Carvalho, A. L., Todo-Bom, A., Faro, C., Pires, E., Verýssimo, P., Purification of a novel aminopeptidase from the pollen of *Parietaria judaica* that alters epithelial integrity and degrades neuropeptides. *J Allergy Clin Immunol* 2006, 118, 878–884.

Cvitanovic, S., Marusic, M., Zekan, L., Koehler-Kubelka, N., Allergy induced by *Parietaria officinalis* pollen in southern Croatia. *Allergy* 1986, 41, 543–545.

D'Amato, G., Baena-Cagnani C E, Cecchi, L., et al., 3 Climate change, air pollution and extreme events leading to increasing prevalence of allergic respiratory diseases. *Multidisciplinary Respiratory Medicine* 2013, 8, 12.

D'Amato, G., Bergmann, K. C., Cecchi, L., et al., Climate change and air pollution: Effects on pollen allergy and other allergic respiratory diseases *Allergo J Int* 2014, 23, 17–23.

D'Amato, G., Cecchi, L., D'Amato, M., Annesi-Maesano, I., Climate change and respiratory diseases, *Eur Respir Rev* 2014, 23, 161–169, doi: 10.1183/09059180.00001714.

D'Amato, G., Dal Bo, S., Bonini, S., Pollen-related allergy in Italy. *Ann Allergy* 1992, 68, 433–437.

D'Amato, G., European airborne pollen types of allergological interest and monthly appearance of pollination in Europe. In: D'Amato, G., Spieksma, F. Th. M., Bonini, S., eds. *Allergenic Pollen and Pollinosis in Europe*. Oxford: Blackwell Sci. Publ., 1991, 66–78.

D'Amato, G., Liccardi, G., Melillo, G., A study on airborne allergenic pollen content of the atmosphere of Naples. *Clin Allergy* 1983, 13, 537–544.

D'Amato, G., Lobefalo, G., Allergenic pollens in the Mediterranean area. *J Allergy Clin Immunol* 1989, 83, 116–122.

D'Amato, G., Ruffilli, A., Ortolani, C., Allergenic significance of Parietaria (Pellitory-of-the wall) pollen. In: D'Amato, G., Spieksma FThM, Bonini, S., editors. *Allergenic Pollen and Pollinosis in Europe.* Oxford: Blackwell Sci. Publ. 1991, 113–118.

D'Amato, G., Ruffilli, A., Sacerdoti, G., Bonini, S., Parietaria pollinosis: a review. Allergy 1992, 47, 443–449.

D'Amato, G., Spieksma FThM, Ickovic, M. R., Allergenic pollen and pollenrelated allergy in Europe. In: Godard Ph, Bousquet, J., Michel FB editors. *Advances in Allergology and Clinical Immunology.* Lancs UK: Parthenon Publ. 1992, 387–390

D'Amato, G., Spieksma FThM. Allergenic pollen in Europe. Grana 1990, 30, 67–70.

D'Amato, G., Spieksma, F. Th. M, Bonini, S., eds. *Allergenic Pollen and Pollinosis in Europe*. Oxford: Blackwell Science, 1991.

D'Amato, G., Spieksma, F., Th.M, Liccardi, G., et al.Pollen-related allergy in Europe. Position Paper of the European Academy of Allergology and Clinical Immunology. *Allergy* 1998, 53, 567–578.

D'Amato, Stephen, T., Holgate, Ruby Pawankar et al. Meteorological conditions, climate change, new emerging factors, and asthma and related allergic disorders. A statement of the World Allergy Organization, *World Allergy Organization Journal* (2015) 8, 25. doi: 10.1186/s40413-015-0073-02

Dahl, A., Strandhede, S. O., Wihl, J. A., Ragweed – an allergy risk in Sweden? *Aerobiologia* 1999, 15, 293–297.

Davies, R. R., Smith, L. P., Forecasting the start and severity of the hay fever season. *Clin Allergy* 1973, 3, 263–267.

Djukanovic, R., Feather, I., Gratziou, C., et al. Effect of natural allergen exposure during the grass pollen season on airways inflammatory cells and asthma symptoms. *Thorax* 1996, 51, 575–581.

Ebner, C., Hirschwehr, R., Baner, L., et al. Identification of allergens in fruits and vegetables. IgE cross reactivities with the important birch pollen allergens Bet v 1 and Bet v 2 (birch profilin). *J Allergy Clin Immunol* 1995, 95, 962–969.

Eder, W., Ege, M. J., von Mutius, E., The Asthma Epidemic. N Engl J Med 2006, 355, 2226–2235.

Emberlin, J. C., Grass, tree and weed pollen. In: Kay, B., editor. *Allergy and Allergic Diseases*. Oxford: Blackwell Scientific Publ., 1997, 845–857.

Eriksson, N. E., Holmen, A., Skin prick test with standardized extracts of inhalant allergens in 7099 adult patients with asthma or rhinitis cross sensitizations and relationship to age, sex, month of birth and year of testing. *J Investig Allergol Clin Immunol* 1996, 6, 36–46.

Florido, J. F., Delgado, P. G., de San Pedro, B. S., Quiralte, J., de Saavedra, J. M., Peralta, V., et al., High levels of *Olea europaea* pollen and relation with clinical findings. *Int Arch Allergy Immunol* 1999, 119, 133–137.

Friedhoff, L. R., Ehrlich-Kantzky, E., Grant, J. H., Meyers, D. A., Marsh, D. G., A study of the human response to *Lolium perenne* (rye) pollen and its components, Lol p 1 and 2 (rye I and rye II). *J Allergy Clin Immunol* 1986, 78, 1190–1201.

Geller-Bernstein, C., Waisel, Y., Lahoz, C., Environment and sensibilization to cypress in Israel. *Allerg Immunol (Paris)* 2000, 32, 92–93.

Gergen, P. J., Turkeltaub, P. C., Kovar, M. G., The prevalence of allergic skin test reactivity to eight common aeroallergens in the, U., S. population: Results from the second National Health and Nutrition Examination Survey. *J Allergy Clin Immunol* 1987, 80, 669–679.

Gioulekas, D., Papakosta, D., Damialis, A., Spieksma, F., Giouleka, P., Patakas, D., Allergenic pollen records (15 years) and sensitization in patients with respiratory allergy in Thessaloniki, Greece. Allergy 2004, 59, 174–184.

Guerra, F., Daza, J. C., Miguel, L., et al. Evolution of pollinosis in our province-10 year clinical results. *Allergy* 1992, 47, 72.

Hemmer, W., Focke, M., Gotz, M., Jarisch, R., Sensitization to *Ficus benjamina*: relationship to natural rubber latex allergy and identification of foods implicated in the Ficus-fruit syndrome. *Clin Exp Allergy* 2004, 34, 1251–1258.

Hemmer, W., Focke, M., Wantke, F., Gotz, M., Jarisch, R., Jager, S., et al. Ash (Fraxinus excelsior)-pollen allergy in central Europe: specific role of pollen panallergens and the major allergen of ash pollen, Fra e 1. *Allergy* 2000, 55, 923–930.

Hidalgo, P. J., Galan, C., Dominguez, E., Male phenology of three species of cupressus: correlation with airborne pollen. *Tree* 2003, 17, 336–344.

Holgate, S. T., Jackson, L., Watson, H. K., Garderton, M. A., Sensitivity to Parietaria pollen in the Southampton area as determined by skin-prick and RAST tests. *Clin Allergy* 1988, 18, 549–556.

Hyde, H. A., Atmospheric pollen and spores in relation to allergy. *Clin Allergy* 1972, 2, 152–179.

Italian Association of Aerobiology. An epidemiological study of *Cupressaceae pollinosis* in Italy. *J Investig Allergol Clin Immunol* 2002, 12, 287–292.

Jager, S., Ragweed (Ambrosia) sensitization rates correlate with the amount of inhaled airborne pollen. A 14-year study in Vienna, Austria. *Aerobiologia* 2000, 16, 149–153.

Kaufman, H. S., Parietaria an unrecognized cause of respiratory allergy in the United States. *Ann Allergy* 1990, 64, 293–296.

Kirmaz, C., Yuksel, H., Bayrak, P., Yilmaz O ¨ . Symptoms of the olive pollen allergy: Do they really occur only in the pollination season? *J Invest Allergol Clin Immunol* 2005, 15, 140–145.

Kortekangas-Savolainen, O., Kalimo, K., Savolainen, J., Allergens of *Ficus benjamina* (weeping fig): unique allergens in sap. *Allergy* 2006, 61, 393–394.

Laaidi, M., Laaidi, K., Besancenot, J. P., Thibaudon, M., Ragweed in France: an invasive plant and its allergenic pollen. *Ann Allergy Asthma Immunol* 2003, 91, 195–201.

Laffer, S., Vrtala, S., Kraft, D., Scheiner, O., cDNA cloning of a major allergen of rye (*Secale cereale*) timothy grass (*Phleum pratense*). *Allergy* 1992, 47, 25.

Liccardi, G., D'Amato, M., D' Amato, G., Oleaceae pollinosis: a review. *Int Arch Allergy Immunol* 1996, 111, 210–217.

Liccardi, G., Lobefalo, G., Russo, M., Manzi, A., D'Amato, G., Evaluation of the age onset of respiratory allergic symptomatology. *Aerobiologia* 1992, 8, 34–376.

Liccardi, G., Russo, M., Mistrello, G., Falagiani, P., D'Amato, M., D'Amato, G., Sensitization to pistachio is common in Parietaria allergy. *Allergy* 1999, 54, 643–645.

Liccardi, G., Visone, A., Russo, M., Saggese, M., D'Amato, M., D'Amato, G., Parietaria pollinosis—Clinical and epidemiological aspects. *Allergy an Asthma Proc* 1996, 17, 23–29.

Mahillon, V., Saussez, S., Michel, O., High incidence of sensitization to ornamental plants in allergic rhinitis. *Allergy* 2006, 61, 1138–1140.

Makra, L., Juhasz, M., Borsos, E., Beczi, R., Meteorological variables connected with airborne ragweed pollen in Southern Hungary. *Int J Biometeorol* 2004, 49, 37–47.

Mandrioli, P., De Nuntiis, P., Ariatti, A., Magnani, R., Cypress in Italy: landscape and pollen monitoring. *All Immunol* 2000, 31, 116–121.

Mandrioli, P., Di Cecco, M., Andina, G., Ragweed pollen: the aeroallergen is spreading in Italy. Aerobiologia 1998, 14, 13–20.

Mari, A., Di Felice, G., Afferni, C., et al. Assessment of skin prick test and serum specific IgE detection in the diagnosis of *Cupressaceae pollinosis*. *J Allergy Clin Immunol* 1996, 98, 21–31.

Martin, B. G., Mansfield, L. E., Nelson, H., S. Cross-allergenicity among the grasses. Ann Allergy 1987, 59, 149–154. Newhouse, C. P., Levetin, E., Correlation of environmental factors with asthma and rhinitis symptoms in Tulsa, OK. *Ann Allergy Asthma Immunol* 2004, 92, 356–366.

Ortolani, C., Fontana, A., Basetti, M., Ciccarelli, M., Pollinosi in Lombardia. G It Allergol Immunol Clin 1991, 1, 515–518. Pace, E., Duro, G., Grutta, S. L., Ferraro, M., Bruno, A., Bousquet, J. et al. Hypoallergenic fragment of Par j 2 increases functional expression of Toll-like receptors in atopic children. *Allergy* 2006, 61, 1459–1466.

Pajno, G. B., Passalacqua, G., Vita, D., Caminiti, L., Parmiani, S., Barberio, G., Sublingual immunotherapy abrogates seasonal bronchial hyper responsiveness in children with Parietaria-induced respiratory allergy: a randomized controlled trial. *Allergy* 2004, 59, 883–887.

Papa, G., Romano, A., Quarantino, D., Di Fonso, M., Viola, M., Artesani MC et al. Prevalence of sensitization to *Cupressus sempervirens*: a 4-year retrospective study. *Sci Total Environ* 2001, 270, 83–87.

Peternel, R., Culig, J., Hrga, I., Hercog, P., Airborne ragweed (*Ambrosia artemisiifolia,* L.,) pollen concentrations in Croatia, 2002–2004. *Aerobiologia*, 2006, 22, 161–168.

Pharm, N. H., Baldo, B. A., Bass, D. J., Cypress pollen allergy-identification of allergens and cross reactivity between divergent species. *Clin Exp Allergy* 1994, 24, 558–565.

Piotrowska, K., Weryszko-Chmielewska, E., Ambrosia pollen in the air of Lublin, Poland. *Aerobiologia* 2006, 22, 151–158.

Polosa, R., Al-Delaimy, W. K., Russo, C., Piccillo, G., Sarva, M., Greater risk of incident asthma cases in adults with Allergic Rhinitis and Effect of Allergen Immunotherapy: A Retrospective Cohort Study. *Respiratory Research* 2005, 6, 153.

Polosa, R., Li Gotti, F., Mangano, G., Paolino, G., Mastruzzo, C., Vancheri, C., et al., Effect of immunotherapy on asthma progression, BHR and sputum eosinophils in allergic rhinitis. *Allergy* 2004, 59, 1224–1228.

Prandini, M., Gherson, G., Zambanini, G., et al., Le pollinosinel VenetoG it. *Allergol Immunol Cli* 1991, 1, 519–522.

Priftanji, A., Gjebrea, E., Shkurti, A., Cupressaceae in Tirana (Albania) 1996–1998, aerobiological data and prevalence of Cupressaceae sensitization in allergic patients. *All Immunol* 2000, 31, 122–124.

Rantio-Lehtimaki, A., Koivikko, A., Kupias, R., Makinen, Y., Pohjola, A., Significance of sampling height of airborne particles for aerobiological information. *Allergy* 1991, 46, 68–76.

Ridolo, E., Albertini, A., Giordano, D., Soliani, L., Usberti, I., Dall'Aglio, P. P., Airborne Pollen Concentrations andthe Incidence of Allergic Asthma and Rhino conjunctivitis in Northern Italy from 1992 to 2003. *Int Arch Allergy Immunol* 2006, 20, 142.

Rodriguez, R., Villalba, M., Batanero, E., Palomares O Salamanca, G., Emerging pollen allergens. *Biomed Pharmacother* 2007 Jan; 61(1), 1–7. Epub 2006 Dec 8.

Ruiz de Clavijo, E., Galan, C., Infante, F., Dominguez, E., Variations of airborne winter pollen in Southern Spain. *Allergology et Inmunology* 1988, 16, 175–179.

Rybncek, O., Jager, S., Ambrosia (ragweed) in Europe. *Allergy Clin Immunol Int* 2001, 13, 60–66.

Schmid, P., Stoger, P., Wuthrich, B., Severe isolated allergy to *Ficus benjamina* after bedroom exposure. *Allergy* 1993, 48, 466–467.

Spieksma FThM, Emberlin, J. C., Hjelmroos, M., Jager, S., Leuschner, R. M., Atmospheric birch (Betula) pollen in Europe: trends and fluctuations in annual quantities and the starting dates of the seasons. *Grana* 1995, 34, 51–57.

Spieksma FThM. Regional European pollen calendars. In: D'Amato, G., Spieksma, F.Th.M., Bonini, S., editors. *Allergenic Pollen and Pollinosis in Europe*. Oxford: Blackwell Sci. Publ., 1991, 49–65.

Subiza, J., Jerez, M., Jimenez, J. A., Narganes, M. J., Cabrera, M., Varela, S., et al., Allergenic pollen pollinosis in Madrid. *J Allergy Clin Immunol* 1995, 96, 15–23.

Taramarcaz, P., Lambelet, C., Clot, B., Keimer, C., Hauser, C., Ragweed (Ambrosia) progression and its health risks: will Switzerland resist this invasion? *Swiss Med Wkly* 2005, 135, 538–548.

Torrigiani Malaspina, T., Cecchi, L., Morabito, M., Onorari, M., Domeneghetti, M. P., Orlandini, S., Influence of Meteorological Conditions on Male Flower Phenology of *Cupressus Sempervirens* and Correlation with Pollen Production in Florence. *Trees–Structure and Function*, 2007, 14.

Touraine, R., Comillon, J., Poumeyrol, B., Pollinose et ambrosia dans la region lyonnaise. Son role dans les maladies par allergic pollinique. *Bull Soc Lyon* 1966, 6, 279–285.

Troise, C., Voltolini, S., Del Buono, G., Negrini, A. C., Allergy to pollens from Betulaceae and Corylaceae in a Mediterranean area (Genoa, Italy). A ten-year retrospective study. *J Investig Allergol Clin Immunol* 1996, 6, 36–46.

Valenta, R., Vrtala, S., Ebner, C., Kraft, D., Scheimer, O., Diagnosis of grass pollen allergy with recombinant timothy grass (*Phleum pratense*) pollen allergens. *Int Arch Allergy Immunol* 1993, 97, 287–294.

Velasco-Jiménez, M. J., Arenas, M., Alcázar, P. et al. Aerobiological and phenological study of Pistacia in Cordoba city (Spain) Total Environ. 2015 Feb 1, 505, 1036-42. doi: 10.1016/j.scitotenv.2014.10.017. Epub 2014 Nov 11.

Villalba, M., Barderas, R., Mas, S., Colas, C., Batanero, E., Rodriguez, R., Amaranthaceae pollens: review of an emerging allergy in the Mediterranean area. *J Investig Allergol Clin Immunol* 2014, 24(6), 371–381, quiz 2 preceding p. 382.

Yankova, R., Zlatev, V., Baltadjieva, D., et al., Quantitative dynamics of Ambrosia pollen grains in Bulgaria. *Aerobiologia* 2000, 16, 299–301.

CHAPTER 10

POLLEN ALLERGY AND METEOROLOGICAL FACTORS

JAE-WON OH

Department of Pediatrics, Division of Allergy and Respiratory Diseases, Hanyang University College of Medicine, Seoul, Korea

CONTENTS

10.1 INTRODUCTION

Pollen grains are amongst the commonest allergens in allergic patients. Pollen allergy is now a public health problem due to its elevated prevalence and associated costs in terms of impaired work fitness, sick leave, consulting physicians and drugs, are very high. In the European Community countries between 8% and 35% of young adults show IgE serum antibodies to grass pollen allergens that are the most commonly encountered. Major pollens involved in rhinitis and asthma besides grass include birch overall in northern countries and ragweed in east-central Europe.

Data about the influence of weather on respiratory allergy are poor and debated. Weather affects asthma directly acting on airways or indirectly, influencing airborne allergens and pollutants levels. The complexity of the aerosol reaching the airways and the several compounds that play a role in this relationship might explain the controversial results of studies conducted so far.

Decrease in air temperature represents an aggravating factor of asthmatic symptoms, regardless of geo-climatic areas under study and of methods of analysis. While results about effects of cold air on asthma are consistent, the role of humidity, wind and rainfall is still debated and studies including these variables showed inconclusive and inconsistent results, maybe because their impact on diffusion of pollen and pollutants is higher than air temperature. Aerobiology is the branch of biology that studies airborne organic particles, including pollen grains and fungal spores and it played a key role in the study of the relationship between allergic diseases and pollen.

10.2 POLLEN AND WEATHER MONITORING

Weather conditions, including rainfall, atmospheric temperature, humidity, wind speed, and wind direction, may alter the concentrations of plant pollens and other allergens, which can subsequently influence the occurrence of allergic diseases such as asthma, allergic rhinitis, allergic conjunctivitis, and even atopic dermatitis. Many studies have demonstrated that CO_2 concentration and increased atmospheric temperature increase pollen concentration.

Most work on the impacts of climate change on aeroallergens can be divided into a number of distinct areas, including impacts on pollen amount, pollen allergenicity, pollen season, plants, and pollen distribution. Metrological factors such as mean temperature, wind speed, humidity, amount of sunlight, and degree-days can directly affect biological and chemical components of this interaction.

The accumulation of daily sunshine, and other impacting meteorology factors such as humidity and precipitation, should be taken into consideration to further improve the accuracy of the modeled start dates and season lengths of birch and oak pollen and develop regression models for pollen prediction. Daily fluctuations in the amount of pollen have to do with a variety of meteorological factors such as temperature, rainfall, and the duration of sunshine. Temperature and rainfall are especially important in determining pollen concentrations, but the relationship is complex and influenced by other variables. At least 10 weather elements that are thought to affect the concentration of pollen are used to develop equations for the pollen forecasts. The elements are: daily mean temperature, rainfall, average wind speed, relative humidity, maximum temperature, minimum temperature, temperature range, continued rainfall hours, accumulated sunshine hours, and accumulated mean temperature. Predictive equations for each pollen species and month are developed based on statistical analyses using observed data with 10 weather elements during the last several years in some countries. Although few observations and estimates were reported regarding season start and length of allergic pollens in the other countries, earlier start dates and rising pollen concentrations have been reported widely in many European countries.

The growing degree hour (GDH) model was used to establish a relationship between start and end dates of pollen production and differential temperature sums using observed hourly temperatures from surrounding meteorology stations. Studies of climate change effects on distributions of allergenic pollens have focused typically on analysis of observed airborne pollen counts and their regression relationships with local meteorological and climatic factors. Observed airborne pollen data for pollen collecting stations at locations representing a wide range of geographic and climatic conditions should be analyzed statistically to identify the trends of start date, season length, and annual mean and peak value of daily concentrations of allergic pollen.

10.3 EFFECTS OF WEATHER ON POLLEN RELEASE/FLIGHT

Pollen season, that is the period during which pollen is present in the air, is related to the flowering season, for pollen has to be previously produced and emitted by mature flowers. Pollen seasons and flowering seasons usually do not fully coincide because of the effects of mid- and/or long-range transport. The onset, duration and intensity (i.e., abundance of pollen grains in the air) of the pollen season vary from year to year. Weather variables, mainly air temperature, sunlight and rainfall, together with CO_2 are among the main factors affecting phenology (that means the times of the appearance of first leaves, first flowers, autumn leaf coloration and so on) and pollen production by plant. In addition weather patterns influence the movement and dispersion of all aeroallergens in the atmosphere through the action of winds, rainfall and depending on the atmospheric stability.

Pollen is released by plants at specific times of the year that depend to varying degrees on temperature, sunlight, and moisture. For example, the timing of flowering and pollen release are closely linked with temperature, while weather patterns influence the movement and dispersion of all aeroallergens in the atmosphere through the action of winds, vertical mixing, and rainfall. Any change in these factors may affect the phenological and quantitative features of the season.

The effect of temperature is stronger on the flowering period of plants, which flower in spring and early summer whereas species that flower in late summer and fall generally are correlated with photoperiod. Then, the former species are more affected by warmer winters and springs, showing an earlier flowering in the last.

The complex relationship between weather, climate and concentration of pollen in the atmosphere play a key role on the allergens level, which patients are exposed to. In order to reduce the exposure to pollen and to improve the measures listed in the subchapter 6.5, it is therefore crucial to provide the patients with a reliable aerobiological forecast. Although quality of weather forecast improved substantially in the last decades, effects of weather variables on aeroallergen load are not completely understood. For instance, rainfall clears the air from pollen, thus reducing the risk of exacerbation of rhinitis and/or asthma; extreme rainfall events, like thunderstorms, are, however, associated with severe/near fatal asthma epidemics. A deeper understanding of the relationship between weather and pollen concentration is the first step for the development of a reliable pollen forecast, able to play a preventative role for pollen-induced symptoms.

10.4 EFFECTS OF WEATHER ON ALLERGEN LOAD AND POLLEN POTENCY

In the last 10 years allergology has changed dramatically, moving from the extracts to a molecular-based diagnosis. This dramatic change prompted a new way to look at the mechanisms linking exposure, sensitization and symptoms of respiratory allergic diseases, involving aerobiology too. Although pollen count has been used for over 50 years for the assessment of allergen exposure both in clinical practice and experimental studies, proof is lacking that pollen count is representative for allergen exposure. In this context, measurement of the allergen content of pollen, the so called "pollen potency," might contribute to improve our knowledge on the relationship between exposure to airborne allergens and allergic sensitization and symptoms. Both climate and weather play a key role in the production, release and bioavailability of pollen-derived allergens.

10.5 ADVICES AND TIPS FOR REDUCING EXPOSURE TO POLLEN

Patients should recognize their allergy symptoms and if they still have not a diagnosis should seek necessary medical help, preferably from an Allergy specialist. It is very important to check and take knowledge the type of pollens that the patient is sensitized.

The patients sensitized to pollens should read their regional Pollen Bulletins to keep themselves properly up-to-date on allergic disease prevention and treatment. This allows them to spot the symptoms, understand the disease better and consequently treat it more efficiently. While knowledge of allergic disease is becoming more and more widespread, it is noted that many allergic patients are under-diagnosis and undertreated.

After diagnosis, the patient should begin treatment during season period, from initial symptoms up to the end of season period. Usually oral anti-histamine medication or/and nasal steroids can help and reduce symptoms on prevention-based treatment, mainly on those suffering of allergic rhinitis. This should be adapted on a case-by-case basis in line with the symptoms in question and always following the physician's instructions.

Certain pollen-allergy patients can benefit from taking anti-allergic vaccines, which are very effective if taken correctly and under the strict supervision of an Allergist. Taking these vaccines can change the course of the allergic disease, which can provide primary prevention of more severe signs, such as asthma.

In conclusion, in the case of pollen allergy, an effective and total avoidance unfortunately is not possible. The other element necessary for the control of an allergic disease is to avoid exposure to the allergens to which the individual is sensitized with pharmacological treatment.

KEYWORDS

- **aeroallergen**
- **allergen**
- **allergy**
- **pollen**
- **pollinosis**
- **weather**

REFERENCES

Beggs, P. J., Adaptation to impacts of climate change on aeroallergens and allergic respiratory diseases. *Int J Environ Res Public Health.* 2010, 7, 3006–3021.

Buters, J. T., Kasche, A., Weichenmeier, I., Schober, W., Klaus, S., Traidl-Hoffmann, C., Menzel, A., Huss-Marp, J., Kramer, U., Behrendt, H., Year-to-year variation in release of Bet v 1 allergen from birch pollen: evidence for geographical differences between West and South Germany. *Int Arch Allergy Immunol.* 2008, 145(2), 122–130.

Buters, J. T., Weichenmeier, I., Ochs, S., et al. The allergen Bet v 1 in fractions of ambient air deviates from birch pollen counts. *Allergy*. 2010 Jul, 65(7), 850–858.

Cecchi, L., From pollen count to pollen potency: the molecular era of aerobiology. *Eur Resp, J.,* 2013, 42(4), 898–900.

D'Amato, G., Cecchi, L., Effects of climate change on environmental factors in respiratory allergic diseases. *Clin Exp Allergy*. 2008, 38, 1264–1274.

D'Amato G., Cecchi, L., Annesi Maesano, I., A trans-disciplinary overview of case reports of thunderstorm-related asthma outbreaks and relapse. *Eur Respir Rev* 2012, 21, 124, 82–87.

Dahl, A., Galan, C., Hajkova, L., Pauling, A., Sikoparija, B., Smith, M., Vokou, D., The onset, course, and intensity of the pollen season. In: *Allergenic Pollen*. Bergman and Sofiev (eds.). Springer, 2012.

De Linares, C., Díaz de la Guardia, C., Nieto Lugilde, D., Alba F Airborne study of grass allergen (Lol p 1) in different-sized particles. *Int Arch Allergy Immunol*. 2010, 152(1), 49–57.

De Linares, C., Nieto-Lugilde, D., Alba, F., Díaz de la Guardia, C., Galán, C., Trigo, M. M., Detection of airborne allergen (Ole e 1) in relation to Olea europaea pollen in S. Spain. *Clin Exp Allergy*. 2007, 37(1), 125–132.

Gina Dapul-Hidalgo, G., Leonard Bielory, L., *Climate Change and Allergic Diseases* 2012, 109, 166–172.

Kim, J. H., Oh, J. W., Lee, H. B., Kim, S. W., Kang, I. J., Kook, M. H., et al. Changes in sensitization rate to weed allergens in children with increased weeds pollen counts in Seoul metropolitan area. *J Korean Med Sci* 2012, 27, 350–355.

Levetin, E., Van de Water, P., Changing pollen types/concentrations/distribution in the United States: fact or fiction? *Curr Allergy Asthma Rep*. 2008, 8(5), 418–424.

Kim, J. H., Oh, J. W., Kim, J. H., Kim, S. W., Jeong, H. R., Park, K. S., Kim, B. S., et al. The impacts of climate change on the changes of allergenic plants. *Allergy Asthma, Respir Dis* 2014, 2(1), 48–58.

Oh, J. W., Lee, H. B., Kang, I. J., Kim, S. W., Park, K. S., Kook, M. H., et al. The revised edition of Korean calendar for allergenic pollens. *Allergy Asthma Immunol Res*. 2012, 4, 5–11.

Schäppi, G. F., Monn, C., Wütrich, B., Wanner, H-A. Anaylsis of allergens in ambient aerosols: comparison of areas subjected to different levels of air pollution. *Aerobiologia* 1996, 12, 185–190.

Schäppi, G. F., Taylor, P. E., Pain, M. C., Cameron, P. A., Dent, A. W., Staff, I. A., Suphioglu, C., Concentrations of major grass group 5 allergens in pollen grains and atmospheric particles: implications for hay fever and allergic asthma sufferers sensitized to grass pollen allergens. *Clin Exp Allergy*. 1999, 29(5), 633–641.

Shea, K. M., Truckner, R. T., Weber, R. W., Peden, D. B., Climate change and allergic disease. *J Allergy Clin Immunol*. 2008, 122, 443–453.

CHAPTER 11

ALLERGIES IN INDIA: A CLINICIAN'S VIEWPOINT

WIQAR SHAIKH[1] and SHIFA WIQAR SHAIKH[2]

[1]*Professor of Medicine, Grant Medical College and Sir J.J. Group of Hospitals, Mumbai, India, E-mail: drwiqar@gmail.com*

[2]*Allergy and Asthma Clinic, Shakti Sadan Coop Housing Society Ground Floor, B-Block, Opp. Navjeevan Society Lamington Road, Mumbai–400007, India*

CONTENTS

11.1 INTRODUCTION

India is a "tropical" country, straddling the Tropic of Cancer in the northern hemisphere (23.4728 N) and has a typical warm and humid climate. Being a large country, with a total area of 3.3 million square kilometers, India has, in fact, been labeled a sub-continent. The term "Tropical Allergy and Asthma," which was first coined by the author (Anonymous, 1986; Coca and Cook, 1923), applies to manifestations of allergy and asthma in a tropical country such as India and which is different when compared to allergy and asthma as seen in the colder, western countries.

Allergic diseases are less common in India as compared to the west. "Atopy," a term first coined by Coca and Cooke in 1923 (Goodman and Gilman, 2014), is derived from the Greek word "Atopos" which means "strange" or "out of place." Atopy is defined as the genetic predisposition to produce increased amounts of IgE levels and developing certain allergic hypersensitivity diseases. In India, the incidence of atopy is 29%. Allergies in India have been analyzed by the authors in a series of studies (Noon, 1911; Scadding and Brostoff, 1986; Shaikh, 1992), which indicate an increase in "atopy" and a change in the allergen positivity pattern over the years. The distribution pattern/incidence of various allergic disorders have remained virtually unchanged in both children and adults. Undoubtedly, naso-bronchial allergies viz. rhinitis and/or asthma are the commonest allergic manifestations in India. An interesting observation is that the male:female ratio in children is 3:1, whereas it is almost 1:1 in adults. A large number of female children who were asymptomatic or may have had subclinical disease in childhood, tend to manifest allergic symptoms when entering adulthood. During adolescence, therefore, watch out for the female child because she may begin to manifest allergic symptoms.

11.2 ASTHMA

Allergic asthma is the commonest allergic manifestation in India and represents approximately 59% of all allergic patients in the country (Shaikh,

1992). Asthma is either under-diagnosed or poorly treated in India. More than 60% of asthmatics in India have associated rhinitis. The concept of the "United Airway Disease" is very relevant in this country and it is imperative that asthmatic patients be scrutinized for allergic rhinitis and vice versa, in patients presenting with allergic rhinitis, asthma must be excluded. In India, asthma, like rhinitis is more often perennial than seasonal. A tropical environment in the country results in stability in temperature and environment throughout the year.

Cough, which is a common manifestation of asthma, is often misdiagnosed as tuberculosis. A patient having chronic cough is usually asked to have a Mantoux test done; this test is positive in the vast majority of Indians and a mistaken diagnosis of tuberculosis is made and the patient subjected to an unnecessary several months of anti-tuberculous therapy. In patients with chronic cough, it is imperative to exclude asthma.

11.3 ALLERGIC RHINITIS

Allergic Rhinitis is the second commonest atopic disease in India and is the manifestation in approximately 56% of all allergy patients in the country (Shaikh, 1992). This figure is true for both, children and adults. Perennial rhinitis and not seasonal rhinitis is usually the norm in India. Rhinitis commonly presents with sneezing, rhinorrhea and nasal blockage. Patients may demonstrate a "Darrier's line," a dark, transverse crease across the middle part of the nose. Darrier's line is a result of repeated rubbing of the nostrils from below upwards with the palm of the hand because of irritation in the nostrils, an action which is termed "the allergic salute." Patients may also present with a "post nasal drip induced cough," a condition which is caused by reverse dripping of allergy induced mucoid secretion into the pharynx, and which is frequently misdiagnosed as a respiratory tract infection including tuberculosis or bronchial asthma.

Another common manifestation of rhinitis is "allergic shiners," which is a pigmented swelling around the lower eyelids and is a result of venous stasis caused by allergic inflammation. "Bunny nose" is yet another sign of allergic rhinitis, in which patients move their nostrils into peculiar positions, to alleviate the itching sensation inside the nostril. On physical examination, allergic rhinitis could manifest with hypertrophic turbinates, a strikingly bluish gray discoloration of the nasal mucosa, deviated nasal septum and nasal polyps.

11.4 DRUG ALLERGIES

In India, non-steroidal anti-inflammatory drugs (NSAID's), antibiotics (such as Penicillins and Cephalosporins) and sulfonamides are the commonest causes of drug allergies. Of these, almost 75% of drug allergies in India are due to NSAID's (Shaikh, 1992). Again, almost 75% of drug allergies in India manifest with a skin rash (Urticaria, angioedema, fixed drug eruption and contact dermatitis). Other manifestations of drug allergies are anaphylaxis, rhinitis and asthma.

There has been an advertisement campaign in India regarding blood tests to detect drug allergies. These blood tests are not scientifically established, are not authentic and are indeed not actually carried out in most cases and the reports are simply typed and delivered. Doctors and patients need to be wary of such advertisements in the lay press.

11.5 ALLERGIC CONJUNCTIVITIS

Allergic conjunctivitis affects approximately 2% of allergy sufferers in India (Shaikh, 1992). In more than two thirds of cases, allergic conjunctivitis is associated with allergic rhinitis. Allergic conjunctivitis and allergic rhinitis often co-exist. The authors have seen innumerable cases where allergic conjunctivitis co-exists with both allergic rhinitis and allergic asthma.

11.6 DERMAL ALLERGIES

Dermal allergies represent approximately 20% of allergic reactions seen in India (Shaikh, 1992). Urticaria/Angioedema is the manifestation in more than half of these patients and the remaining are allergic contact dermatitis and atopic eczema. In Indian children, the incidence of atopic eczema, as expected, is much higher when compared with adults (22% in children and

2% in adults). Dermal manifestations represent approximately 75% of all drug allergies seen in India.

Dermographism is a condition that is often misdiagnosed as Urticaria. Patients present with an itchy skin rash and a simple scratch on the forearm, elicits a linear, wheal and flare reaction. Dermographism literally means "the ability to write on the skin." Management of Dermographism is on similar lines as Urticaria.

Contact dermatitis is a type IV delayed hypersensitivity mediated by T-delayed type hypersensitivity (T-DTH) lymphocytes. The site of the reaction provides a clue to the causative allergen. An area of contact dermatitis on the forehead could be due to the adhesive in the "bindi," a reaction on the wrist could be due to nickel in the watch, and again due to nickel on the tips of the fingers in coin-handlers. Artificial jewelry which also contains nickel, could lead to reactions in the part of the body where the artificially jewelry is worn.

Atopic eczema is commonly seen in infants and young children. Typical eczematous lesions are seen on the cheeks, forehead and flexural surfaces such as the ante-cubital fossa and the popliteal fossa.

11.7 INVESTIGATIONS FOR ALLERGIC DISEASES SERUM IGE LEVELS

In our studies, total serum IgE levels were found to be elevated in all patients manifesting allergies (Shaikh, 1992), except in patients having allergic contact dermatitis. Being a delayed type hypersensitivity and mediated through T-DTH cells, serum IgE levels were not done in allergic contact dermatitis. As has been reported in international literature, serum IgE levels were found to be the highest in patients with atopic dermatitis.

In India, specific IgE kits to individual allergens are available from various manufacturers who import these kits from abroad. Unfortunately, there is complete lack of organized control over these so called "blood tests" to diagnose allergic triggers. "Why do painful skin tests when we can diagnose your allergies with a small quantity of blood" is the slogan put out by several laboratories who serve as franchises to the manufacturers. Shockingly enough, the clinician is resultantly omitted, the patient's history and physical examination is ignored, the diagnosis of an allergic etiology is mistakenly made and using a blood sample, a report is generated. This practice is termed "the remote practice of allergy" and has been condemned by reputed allergy organizations such as the American Academy of Allergy, Asthma and Immunology (Shaikh, 1993). We have seen several non-allergic individuals in whom these tests have been done, such as chronic renal failure, eczema craquele, allergic contact dermatitis, Chronic Obstructive Pulmonary Disease (COPD), etc. What is worse we have seen positive tests to allergens not existing in India, but then these companies hide behind the so called "cross reactivity" which in reality is not "true reactivity." We have compared specific IgE levels to individual allergens in one of our studies and found the skin prick tests to be more sensitive and reliable (Shaikh, 1995).

11.8 SKIN PRICK TESTS

Skin prick tests (SPT) are an important investigation in allergic disorders, particularly to formulate a strategy for avoidance measures and for specific immunotherapy (SIT). The authors believe in doing the SPT in view of its simplicity, reliability and reproducibility. Rather surprisingly, in several clinics in India, the intradermal skin test and the scratch tests are still being used. The intradermal test requires an amount of 0.1 ml to be injected using a tuberculin syringe, is an operator dependent procedure and therefore, not standardized. The scratch test is a less sensitive test when compared to SPT and is often considered more painful by patients. Also, anaphylactic reactions, which are often reported during intradermal testing, are virtually unknown with SPT. An amount of 0.04 mL of allergen enters the intradermal area in the SPT and in trained hands, it is reliable and reproducible. The SPT is therefore, the gold standard in allergy testing.

In the western countries, pollen allergens have shown a positivity rate of approximately 20%; however, in our studies, the positivity rate for pollen allergens is about 9% (Shaikh, 1992). The commonest pollen allergens in India are *parthenium hysterophoris*, *cynodon dactylon* and *cocos nucifera*. Alternaria and Aspergillus species are the commonest fungi (mold) allergens. *Parthenium hysterophorus* is positive in more than 17% of Indian allergy patients. Parthenium, also known as "Congress grass" is a wild weed, which is not native to India. It was introduced accidentally in this country through wheat aid from the USA in the 1960's. It found a rather conducive, tropical environment for growth and has since, spread to several parts of the country. Parthenium is a common cause of asthma, rhinitis and air-borne contact dermatitis (ABCD) in India. In fact, ABCD is a particularly disfiguring condition manifesting with a severe, itchy dermatitis of the exposed areas of the body, such as the face, neck, hands and feet. In ABCD, the face particularly, presents with a ghost-like appearance.

More than 50% of allergy sufferers in India are skin test positive to three common household insects viz. mosquito, housefly and cockroach. Insect control (pest control) is an extremely important avoidance measure in this country. Similarly, pets, such as cats and dogs are positive on more than 33% of allergy sufferers. In western countries, *D. pteronyssinus* is the common dust mite whereas in India, *D. farinae* is more common. More than 75% patients are positive to *D. farinae* and indeed, it has the highest positivity rate amongst all allergens in this country. It must be therefore emphasized that India is *D. farinae* country (Shaikh, 1992).

Amongst food allergens, the commonest positive allergens in western countries such as milk, eggs, meat and wheat are much less positive in India. The highest positivity rates in this country are seen with peanuts (ground nuts), chocolate, fish and coconut. A high positivity rate (almost 19%) is seen with soya bean and it must be emphasized that the general understanding that soya milk is less allergenic than cow or buffalo milk is really a myth. Approximately 7% of Indian allergy sufferers are positive to rice; indeed, rice has rarely, if ever been reported from other countries (except Japan). A quantum increase in the incidence of cocoa (chocolate) allergy is seen in this country and cocoa is now the second most common food allergen in India. Interestingly enough, the SPT positivity rates for various allergens in India are remarkably similar in both adults and children. The authors believe that in this country, the vast majority of patients react to artificial colors in foods and to food preservatives. It is recommended that both these should be eliminated from the diet of allergic individuals.

In India, it must be strongly emphasized that allergens such as Silver Birch, London Plane, Pine, Ragweed, etc. do not exist in this country. The availability of such allergens for both specific IgE and SPT as well as the fact that these are being used on Indian patients is not justifiable.

11.9 PATCH TEST

A patch test is done to confirm the trigger factors in allergic contact dermatitis. A patch containing the appropriate allergen is applied to the back of the patient is removed after 72 hours and the reactions graded from 1 to 4.

The two common allergens causing contact dermatitis in India are nickel sulphate (40%) and *Parthenium hysterophorus* (38%) (Shaikh, 1992). Nickel sulphate contact allergy is seen with artificial jewelry, watches and in coin handlers.

11.10 SPIROMETRY

Pulmonary function tests using a spirometer are an essential investigational tool for patients having allergic asthma as also in those with allergic rhinitis (to exclude asthma). A spirometer is useful in assessing the severity of the illness as well as the reversibility with bronchodilators. India requires mass production of low cost spirometers, which could be particularly used in rural and semi-rural areas. Low cost peak expiratory flow meters are available in India; however, peak expiratory flow rates are not a reliable substitute for spirometry.

11.11 NASAL FLOW RATES

Assessment of the "Peak Nasal Inspiratory Flow Rate" (PNIFR) using the Youlten's Peak Inspiratory Flow Meter is essential in assessing the severity of nasal blockage in allergic rhinitis as well as reversibility following medication. PNIFR is a simple but reliable technique when compared to rhinomanometry.

11.12 MANAGEMENT OF ALLERGIES IN INDIA

Management of allergic diseases is based on a combination of avoidance measures, pharmacotherapy and specific immunotherapy (SIT).

11.13 AVOIDANCE

Avoidance measures are the frontline management of allergic diseases. The list of avoidance measures needs to be tailor-made for an individual patient, depending upon a detailed history, careful physical examination and the results of the skin prick test. Avoidance measures include food avoidance, possible changes in the house and/or workplace, as also avoidance of certain drugs. Compliance to avoidance measures results in satisfactory control of allergy symptoms.

11.14 PHARMACOTHERAPY

Medications in allergic diseases would depend upon the manifestation or a combination of manifestations. In allergic rhinitis, nasal sprays should be the mainstay of management. Nasal sprays are undoubtedly more effective than oral medications in allergic rhinitis. A combination of nasal corticosteroid (Budesonide), a local anti-histamine (Azelastine) and a mast cell stabilizer cum local anti-histamine (Olopatadine) is more effective than any of them alone. In asthma, the authors prefer to use a combination of inhaled bronchodilator (Salbutamol) with an inhaled corticosteroid (Budesonide) in exacerbated/unstable asthmatics. In stable asthma and in those who need maintenance medications, a combination of inhaled Formoterol (a dual, short and long acting bronchodilator) and Budesonide is effective. The authors believe in using Budesonide, because it is a safe and effective corticosteroid. The authors do not use Beclomethasone because the first author reported a series of cases of Beclomethasone induced tuberculosis (Shaikh, 1996). It must be emphasized that the concept of the "United Airway Disease" needs to be clearly understood and that in every asthmatic patient, the presence of rhinitis must be excluded. If asthma alone is treated and rhinitis, if exists, is ignored, the results of treatment are expected to be unsatisfactory. The authors prefer to use dry powder inhalers because of ease of use. It is imperative to spend time with patients and impart appropriate training in the use of nasal sprays and inhalers. Errors are frequently observed when patients are asked in the clinic to demonstrate the correct method of using nasal sprays and inhalers and this results in inadequate control of symptoms.

An interesting study published by the first author concluded that in asthma with rhinitis, exhaling a metered dose inhaled corticosteroid (ICS) through the nose results in improvement in symptoms of rhinitis (Shaikh, 1997). Also, in another study, ephedrine saline nasal wash was shown by the first author to be effective treatment for allergic rhinitis (Shaikh, 1997a).

There are several misconceptions in India, regarding inhalers, as also about corticosteroids. The common refrain regarding inhaled medications is that "they dry up the lungs," "they destroy the lungs" and "they are as addictive as alcohol and smoking." Corticosteroids or as they are commonly called "steroids" are possibly the most feared drugs in India. Patients frequently ask whether the drugs they are being prescribed contain steroids. It is mandatory that every patient be educated regarding the safety of nasal sprays and inhalers and particularly about the efficacy and safety of ICS. It is surprising that several prescriptions for nasal sprays and inhalers specify a short period of usage, such as 10 days. Also, despite the fact that allergy and asthma are now accepted as diseases of chronic inflammation, several patients are yet prescribed a stand-alone bronchodilator. This practice could lead to acute exacerbations of asthma because the inflammatory reaction is left untreated.

Oral medications have no role for the authors in the management of naso-bronchial allergies. However, oral anti-histamines are the mainstay of treatment of dermal allergies such as urticaria and atopic eczema. A combination of anti-histamines is preferable to a single anti-histamine and caution should be exercised when using higher doses of anti-histamines, in view of side effects. Also, higher doses of anti-histamines are not licensed in India. The authors prefer non-sedating anti-histamines to sedating anti-histamines. Oral corticosteroids may have to be used, particularly in chronic urticaria, ABCD and atopic eczema. The authors prefer Deflazacort, a bone friendly and women friendly corticosteroid. Food allergies are, as yet, treated only through avoidance. The first author has shown that cetirizine is effective in food (egg) allergy (Shaikh, 1999).

The authors do not prefer to use Montelukast (Coca and Cook, 1923), since studies have equated it to a placebo, as also because of side-effects such as psycho-somatic manifestations (including suicidal tendencies), Churg-Strauss vasculitis, angioedema, liver injury, etc. The authors also do not use Omalizumab (Coca and Cook, 1923), a chimeric anti-IgE antibody in allergy management. Besides the cost factor, Omalizumab has several adverse effects such as anaphylaxis, Churg Strauss vasculitis, thrombocytopenia, cardiovascular events, etc. IgE is important in tumor surveillance and the effect of either elimination or drastic reduction of IgE on the incidence of malignancies can only be speculated. Besides, in a tropical country such as India, the role of IgE in parasitic infestations is indispensable. Therefore, the elimination or drastic reduction of IgE is questionable. Finally, following administration of Omalizumab, IgE returns to normal within a year which makes it a short-term therapy with no long term benefits.

It is rather surprising that Diethylcarbamazine Citrate (DECC) is extensively used in allergy treatment in India. An elevated eosinophil count in a given patient will almost certainly be treated with DECC. Pharmacology literature however, is clear that "filariasis" is the only indication for treatment with DECC (Shaikh, 2001). It must therefore emphasized that allergic eosinophilia is not an indication for DECC and this practice must be abandoned.

11.15 SPECIFIC IMMUNOTHERAPY

Vaccination for allergic diseases which is termed as *specific immunotherapy* (SIT) was introduced in 1911 by Leonard Noon at the St. Mary's Hospital in London, UK (Shaikh, 2005). Since then SIT has evolved and is now the cornerstone in the management of several allergic manifestations. SIT is the only disease modifying treatment available for allergic diseases. SIT was earlier available only as subcutaneous immunotherapy (SCIT), but this form of treatment had adverse effects such as anaphylaxis and mortality. Sublingual immunotherapy (SLIT) has become a more popular form of SIT (Shaikh, 2006). Systemic adverse effects with SLIT are rare and the major advantage is ease of use; the patient can self-medicate and does not need to visit a doctor as is the case with SCIT. Both SCIT and SLIT are effective *disease modifying drugs* (DMDs).

The clinical benefits of SIT manifest after at least one year of continuous use and literature recommends that SIT should not be discontinued up to at least 3 years after initiation. Indeed, the authors prefer to continue SIT for 5 to 7 years for maximum, long-term benefits. Our study concluded that SCIT could have beneficial effects for up to 27 years (Shaikh, 1998). It is a matter of serious concern that SIT is discontinued in several patients within a few months of initiation. Inappropriate practice of SIT has led to a decline in the faith of both patients and doctors in the specialty of allergy and in SIT as an effective and beneficial form of treatment.

SIT has been found to be safe during pregnancy. Two different studies from our clinic have shown that both SCIT and SLIT are safe during pregnancy (Shaikh, 2006, 2008) and should not only be continued in a pregnant patient but could also be initiated for the first time during pregnancy.

SIT when combined with avoidance measures and pharmacotherapy is more beneficial to patients than SIT alone. A study conducted in our clinic compared SIT to an ICS (budesonide) and found that with SIT the improvement was slow but sustained even after SIT was discontinued (Shaikh, 2009). On the other hand, budesonide resulted in rapid relief on initiation and on discontinuation resulted in equally rapid deterioration. The implication of this study is that SIT when combined with budesonide provides rapid and sustained relief.

Certain principles should be adhered to when prescribing SIT. The authors do not prescribe SIT in children below 6 years of age, which is in fact the universal recommendation. SIT should be used only in allergic rhinitis, allergic asthma and allergic conjunctivitis. SIT has no role in treating dermal allergies. There is no role for SIT in allergic contact dermatitis and its use in this condition needs to be condemned. SIT should be used only for pollen, dust and dust mites and insects. SIT has no role in the management of food allergies. Also, fungal allergens should not be mixed with other allergens in an SIT prescription because of incompatibility. The SIT prescription should not contain a mixture of more than 5 or 6 allergens and indeed, the lesser the number of allergens, the more effective is SIT likely to be. Patients need to be appropriately counseled in the use of SIT and should be instructed regarding appropriate refrigeration. The authors prefer to give patients a detailed instruction sheet and an appropriate timetable for SIT as also the date for the next order for SIT.

11.16 COMPLIANCE

Compliance to therapy is extremely important in allergic diseases. A study on this essential aspect of management was published by the authors (Shaikh, 2012). Interestingly enough, compliance in India was least with nasal sprays (62%) and highest with SLIT (84%). The possible reasons for better compliance with SLIT as compared to oral medications, nasal sprays and dry powder inhalers are two. One, the novelty of SLIT when compared with other therapeutic options and two, there is an emotive faith in vaccines which encouraged patients to take SLIT more regularly.

KEYWORDS

- **allergy**
- **asthma**
- **immunotherapy**
- **India**
- **rhinitis**
- **tropical**

REFERENCES

Anonymous, American Academy of Allergy, Asthma and Immunology. Position Statement—Remote practice of Allergy. *J. Allergy Clin Immunol* 1986, 77, 651.

Coca, A. F., Cook, R. A., On the classification of the phenomena of hypersensitiveness. *J. Immunol* 1923, 8, 163–182.

Goodman and Gilman. *Manual of Pharmacology and Therapeutics*. McGraw Hill Education, 2nd edition, 2014, 1321.

Noon, L., Prophylactic inoculation against hay fever. *Lancet* 1911, 1, 1572–1573.

Scadding, G. K., Brostoff, J., Low dose sublingual immunotherapy in patients with allergic rhinitis due to hose dust mite. *Clin. Allergy* 1986, 16(5), 483–491.

Shaikh, W. A. (ed.). *Allergy and Asthma: A Tropical View*. IJCP Group Publication 2001.

Shaikh, W. A. (ed.). *Principles and Practice of Tropical Allergy and Asthma*. Vikas Medical Publications, Bombay. 2006.

Shaikh, W. A., A retrospective study on the safety of immunotherapy in pregnancy. *Clinical and Experimental Allergy*, October 1993, 23, 857–860.

Shaikh, W. A., Allergies and Asthma in India: An analysis of 2467 patients seen over a six year period. *Indian Journal of Clinical Practice*, May 1998, 8(12), 23–26, 46–47.

Shaikh, W. A., Allergies in India–An analysis of 1619 patients attending an Allergy Clinic in Bombay. *International Review of Allergology and Clinical Immunology*. 1997, 3(2), 101–104.

Shaikh, W. A., Cetirizine–effective treatment in food (egg) allergy. *Allergy* (European Journal of Allergy and Clinical Immunology), April 1996, 51(4), 275–276.

Shaikh, W. A., Ephedrine-saline nasal wash in allergic rhinitis. *Journal of Allergy and Clinical Immunology*, November 1995, 96(5), part 1, 597–600.

Shaikh, W. A., Exhaling a budesonide inhaler through the nose results in a significant reduction in dosage requirement of budesonide nasal spray in patients having asthma with rhinitis. *Journal of Investigational Allergology and Clinical Immunology*, January–February 1999, 9(1), 45–49.

Shaikh, W. A., Immunotherapy versus inhaled budesonide in bronchial asthma–an open, parallel, comparative trial. Clinical and Experimental Allergy, November 1997, 27(11), 1279–1284.

Shaikh, W. A., Long-term efficacy of House Dust Mite Immunotherapy in Bronchial Asthma: A 15 year follow-up study. *Allergology International* (Japan). 2005, 54(3), 443–449.

Shaikh, W. A., Pulmonary Tuberculosis in patients on inhaled Beclomethasone. *Allergy* (European Journal of Allergy and Clinical Immunology), August 1992, 47(1), 327–330.

Shaikh, W. A., Shaikh, S. W., A prospective study on the safety of sublingual immunotherapy in pregnancy. Dr. Shifa Wiqar Shaikh. *Allergy* (European Journal of Allergy and Clinical Immunology), 67, 2012 (early view – published April 5, 2012).

Shaikh, W. A., Shaikh, S. W., Allergies in India: A study on medication compliance. *Journal of the Indian Medical Association*. 2009 July, 107, 462–463.

Shaikh, W. A., Shaikh, S. W., Allergies in India: an analysis of 3389 patients attending an allergy clinic in Mumbai, India. *Journal of the Indian Medical Association*. 2008 April, 106, 220–224.

Shaikh, W. A., Shaikh, S. W., Skin prick test–more reliable than estimation of specific IgE in allergy diagnosis. *Journal of the Indian Medical Association*. 2006 October, 104(10), 592–595.

PART IV

ALLERGY IN CHILDREN

CHAPTER 12

ALLERGIC RHINITIS IN CHILDREN

MAJOR K. NAGARAJU

Paediatric Allergist, Saveetha Medical College and Hospital, Consultant Paeditric Allergist, Apollo Children's Hospital, Director, VN Allergy and Asthma Research Centre, Chennai, India

CONTENTS

ABSTRACT

Allergic rhinitis (AR) is a common chronic disease in childhood, however patients and physicians often overlook it. It can present as part of the atopic spectrum of disorders and can affect not only the nose but also its connections, manifesting often with a multiplicity of symptoms, including associated comorbidities. If uncontrolled or inappropriately treated, AR can severely impair quality of life for children and their families. AR is associated with bronchial asthma and is a risk factor for asthma development and a major factor in exacerbations.

Diagnosis of AR is largely clinical with history, thorough physical examination, in the absence of upper respiratory tract infection and structural abnormalities of nose playing an important role. Skin tests are the most accurate diagnostic tool and are regarded as the gold standard for detection of IgE antibodies to specific allergic triggers. Prick or puncture tests are the most convenient, least expensive and best screening method for detecting IgE mediated allergies. Allergen-specific IgE antibodies are more expensive and are used as a back-up diagnostic tests. Standardized allergen extracts should be used for allergy diagnostic tests.

Management is largely based on avoidance of the triggering allergen(s), the use of second-generation non-sedative antihistamines for mild disease, and of non-systemically bio-available nasal steroids for moderate/severe disease. Allergen immunotherapy is the only treatment modality potentially able to alter long term not only disease severity, but also progression. Education of patients, caretakers and the practitioners about the nature of AR, the possible need for long-term therapy and the optimal use of the drugs, is vital in the management.

12.1 INTRODUCTION

Allergic disorders including allergic rhinitis (AR) are common disorders affecting children and adolescents. The International Study of Asthma and Allergies in Childhood (ISAAC) phase three studies documented the prevalence of rhinitis in 6- to 7-year-old children at 8.5% and for 13- to 14-year-old children it was 14.6%. The prevalence from the children in Indian subcontinent was estimated to be 26.6% (6- to 7-year-old) and 15.1% (13- to 14-year-old). The ISAAC study also showed that the incidence of AR increases by 1.43 percent per year in India.

Patients and physicians often overlook the burden of AR, as it is frequently believed to be a common cold. Along with the physical symptoms,

AR severely impacts the social well being of a child by having an impact on the psychological health. The financial burden and morbidity associated with this disorder if left undetected, places further emphasis on early diagnosis. Additionally, progression of pediatric AR to asthma is frequent and part of the widely accepted phenomenon 'atopic march.' Thus, early diagnosis and an appropriate treatment strategy including allergen immunotherapy (AIT) in the suitable candidates may have a higher chance to alter the natural progression of AR.

12.2 DEFINITIONS

Allergic rhinitis is defined as an IgE mediated inflammation of the nasal epithelium and is characterized by at least any of the two nasal symptoms: rhinorrhea, blockage, sneezing or itching. AR is the commonest form of rhinitis and about two-thirds of children with rhinitis will present with allergic rhinitis. Their symptoms are caused by exposure to an allergen to which a patient is sensitized. A diagnosis of AR is based on the rhinitis symptoms in the presence of sensitization. Sensitization can be determined by demonstrating specific IgE reactivity to a relevant allergen with a positive skin test or raised serum specific IgE levels. The common implicated allergens include house dust mite, grass pollen, tree pollen, weed pollens, animal dander and molds.

12.3 PATHOPHYSIOLOGY

AR occurs in patients with a genetic predisposition to developing allergies. Other risk factors for allergic rhinitis include high socioeconomic status, environmental pollution, no older siblings, late entry into nursery or preschool education (e.g., at age 4 years and older), heavy maternal smoking during the first year of life, exposure to indoor allergens such as animal dander and dust mites, high concentrations in serum of IgE (>100 IU/mL before age 6 years) (Figures 12.1–12.11).

Individuals who have inherited the potential to develop IgE-mediated, or "allergic," responses on repeated exposure to aeroallergens

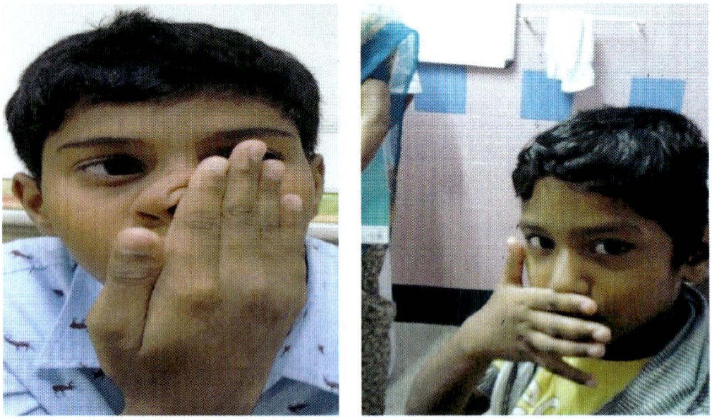

FIGURES 12.1–12.2 Allergic salute: (Rubbing of the tip of nose to relieve itching of the nose.)

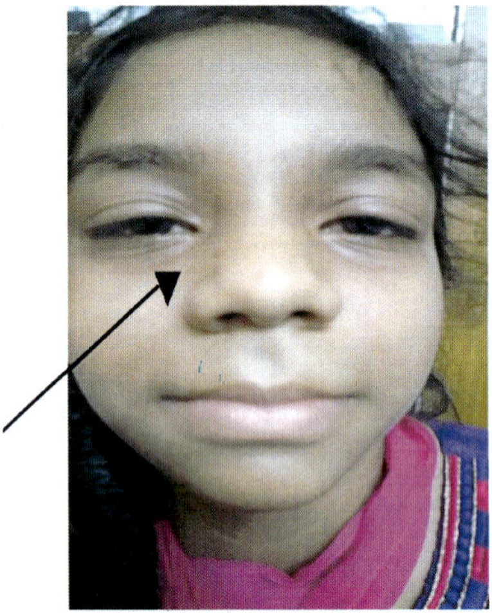

FIGURE 12.3 Dennies–Morgan Folds (creases in lower eyelid due to Müller muscle spasm).

causes B cell activation and maturation into plasma cells, which produce specific IgE antibodies. The IgE binds to specific receptors on the surface of basophils and mast cells. When cell bound specific IgE is cross-linked by the sensitizing allergen, the cells release or generate chemical mediators (including histamine), which produce the allergic symptoms.

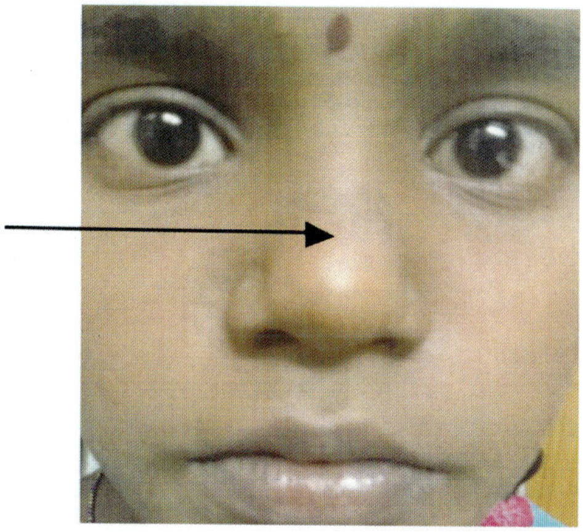

FIGURE 12.4 Allergic line (dark line between cartilaginous and bony portion of nasal septum due to constant upward pressing over the nose due to nasal block).

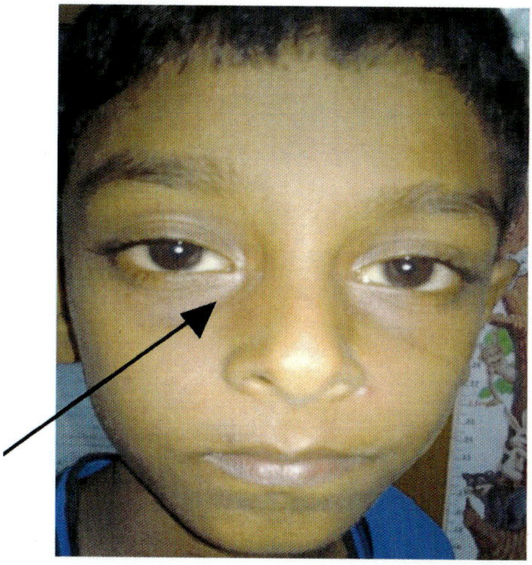

FIGURE 12.5 Allergic Shiners (Bluish black discoloration of lower eyelids due to venous stasis because of nasal block in alveolar tissues of lower orbital palpebral grooves by edematous allergic mucous membrane of nose).

12.4 CLINICAL FEATURES

Symptoms of allergic rhinitis are often ignored or mistakenly attributed to a respiratory infection. Classic symptoms of allergic rhinitis include:

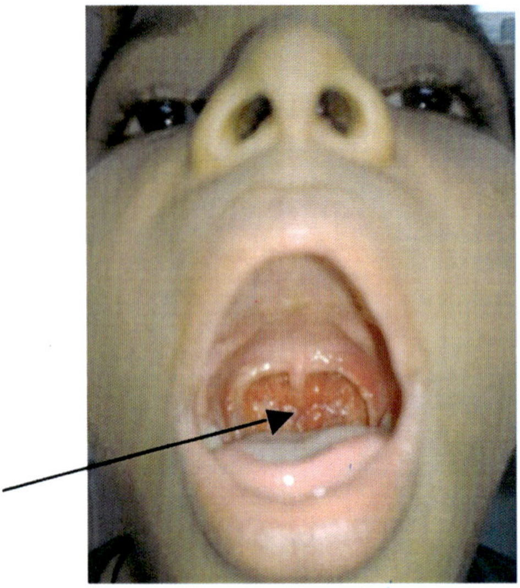

FIGURE 12.6 Cobble stone Pharynx (pharyngeal lymphoid hyperplasia due to constant post nasal drip).

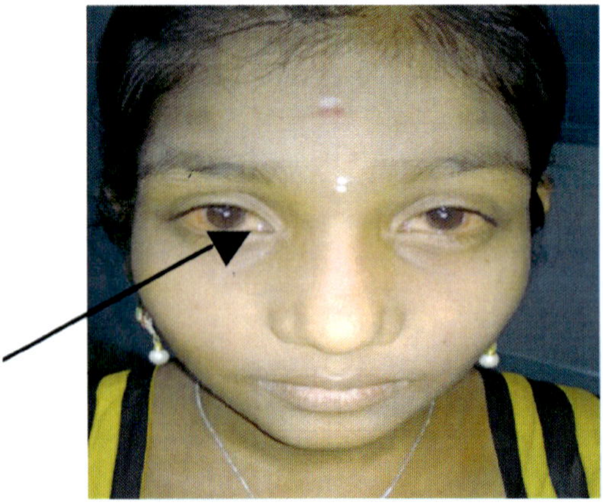

FIGURE 12.7 Allergic Conjunctivitis.

- intermittent/persistent congestion;
- sneezing;
- itching (nasal);
- rhinorrhea.

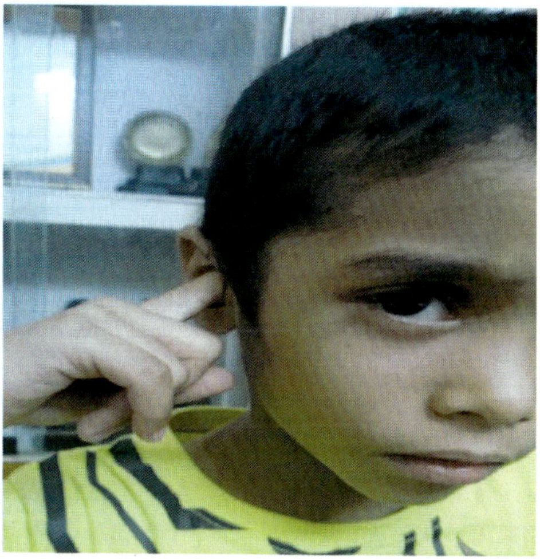

FIGURE 12.8 Shacking the external auditor canal to relieve the block in the middle ear due to *Eustachian tube* obstruction.

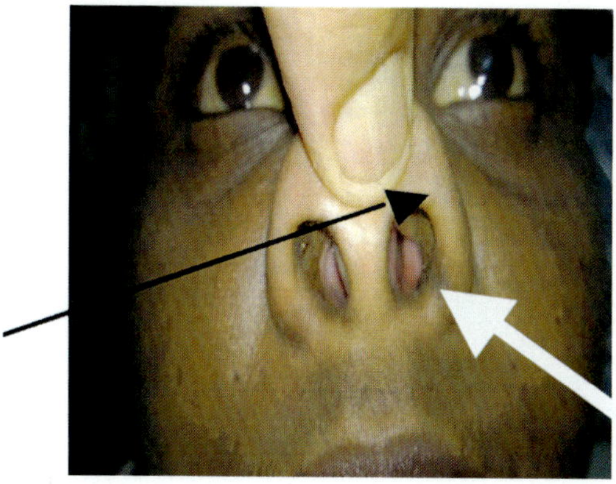

FIGURE 12.9 Allergic gape (child is breathing through the mouth due to severe nasal block).

The symptoms are precipitated by allergen exposure and may last for hours. The symptoms may be less clear in young children. Nasal congestion leading to obstruction is recognized in most patient surveys as the most bothersome symptom identified by sufferers of allergic rhinitis. It is not

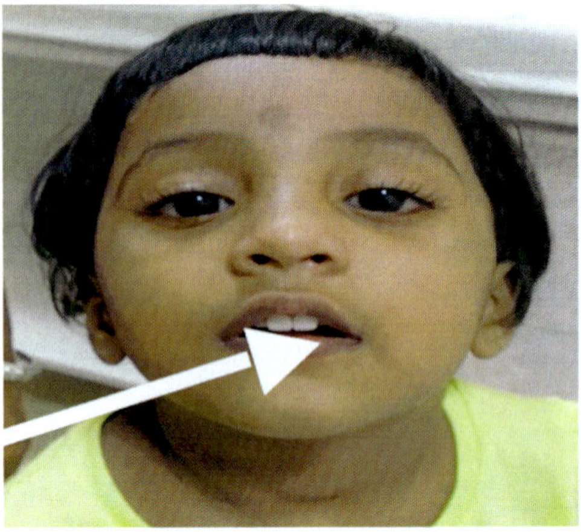

FIGURE 12.10 Method of examination of nose in a child (Pale Nasal mucosa due to allergic rhinitis).

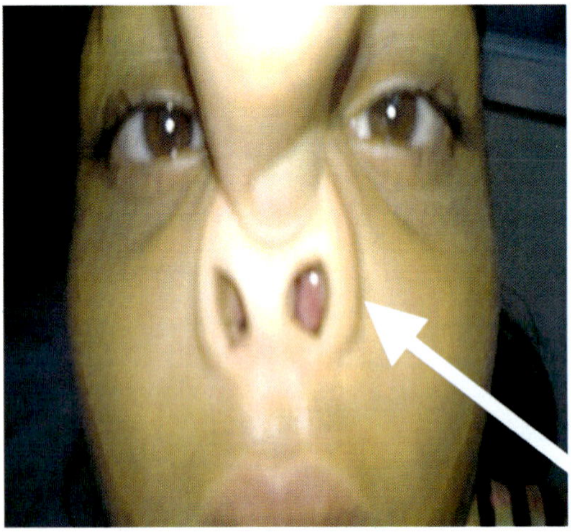

FIGURE 12.11 Hypertrophied inferior turbinate left.

always recognized in patients, especially those who have had the disease many years and accept a degree of obstruction as normal. All the symptoms have a negative impact on the quality of life. Table 12.1 gives the overview of the symptoms and signs associated with allergic rhinitis in children.

TABLE 12.1 Symptoms and Signs Associated with Allergic Rhinitis

Body Part	Symptom	Signs
Face	Mouth breathing, dryness of facial skin, facial pain.	Allergic shiners, allergic salute, allergic mannerisms, Dennies lines, allergic gape, allergic line, sniffling, long face syndrome, dental malocclusions.
Eyes	Itching, burning, swelling, increased tears, light pain, foreign body sensation.	Conjunctivitis, hyperemia, chemosis, long silky eyelashes, lower lid edema.
Nose	Running Nose, Watery/thick secretions, nasal itching, nasal block, nasal voice, heaviness of head, headache.	Pale nasal mucosa, hypertrophied turbinates, nasal polyps, hyper nasality, epistaxis (pricking of the nose), lateral fold in the lower nasal part.
Mouth	Dryness of mouth due to mouth breathing.	Dry lips, chapped lips, persistent mouth breathing.
Throat	Itching, burning, difficulty in swallowing, dryness, post nasal drip with throat clearing sounds	Cobble stone pharynx, allergic cluck.
Ears	Itching, blocking sensation, ear fullness, hard of hearing, watery/mucoid/pus discharge, otalgia, tinnitus, giddiness.	Serous otitis media (Glue ear).
Skin	Itching, burning, dryness of skin, often associated with eczema, swelling.	Flexural ulcers, urticarial rashes, dry skin, dermographism if associated with atopic rashes, urticarial dermatitis.
Chest	Cough, with or without sputum, difficulty in breathing.	Wheezing, accessory muscle use if associated with asthma.

12.5 CLASSIFICATION OF ALLERGIC RHINITIS

Allergic rhinitis can be seasonal or perennial, according to the relevant allergen. Seasonal AR is caused by a hypersensitivity reaction mediated by IgE to seasonal aeroallergens like pollens (i.e., outdoor allergens). Perennial AR on the other hand is due to allergens to which exposure may be present throughout the year; such as mites, mold, and animal dander (i.e., indoor allergens).

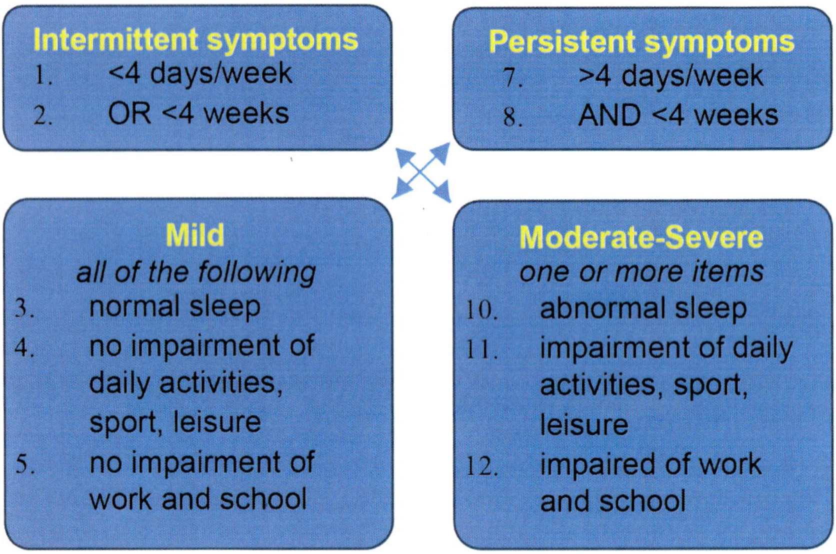

FIGURE 12.12 Allergic rhinitis and its impact on asthma (ARIA) classification of allergic rhinitis.

The distinction between seasonal and perennial is not globally applicable, and therefore, the Allergic Rhinitis and its Impact on Asthma (ARIA) group have revised it. Based on duration of symptoms, ARIA subdivides AR into intermittent or persistent (Figure 12.12).

Both approaches have their value, seasonal–perennial is useful for describing specific seasonal relationships with allergen exposure, whilst the ARIA approach is useful both for describing how the rhinitis manifests in terms of symptoms, its effects on quality of life and suggests the treatment approach. ARIA classification also usefully divides AR severity into mild, moderate and severe according to its impact on quality of life.

12.6 CO-MORBIDITIES OF ALLERGIC RHINITIS

Multiple co-morbidities commonly exist in patients with AR. The patients frequently have symptoms of other allergic diseases, such as atopic dermatitis, conjunctivitis and asthma. More than 40% of patients with AR have asthma, and more than 80% of asthmatic patients suffer concomitant rhinitis. Concomitant AR with asthma also increases the risk of asthma exacerbations and hospitalization.

12.6.1 ASTHMA

Progression from AR to asthma can occur and is described as the "allergic" or "atopic march." Although AR usually precedes asthma (or appears simultaneously), the opposite can be observed, often in preschoolers. In fact, in children, atopic dermatitis usually represents the first step of the atopic march, followed by allergic respiratory symptoms. In a recently published study, all patients, who presented with moderate-to-severe persistent AR, developed asthma symptoms. These results strongly indicate that the persistence of AR may be an important factor that increases the risk of asthma development in children.

12.6.2 SINUSITIS

Literature also supports a link between AR and sinusitis; 25–30% of individuals with acute sinusitis have AR, as do 40–67% of those with unilateral chronic sinusitis and up to 80% with chronic bilateral sinusitis. Other co-morbidities that are observed with increased frequency in patients with AR include nasal polyposis, upper respiratory infections, otitis media with effusion, breathing through the mouth, sleep disorders, decreased quality of life, and impaired learning and attention in children.

AR is also associated with an increased economic burden, it has been demonstrated that patients with AR have two-fold increases in medication costs and 1.8 times the number of visits to health practitioners when compared with matched controls.

12.6.3 QUALITY OF LIFE

Up to 88% of children with AR have sleep problems, leading to daytime fatigue and somnolence. These are accompanied by disorders of learning performance, behavior and attention. Children in the USA miss about

2 million school days a year because of AR. They might also be unable to take part in family or social events, resulting in emotional disturbances that manifest as anger, sadness, frustration, and withdrawal. In the UK, performance in school examinations taken by children aged 15–16 years is worsened by allergic rhinitis, particularly if antihistamines that cause sedation are used. Such studies may be unavailable in the developing countries; however, clinically these problems are found to be similar as compared to the developed countries. Furthermore, to strengthen the relationship, it has also been shown that management of allergic rhinitis in children may be accompanied by improvement of attention.

12.7 DIAGNOSIS

The diagnosis of allergic rhinitis is mainly made by clinical history (recurrence of same symptoms when exposure to same allergen), thorough physical examination, in the absence of upper respiratory tract infection, absence of structural abnormalities of nose, and a small number of IgE sensitization tests (SPT or specific IgE).

12.7.1 MEDICAL HISTORY AND PHYSICAL EXAMINATION

Clinical history remains the cornerstone for diagnosing and characterizing rhinitis in children. It is most important to identify a temporal association between symptoms suggestive of allergy and allergen exposures. Seasonal rhinitis is more commonly associated with outdoor pollen allergens, while indoor allergens are associated with perennial rhinitis. The following components can be helpful to take a history of allergies:

- Present illness and symptoms: age of onset, suspected cause, specific situations, locations, seasonal pattern, frequency, duration, relation to specific triggers or activities, exposures, eating, emotions, menstrual period, time of day
- Environmental history: use of air conditioning, detergents, carpets and sources of specific allergens or irritants at home
- Occupations and exposures to allergens or irritants
- Personal active or passive tobacco exposure

- Review of previous evaluations and treatments, current management and response to prior therapy
- Impact of illness: number of lost days from school, social adjustments, limitation of activities, presence of nocturnal symptoms, frequency of unscheduled physician's visits, emergency room visits or hospitalizations, fatigue, sleep disturbances, low self-esteem, shyness, depression, anxiety, hyperactivity, learning and attention problems, absenteeism.
- Presence of other organ-related diseases and medications
- Past medical history
- Prior drug or food allergies and intolerances
- Family history of allergy

The medical history is supplemented by an in-detail physical examination of the respiratory tract (including nose and chest), eyes, ears, and skin.

12.7.2 INVESTIGATIONS

12.7.2.1 In Vivo Testing

Skin tests are the most accurate diagnostic tool and are regarded as the gold standard for detection of IgE antibodies to specific allergic triggers. They are convenient, simple, biologically relevant, reproducible, easy and rapid to perform, with low cost and high sensitivity. However, they require a degree of training and experience to interpret the results and correlate them with the clinical history and physical findings. In addition, they must be performed in allergist clinics with emergency equipment available for the treatment of anaphylaxis.

Standardized, high quality extracts are required for optimal testing. A positive control (histamine) and a negative control (saline diluent) should always be included in the test. These controls help to avoid misinterpretation due to false negative and false positive results. Skin tests may be performed at any age, but reactions are less pronounced in small children. Medications such as antihistamines, topical high-potency corticosteroids, tricyclic antidepressants and some tranquilizers reduce skin reactivity and may cause false negative results, while dermatographism is the most common cause of false positive results.

Positive skin tests determine only sensitizations and not allergenicity of the extracts. All reactions should be correlated with the clinical history.

12.7.2.1.1 Types of Skin Tests

12.7.2.1.1.1 Epicutaneous

Prick or puncture tests (Figures 12.13 and 12.14) are the most convenient, least expensive and best screening method for detecting IgE mediated allergies. They are highly reproducible when carried out by trained personnel. Wheal diameter is measured 15–20 min after the test and a wheal size of 3 mm is generally considered to be positive. Results must be reported in millimeters (mm) to avoid the risk of confusing interpretations by other allergists. Prick tests are more specific and safe, but less sensitive than intracutaneous tests.

12.7.2.1.1.2 Intracutaneous

Intracutaneous are generally used when Epicutaneous tests are negative, despite an adequate history of exposure and symptoms. They are 10,000 times more sensitive than prick tests, show higher rates of false positives, and pose a greater risk of systemic reactions.

12.7.2.1.2 Nasal Challenge Tests

They are indicated when no other diagnostic methods are available, when the results of previous screening tests are not conclusive, and the benefit

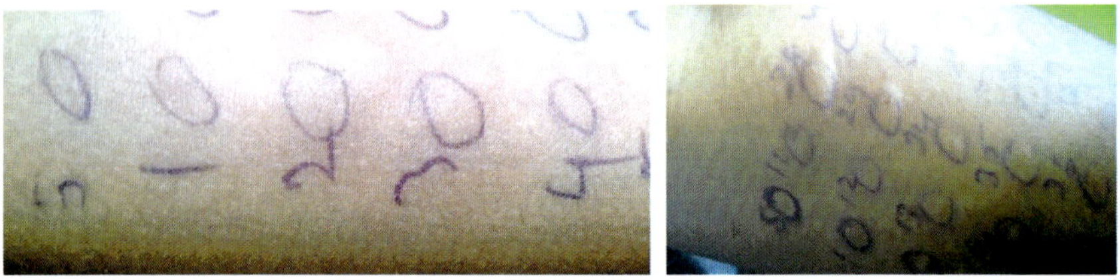

FIGURES 12.13–12.14 Allergy skin Prick test – Reaction.

of the test results outweighs the risk involved. Keeping in mind of the complexities involved these tests should only be performed by trained allergists.

12.7.2.2 In Vitro Testing

12.7.2.2.1 Total Serum IgE

Total serum IgE has been used as a marker for atopy. However, approximately half of allergic patients have a total IgE within the normal range. Therefore, the measurement of total serum IgE has little value in assessing allergic aetiology of rhinitis in childhood.

12.7.2.2.2 Allergen-Specific IgE Antibody

Allergen-specific IgE antibody is the most important serological marker used in the diagnosis of allergic disease to confirm sensitization in an individual who has a positive history of exposure. They are especially indicated in patients with extensive skin inflammation, those who cannot abstain from antihistamine therapy, who are uncooperative, or who have a high risk of anaphylaxis. They are more expensive than skin tests and require longer obtaining the results.

Since quality assurance is of paramount importance when in vitro assays are used for diagnostic purposes, the ideal situation would be to refer patients (or send their serum samples) to certified laboratories that use a third generation IgE antibody assay to report quantitative results.

12.7.2.2.3 Component Resolved Diagnostics

Recent studies employing a molecular diagnostic approach suggest that measurement of IgE response to specific allergenic components may be more useful in determining clinically relevant sensitization.

12.7.2.3 Other Tests

12.7.2.3.1 Radiographic Studies

Radiographic studies are not needed to establish the diagnosis of allergic rhinitis; they can be helpful for evaluating possible structural abnormalities or to help detect complications or comorbid conditions, such as sinusitis or adenoid hypertrophy.

12.7.2.3.2 Peak Nasal Inspiratory Flow Rate

Peak nasal inspiratory flow is an easy and inexpensive means of measuring nasal obstruction and correlates significantly with severity of symptoms scores. The normal peak nasal inspiratory flow rate (PNIFR) is 100–300 L/min. A PNIFR below 100 L/min is suggestive of nasal obstruction. The PNIFR can be used to assess the efficacy of intranasal steroids.

12.7.2.3.3 Rhinomanometry

Rhinomanometry is a measurement of nasal resistance to airflow. This requires expensive equipment as well as trained personnel; therefore it remains as research tool.

12.7.2.3.4 Spirometry

All patients of allergic rhinitis should undergo spirometry to exclude latent asthma.

12.8 TREATMENT

Medications for allergic rhinitis will help the patient in controlling their symptoms and improving quality of life. The goal of management is to achieve optimal symptom control. Therapeutic options include:

- parent and patient education,
- allergen avoidance,
- nasal irrigation,
- pharmacotherapy, and
- alergen specific immunotherapy.

12.8.1 PARENT AND PATIENT EDUCATION

Parents and patients (late childhood/adolescents) should be educated about the nature of allergic disease, the likelihood of disease progression, and the need for treatment. Concerns about safety of the treatment modalities used should be adequately discussed. Medical treatment aims to either reduce symptoms or alter the immune system to induce tolerance, or both of these. Information on the aims of treatment, probable benefits, dosing schedule and possible side-effects should be provided to prevent false expectations and enhance adherence to the prescribed regimen. Techniques to be used for medicine delivery should be well demonstrated and discussed; this can help in reducing medication errors. Patients should be informed about factors that aggravate nasal symptoms because avoidance of these could alleviate them.

12.8.2 ALLERGEN/IRRITANT AVOIDANCE

The first therapeutic approach is avoiding the allergen/irritant responsible for causing the symptoms. The avoidance of the allergen/irritant has been proven to result in improvement in symptoms of allergic rhinitis and reduction of the need for drugs. The beneficial effect of environmental control may take from days to weeks. In most cases, complete avoidance of the allergen is not feasible due to practical and/or economic reasons. Appropriate allergen-avoidance measures should be considered along with pharmacologic treatment. A range of inhalant allergens has been associated with allergic rhinitis, of which house dust mite is the more common and most investigated allergen. Although the general consensus is that allergen avoidance should lead to an improvement of symptoms, the interventions should be aimed at multiple modalities and not on single strategies.

For house dust mite the major strategies include, regularly washing bedding (every 1–2 weeks) at 55–60°C, if possible, to kill mites; washing pillows in hot water (55–60°C) and encasing pillows and mattresses with protective coverings that have a pore size of 6 mm or less; reducing indoor relative humidity to below 50% and avoid damp housing conditions. For pollen, avoiding contact with them during the pollen season by keeping windows closed and using air-conditioning where possible is advised.

12.8.3 NASAL IRRIGATION

Nasal irrigation with saline is an inexpensive treatment for allergic rhinitis. It is associated with improvement in nasal itching and congestion, rhinorrhea, and sneezing along with reduced the need for antihistamines. The procedure is associated with improved mucociliary function, reduced mucosal oedema and decreased inflammatory mediators. Irrigation is generally well tolerated in children because of the preference towards finer sprays. Commercially available pediatric irrigation kits contain a nasal irrigation bottle and sachets of measured sodium chloride for adding to warm water. Alternatively, a small syringe or a bulb applicator may be used. Ideally, douching may be incorporated into a daily bathing regimen and should be continued while symptoms persist.

12.8.4 PHARMACOTHERAPY

Drugs available for treating allergic rhinitis in children are oral or intranasal antihistamines, intranasal corticosteroids, and leukotriene receptor antagonists. Approach to therapy for pediatric allergic rhinitis as recommended by the European Academy of Allergy and Clinical Immunology (EAACI) has been outlined in Figure.12.19.

While considering pharmacological treatment, the following factors are to be considered:

- age of the patient;
- severity of the disease;
- safety of the drug;

- efficacy of the drug;
- cost-effectiveness of the drug;
- compliance.

12.8.4.1 Oral H1 Antihistamines

Oral antihistamines are the most commonly used medications in childhood allergic rhinitis.

The **first generation antihistamines** are generally not recommended due to sedative effect, cognitive impairment, which lead to poor school performance, tachyphylaxis and cause anti-cholinergic side effects. First generation antihistamines have long half-life with bed-time dose can cause sedation in day time.

Newer, **second-generation anti-histamines** have now become the first-line therapy for children with allergic rhinitis. Second generation antihistamines have greater selectivity for peripheral H1 receptors with an additional anti-inflammatory effect. Second generation H1 antihistamines, such as cetirizine, levocitirizine, Fexofenadine, desloratidine, and loratadine, have fewer side effects than earlier formulations; in particular they are less sedating, faster acting, and have a longer duration of action. Cetirizine, Levocetirizine, and Desloratadine are indicated from 6 months of age in children, however, Loratadine and Fexofenadine, are indicated from 2 years of age. As for the efficacy is concerned, all these agents have equally effective even though cetirizine group shows little sedation in certain children. Cetirizine and fexofenadine differ from other antihistamines as they are not metabolized in the liver, but they are mainly excreted unchanged in the urine or in the faces.

In a large international Observational Survey in Children with Allergic Rhinitis (OSCAR) which recruited 4581 patients (3048 with AR), it was documented that second-generation antihistamines have a better risk:benefit ratio than first-generation antihistamines. Furthermore, levocetirizine and fexofenadine were perceived by parents and physicians to produce significantly higher treatment satisfaction than the majority of the other antihistamines with respect to overall efficacy and tolerability, and impact on the child's sleep and school activities.

An open label study in 62 patients indicated that levocetirizine 5 mg for 6 months reliably controlled persistent rhinitis, and showed a trend to be more effective for reduction of symptoms, improvement of QOL and decreasing nasal inflammation, when administered as long-term continuous therapy rather than as on-demand therapy.

12.8.4.2 Intranasal Antihistamines

Intranasal H1-antihistamines are effective in reducing itching, sneezing, runny nose and nasal congestion. They are effective within minutes of administration.

Azelastine nasal spray 0.15%, a topical second-generation antihistamine, was approved for use in patients above 5 years of age and older with seasonal allergic rhinitis and it is well-tolerated. Because of side effects such as mild somnolence or bad taste in some patients, Azelastine nasal spray not recommending in children. Combination of H1 antihistamine with azelastine is not recommended in children.

Olopatadine 0.6% is another intranasal H1 antihistamine approved for children with Seasonal Allergic Rhinitis above 6 years. Found to be effective even in Allergic Conjunctivitis also. In clinical trials, it is demonstrated few side effects like bitter taste, headache and pharyngolaryngeal pain. Few other studies demonstrated similar efficacy and side effect profile in children between 2 and 6 years.

12.8.4.3 Intranasal Steroids

Data from meta-analyses have documented that intranasal corticosteroids are the most effective therapeutic agents for allergic rhinitis. They are the first line of treatment for moderate to severe allergic rhinitis and in nasal blocker. They are very effective in improving all symptoms of allergic rhinitis like sneezing, running nose, nasal congestion and itching, as well as ocular symptoms. If nasal congestion is the predominant symptom, intranasal steroid is the first line of therapy. For the ocular symptoms of allergy, intranasal steroids appear to be at least as effective as oral antihistamines.

In a recent consensus paper, the American College of Allergy, Asthma and Immunology listed intranasal steroids as the most effective therapy in controlling the symptoms of allergic rhinitis. Due to their mechanism of action efficacy usually appears after 7–8 hours of dosing but maximum efficacy may take up to 2 weeks. Quality of life score improvement with intranasal steroids better than oral and topical H1 antihistamines.

The current intranasal preparations are well tolerated and can be used on a long-term basis without atrophy of the mucosa. Therapy failure is often due to poor compliance or wrong technique of administration of the drug. The most frequently reported adverse effects include: nasal stuffiness, dry nose, dry mouth, minimal nasal bleeding, sneezing, irritation of the nose and throat, nausea, headache, and dizziness. These reactions are more frequent with the older agents but several of those products have been reformulated as aqueous (AQ) preparations to reduce adverse effects. Although extremely rare, children receiving long-term therapy should also be monitored for nasal septum perforation, which is very rare and can be due to prolonged use with wrong technique. Localized infections of the nose and pharynx with *Candida albicans* are infrequent (Figures 12.15–12.17).

One of the greatest concerns for most families is the effect of long-term steroid use on growth. Evidence shows that the long-term use of intranasal steroids is free of the concerns associated with growth. Patients receiving only intranasal steroids appear to be at low risk of developing hypothalamic-pituitary-adrenal axis (HPAA) suppression because of the low systemic bioavailability and the use of low doses. The need for continuation of therapy and technique is to be evaluated in every consultation. Current intranasal preparations can be used on long-term basis and are well tolerated. Evaluate the child for technique and need for intranasal steroid during every visit. Choose an intranasal steroid with low systemic bioavailability at a minimum dose required to achieve symptom control (Table 12.2).

12.8.4.4 Cromones

The chromone sodium cromoglycate is less effective than antihistamines and corticosteroids. Nedocromil sodium seems to have only slightly

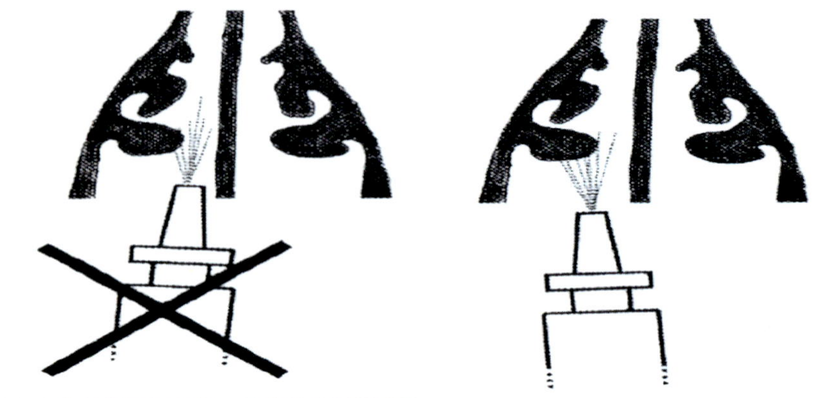

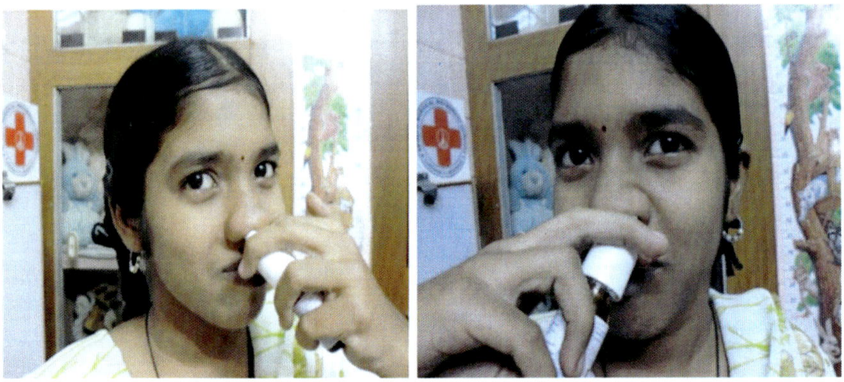

FIGURES 12.15–12.16 Correct method of usage of intranasal steroid spray.

greater efficacy and a more rapid onset of action compared to disodium chromoglycolate. Therefore, cromones are not considered a major therapeutic option in the treatment of allergic rhinitis. Additionally frequent dosing may hamper compliance in patients.

12.8.4.5 Decongestants

Nasal decongestants (xylometazoline, oxy-metazoline) are effective in controlling nasal obstruction. Intranasal decongestants are to be used short periods only. Prolonged use (>10 days) of intranasal decongestants may

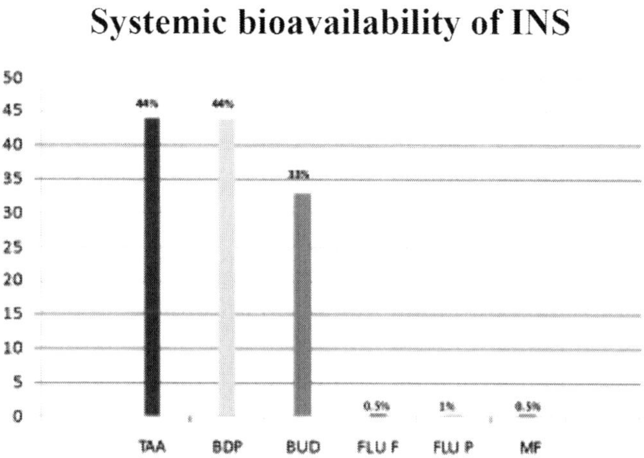

FIGURE 12.17 Bioavailability of Various Intranasal Steroids (*Adapted from Eli O. Meltzer. The Role of Nasal Corticosteroids in the Treatment of Rhinitis. Immunology and Allergy Clinics of North America. Michael A. Kaliner August 2011, vol. 31, pp. 545–560. Used with permission from Elsevier.)

lead to tachyphylaxis, a rebound swelling of the nasal mucosa and leads to "drug-induced rhinitis" (rhinitis medicamentosa). Hence not recommended in small children.

Oral decongestants such as ephedrine, phenylephrine, and phenylpropanolamine (banned in some countries including the USA) and pseudoephedrine are available oral decongestants. These drugs are commonly used as cough and cold syrups along with first generation antihistamines. Due to systemic side effects like irritability, dizziness, headache, tremor and insomnia as well as tachycardia and hypertension, these drugs are not recommended in children with allergic rhinitis.

12.8.4.6 Leukotriene Receptor Antagonist

Montelukast was found to improve nasal and bronchial symptoms. Leukotriene receptor antagonists are more effective than placebo, equivalent to intranasal glucocorticosteroids for treating seasonal allergic rhinitis. Montelukast is effective in allergic rhinitis associated with other comorbid conditions like asthma, urticaria, etc. The addition of an antihistamine to montelukast does not appear to have added benefit in some studies.

12.8.4.7 Ipratropium Bromide

The anticholinergic intranasal agent ipratropium bromide is effective in severe intractable rhinorrhea due to allergic rhinitis or vasomotor rhinitis. It has no effect on nasal block or nasal itching. Therefore ipratropium nasal spray is not effective in the vast majority of cases of AR. Side effects include mild intermittent nose bleeds and nasal dryness. It is recommended for above 5 years old children, if required.

12.8.4.8 Alternative Therapies

Alternative treatment modalities such as acupuncture, homeopathy, siddha medicine, phototherapeutics, and bio resonance are not sufficiently validated and therefore are not recommended.

The daily dosage of the different drugs are mentioned in Table 12.2, along with advantages and disadvantages of individual pharmacotherapy options discussed in Table 12.3.

12.8.5 ALLERGEN-SPECIFIC IMMUNOTHERAPY (AIT)

AIT is the administration of increasing doses of allergen extract to an allergic patient to ameliorate the symptoms associated with the subsequent exposure to the causative allergen and was introduced on an empirical basis about one hundred years ago. In the last 20 years there has been an impressive development in the field of allergen immunotherapy. AIT induces clinical and immunologic tolerance thereby preventing the progression of the disease and halt the atopic march and improving the quality of life. It also prevents development of neosensitization to allergen. Immunotherapy has demonstrated short-term and long-term benefits and it provides sustained long-term benefit after treatment completion. The routes of administration commonly used

TABLE 12.2 Daily Dosages of Various Medicines According to Patient Age

Agent	Daily Dosage	Age
Antihistamines		
Cetirizine	5 or 10 mg q.d.	>12 years
	5 or 10 mg q.d.	6–11 years
	2.5 mg (1D2 tsp of syrup) q.d. or bid	2–5 years
	Maximum dose: 5 mg q.d. (syrup or chewable tablet)	6–23 months
	2.5 mg (1D2 tsp of syrup) q.d.	
	Maximum dose: 2.5 mg (1D2 tsp of syrup) b.i.d.	
Levocetirizine	1.25 mg q.d. or 2.5 mL of syrup 2.5 mg q.d. or 5 mL of syrup	6 months to 5 years 6–11 years
	(5 mL – 2.5 mg)	>12 years
	5 mg q.d. or 1o ml of solution	
Desloratadine	Tablets: 5 mg q.d.	>12 years to 6 11 years
	Syrup: 2.5 mg in 5 mL (1 tsp) or 2.5 mg q.d. Syrup: 1.25 mg in 2.5 mL (1D 2 tsp) q.d. Syrup: 1.0 mg in 2.0 mL q.d.	1–5 years 6–11 months
Loratadine	10 mg q.d.	>12 years
	5 mg q.d. (5 mL syrup = 5mg)	2 – 12 years
Fexofenadine	180 mg q.d. or 60 mg b.i.d.	>12 years
	30 mg b.i.d. or 5 ml b.i.d. (30 mg – 5 mL)	2–11 years
Intranasal steroids		
Fluticasone propionate	Start dose: 50 mg each nostril/nostril q.d.; increase to 100 mg each nostril q.d.	>4 years through adolescence
	Maximum dose: 200 mg/nostril q.d. (each spray – 50 mg)	
Mometasone furoate	2 sprays in each nostril (100 μg/nostril) q.d.	>12 years
	Maintenance dose: one spray each nostril	
	One spray each nostril (50 μg/nostril) q.d.	2–11 yr
	Each spray contains – 50 mg	

TABLE 12.2 (Continued)

Agent	Daily Dosage	Age
Fluticasone furoate	2 sprays each nostril (110 mg) q.d.	>12 years
	One spray each nostril (55 mg) q.d.	2–12 years
Budesonide aqueous preparation	Initial 2 sprays each nostril and reduce to one spray each nostril q.d. (each spray – 100 mgs)	>6 years and adolescents
	Each spray (32 mg) – 4 sprays each nostril q.d.	>12 years
	2 sprays each nostril q.d.	6–11 years
Triamcinolone acetonide aqueous	110 μg/nostril q.d /nostril q.d to b.i.d.	>12 years to 6–11 years
	110 μg/nostril q.d. (2 sprays each nostril)	2–5 years
	1 spray each nostril q.d. each spray – 55 mg.	
Leukotriene-receptor antagonist		
Montelukast	10 mg q.d.	15 years and more 5–14 years
	5 mg (chewable tablet) q.d.	2–4 years
	4 mg (chewable tablet or packet of oral granules) q.d.	6–23 months
	4 mg (packet of oral granules) q.d.	

Note: q.d.: once daily; b.i.d.: twice-daily; t.i.d.: three times per day.

TABLE 12.3 Advantages and Disadvantages of Pharmacotherapy

Advantages	Disadvantages
Inhaled Nasal Steroids	*Inhaled Nasal Steroids*
• Most potent anti-inflammatory treatment; • Strong suppression of all nasal symptoms; • Good effect on conjunctival symptoms; • Superior to other available pharmacological treatments; • Clinically relevant improvement of quality of life; • Low bioavailability with recent molecules such as fluticazone and Memotazone.	• Reduction of symptoms could take several days to weeks; • Faulty technique can leads to treatment failure or adverse events such as epistaxis (in 10–15% of patients); • Steroid phobia (for some patients and parents); • Nausea/vomiting can occur due to if drug enters the pharynx.

TABLE 12.3 (Continued)

Advantages	Disadvantages
Oral Antihistamines	*Oral Antihistamines*
• Effective for nasal symptoms of itch, sneezing, and rhinorrhea; • Reduction of conjunctival, oral, and skin symptoms; • Rapid onset of action (within 1 h); • Few interactions with drugs or alcohol.	• Regular treatment is more effective than on-demand therapy; • Modest effect on nasal congestion; • Sedation still happens in some patients.
Intra Nasal Antihistamines	*Intra Nasal Antihistamines*
• Effective and safe treatment for nasal itch, sneezing, and rhinorrhea. • Rapid onset of action (within 15 min) Disadvantages: neglect of systemic nature of allergic rhinitis; sparse	• Neglect of systemic nature of allergic rhinitis; • Sparse effects on co-morbid conditions (e.g., conjunctival symptoms)
Chromones	*Chromones*
• Safe treatment with effect on nasal symptoms related to allergic rhinitis.	• Several applications per day; • Weak effect on symptoms of AR
Antileukotrienes (Montelukast)	*Antileukotrienes (Montelukast)*
• Effective for nasal obstruction, rhinorrhea, and conjunctival symptoms; • Effective for bronchial symptoms in patients with allergic rhinitis; • Generally well tolerated.	• Not consistently effective; • Occasional reports of adverse events, such as headache, gastrointestinal symptoms, hyperactivity, rash.
Oral Decongestants	*Oral Decongestants*
• Reduces nasal obstruction • Available in combination with an antihistamine	• Frequent reports of side-effects, such as hypertension, insomnia, agitation, and tachycardia.
Nasal Decongestants	*Nasal Decongestants*
• Advantages: potent vasoconstrictive agents acting on nasal congestion only; rapid onset of action (within 10 min)	• Overuse by patients is common; • Rhinitis medicamentosa after prolonged use > 10–14 days. • Occasional adverse events (e.g., nasal irritation and increased rhinorrhea)

TABLE 12.3 (Continued)

Advantages	Disadvantages
Intra nasal anticholinergics (Ipatropium)	*Intra nasal anticholinergics (Ipatropium)*
• Good effect on rhinorrhea.	• Three applications per day; • Occasional reports of adverse events such as dry nose, epistaxis, urinary retention, and glaucoma.
Systemic steroids	*Systemic steroids*
• Most potent rescue treatment, with beneficial effects for all symptoms, including nasal obstruction; systemic anti-inflammatory treatment in some countries.	• More adverse events related to oral corticosteroid treatment; rarely indicated; only for short-term use.

are the subcutaneous immunotherapy (SCIT) and sublingual immunotherapy (SLIT). SLIT therapies are available either as tablets or drops (liquid).

12.8.5.1 Indications and Contraindications

There should be a clear history of AR with evidence of clinically relevant sensitizations, not responding adequately to pharmacotherapy. AIT should be performed with a standardized allergen extract or preparation registered or approved by the authorities. A physician should initiate therapy with training in the diagnostic procedures, treatment and follow-up of allergic rhinitis children. Significant concurrent disease, impaired lung function and severe asthma are contraindications.

12.8.5.2 Subcutaneous Injection Immunotherapy (SCIT)

SCIT entails repeated injections with allergen extracts and represents the standard modality of immunotherapy. The 2007 Cochrane systematic review of SCIT in AR demonstrates that it is effective although there were no accepted studies that were conducted exclusively in children. Subcutaneous injection immunotherapy has been associated with systemic reactions but it is generally well tolerated in children. There are also some non-blinded data to suggest that SCIT may alter the natural history of allergic disease in childhood. Factors associated with severe adverse effects are unstable asthma, elevated allergen exposure during therapy, concomitant diseases such as severe infections and inexperienced healthcare staff. Pre treatment with antihistamine may reduce the rate of adverse effects of SCIT. Also, pre treatment with anti-IgE has been used to reduce the rate of adverse reactions associated with up dosing with SCIT. Patients should only be given subcutaneous allergen immunotherapy in clinics supervised by doctors who are trained and skilled in adjustment of doses of immunotherapy. There are no pediatric data addressing the question of how long SCIT should be continued although adult data would suggest that 3 years is sufficient at least for pollens.

12.8.5.3 Sublingual Immunotherapy (SLIT)

The effectiveness of SLIT for AR has been evaluated in a number of systematic reviews. The 2011 review demonstrates its effectiveness for pollen and house dust mite-driven rhinitis. This review highlights the considerable heterogeneity between studies, not all preparations seem to be effective. Both continuous and co seasonal protocols have been described, both seem to be effective although the latter may take longer to impact on the symptoms. There are also some non-blinded data to suggest that SLIT may prevent the development of asthma. Two commercial grass products have received authorization for patients at least 5 years of age. It seems to be safer than subcutaneous immunotherapy because side-effects are usually restricted to the upper airways and gastrointestinal tract; rare anaphylactic episodes, but no deaths, have been reported. Although perceived to be a convenient therapy, there is concern about compliance with SLIT with sales data suggesting 44% compliance in the first year, 28% in second year and 13% in the third year although regular clinic contact may improve this. Again, adult data would suggest that 3 years of SLIT is sufficient, at least for pollens.

12.8.5.4 Health Economics

Pharmacoeconomic models based on data provided by clinical trials and meta-analyses indicate that AIT is cost-efficient. One of the few real patient cohort studies to investigate cost-effectiveness of SCIT was performed in US children with allergic rhinitis; patients in the SCIT group incurred 33% lower healthcare costs.

12.8.5.5 Other Routes

Thirteen out of fourteen controlled studies presently available agree on the clinical effectiveness of local nasal immunotherapy (LNIT) in reducing symptoms of pollen- and mite-induced rhinitis and the specific nasal reactivity (Figure 12.18). The majority of the clinical studies have been conducted in adult patients. Oral immunotherapy and bronchial immunotherapy are presently not sufficiently supported by experimental evidence.

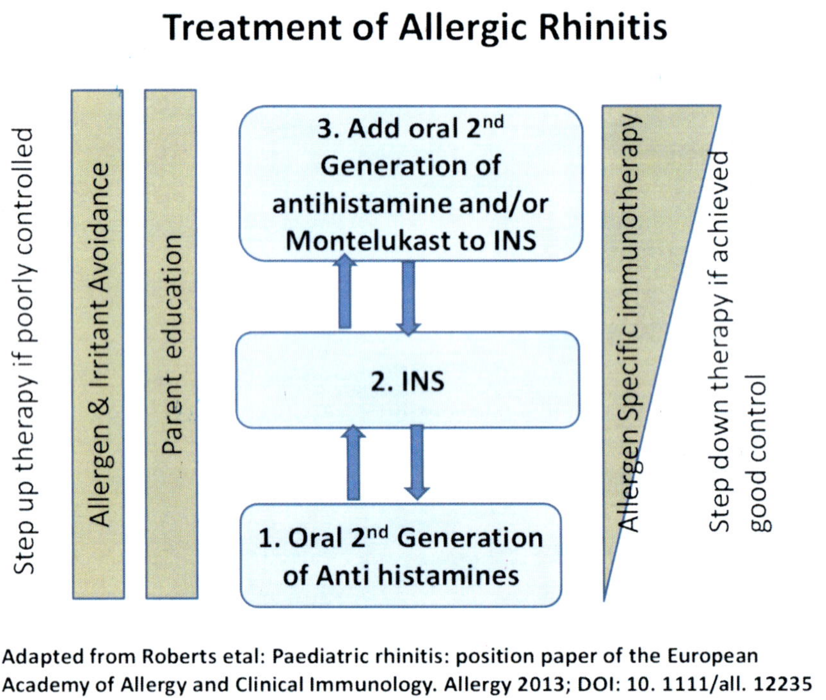

FIGURE 12.18 Approach to therapy for pediatric allergic rhinitis (1, 2 and 3 are potential entry points into therapeutic approach depending on the severity of the rhinitis symptoms).

Clinical trials with Intra lymphatic IT and Epicutaneous IT for AR are promising.

12.9 CONCLUSIONS

AR is a large and growing burden on the pediatric population. Early appropriate diagnosis and effective management is vital to avoid educational, social, and emotional problems in children. Allergen avoidance is an ideal, though often impractical therapy for AR. In most cases, pharmacotherapy will be the major intervention with antihistamines and intranasal steroids being the first-line agents. First-generation antihistamines should be avoided because of their poor side-effect profiles. In children with persistent symptoms and in nasal blockers, intranasal steroids are an effective therapeutic option and newer agents exhibit no meaningful systemic effects. Several other medication classes, including decongestants, antileukotrienes, and anticholinergics, are available as adjuncts to antihistamine and steroid treatment. Furthermore, immunotherapy is an effective, disease-modifying strategy. In all pediatric cases, finding an effective, convenient treatment regimen, devoid of sedative or cognitive side effects, should be the clinical goal.

KEYWORDS

- **allergen immunotherapy**
- **allergic rhinitis**
- **antihistamines**
- **atopic march**
- **intranasal corticosteroids**
- **quality of life**
- **serum-specific IgE**
- **skin test**
- **type1 hypersensitivity**

REFERENCES

Aït-Khaled, N., Pearce, N., Anderson, H. R., Ellwood, P., Montefort, S., Shah, J., ISAAC Phase Three Study Group. Global map of the prevalence of symptoms of rhinoconjunctivitis in children: the International Study of Asthma and Allergies in Childhood (ISAAC) phase three. *Allergy* 2009, 64, 123–148.

Angier, E., Willington, J., Scadding, G., Holmes, S., Walker, S., British Society for Allergy and Clinical Immunology (BSACI) Standards of Care Committee. Management of allergic and non-allergic rhinitis: a primary care summary of the BSACI guideline. *Prim Care Respir J.* 2010 Sep, 19(3), 217–222

Barr, J. G., Al-Reefy, H., Fox, A. T., Hopkins C. Allergic rhinitis in children. *BMJ.* 2014, 349, g41–53.

Bousquet, J., Khaltaev, N., Cruz, A. A., Denburg, J., Fokkens, W. J., Togias, A., et al. Allergic rhinitis and its impact on asthma (ARIA). *Allergy* 2008, 63, 990–996.

Bousquet, J., Van Cauwenberge, P., Bachert, C., Canonica, G. W., Demoly, P., Durham, S. R., et al. European Academy of Allergy and Clinical Immunology (EAACI); Allergic Rhinitis and its Impact on Asthma (ARIA). Requirements for medications commonly used in the treatment of allergic rhinitis. *Allergy* 2003, 58, 192–197

Brozek, J. L., Bousquet, J., Baena-Cagnani, C. E., Bonini, S., Canonica, G. W., Casale, T. B., et al. Global Allergy and Asthma European Network; Grading of Recommendations Assessment, Development and Evaluation Working Group. Allergic Rhinitis and its Impact on Asthma (ARIA) guidelines: 2010 revision. *J Allergy Clin Immunol* 2010, 126, 466–476.

Burgess, J. A., Walters, E. H., Byrnes, G. B., Matheson, M. C., Jenkins, M. A., Wharton, C. L., et al. Childhood allergic rhinitis predicts asthma incidence and persistence to middle age: a longitudinal study. *J Allergy Clin Immunol* 2007, 120, 863–869.

Canonica, G. W., Fumagalli, F., Guerra, L., Baiardini, I., Compalati, E., Rogkakou, A., et al; Global Allergy and Asthma European Network. Levocetirizine in persistent allergic rhinitis: continuous or on-demand use? A pilot study. *Curr Med Res Opin. 2008*, 24(10), 2829–2839.

Ciprandi, G., Cirillo, I., Vizzaccaro, A., Tosca, M., Passalacqua, G., Pallestrini, E., et al. Seasonal and perennial allergic rhinitis: is this classification adherent to real life? *Allergy* 2005, 60, 882–887.

Di Cara, G., Carelli, A., Latini, A., Panfili, E., Bizzarri, I., Ciprandi, G., et al. Severity of allergic rhinitis and asthma development in children. *World Allergy Organ J.* 2015, 8(1), 13.

Eli O Meltzer. The Role of Nasal Corticosteroids in the treatment of Rhinitis. Immunology and Allergy clinics of North America. Michael A. Kaliner August 2011, 31, 545–560.

Ferrer, M., Morais-Almeida, M., Guizova, M., Khanferyan R. Evaluation of treatment satisfaction in children with allergic disease treated with an antihistamine: an international, non-interventional, retrospective study. *Clin Drug Investig.* 2010, 30(1), 15–34

Greiner, A. N., Hellings, P. W., Rotiroti, G., Scadding GK. Allergic rhinitis. *Lancet.* 2011, 378(9809), 2112–2122.

Hofmaier S. Allergic airway diseases in childhood: An update. *Pediatr Allergy Immunol* 2015, 25, 810–816.

Høst, A., Andrae, S., Charkin, S., Diaz-Vázquez, C., Dreborg, S., Eigenmann, P. A., et al. Allergy testing in children: why, who, when and how? *Allergy* 2003, 58, 559–569.

James, L. K., Durham SR. Update on mechanisms of allergen injection immunotherapy. *Clin Exp Allergy* 2008, 38, 1074–1088.

Jáuregui, I., Mullol, J., Dávila, I., Ferrer, M., Bartra, J., del Cuvillo, A., et al. Allergic rhinitis and School Performance. *J Investig Allergol Clin Immunol* 2009, 19S(1), 32–39.

Kim, D. K., Rhee, C. S., Han, D. H., Won, T. B., Kim, D. Y., Kim, J. W. Treatment of allergic rhinitis is associated with improved attention performance in children: the Allergic Rhinitis Cohort Study for Kids (ARCO-Kids). *PLoS One.* 2014, 9(10), e109–145.

Kim, J. M., Lin, S. Y., Suarez-Cuervo, C., Chelladurai, Y., Ramanathan, M., Segal, J. B., et al. Allergen-specific immunotherapy for pediatric asthma and rhinoconjunctivitis: a systematic review. *Pediatrics.* 2013, 131(6), 1155–1167.

Mallol, J., Crane, J., von Mutius, E., Odhiambo, J., Keil, U., Stewart, A., ISAAC Phase Three Study Group. The International Study of Asthma and Allergies in Childhood (ISAAC) phase three: a global synthesis. *Allergol Immunopathol (Madr)* 2013, 41, 73–85.

Meltzer, E. O. Quality of life in adults and children with allergic rhinitis. *J Allergy Clin Immunol* 2001, 108(1 Suppl), S45–53.

Nagaraju, K. Allergen Specific Immunotherapy, Allergic Disorders, *Indian Journal of Practical Pediatrics* 2013, 15(3), 212–216.

Nagaraju, K. Clinical features and Diagnosis of Allergic rhinitis. In: *Manual of Pediatric Allergy*. Major K Nagaraju (eds.) 1st edition, Jaypee, The Health Science Publishers: New Delhi, pp. 97–105.

Nagaraju, K. Treatment of Allergic rhinitis. In: *Manual of Pediatric Allergy*. Major K. Nagaraju (eds.). 1st edition, Jaypee, The Health Science Publishers: New Delhi, pp. 106–113.

Portnoy, J. M., Van Osdol, T., Williams, P. B. Evidence-based strategies for treatment of allergic rhinitis. *Curr Allergy Asthma Rep.* 2004, 4(6), 439–446.

Roberts, G., Xatzipsalti, M., Borrego, L. M., Custovic, A., Halken, S., Hellings, P. W., et al. Pediatric rhinitis: position paper of the European Academy of Allergy and Clinical Immunology. *Allergy*. 2013, 68(9), 1102–1116.

Rotiroti, G., Roberts, G., Scadding GK. Rhinitis in children: common clinical presentations and differential diagnoses. *Pediatr Allergy Immunol.* 2015, 26(2), 103–110.

Rotiroti, G., Scadding GK. Allergic rhinitis – an overview of a common disease. *Paed & Child Health* 2012, 22, 7.

Scadding, G. K. Optimal management of allergic rhinitis. *Arch Dis Child* 2015, 100, 576–582.

Schad, C. A., Skoner DP. Antihistamines in the pediatric population: achieving optimal outcomes when treating seasonal allergic rhinitis and chronic urticaria. *Allergy Asthma Proc.* 2008, 29(1), 7–13.

Simons FER on Behalf of the Early Prevention of Asthma in Atopic Children (EPPAC) Study Group. Safety of levocetirizine treatment in young atopic children: An 18 months study. *Pediatr Allergy Immunol.* 2007, 18(6), 535–542.

Skoner, D. P. Allergic rhinitis: definition, epidemiology, pathophysiology, detection, and diagnosis. *J Allergy Clin Immunol* 2001, 108(1 Suppl), S2–8.

Weiner, J. M., Abramson, M. J., Puy, R. M. Intranasal corticosteroids versus oral H1 receptor antagonists in allergic rhinitis: systematic review of randomized controlled trials. *BMJ* 1998, 317, 1624–1629.

Wilson, A. M., O'Byrne, P. M., Parameswaran, K. Leukotriene receptor antagonists for allergic rhinitis: a systematic review and meta-analysis. *Am J Med* 2004, 116, 338–344.

World Allergy Organization (WAO) website: http://www.worldallergy.org/professional/allergic_diseases_center/ rhinitis/rhinitis_indepth.php accessed on July 30, 2015.

World Allergy Organization (WAO). White book on allergy. 2011.

Yanez, A., Rodrigo, G. J. Intranasal corticosteroids versus topical H1 receptor antagonists for the treatment of allergic rhinitis: a systematic review with meta-analysis. *Ann Allergy Asthma Immunol* 2002, 89, 479–484.

CHAPTER 13

CURRENT CONSENSUS ON CHILDHOOD ASTHMA

H. PARAMESH

Pediatric Pulmonologist and Environmentalist and Chairman, Lakeside Center for Health Promotion, Bangalore, India

CONTENTS

13.1 INTRODUCTION

Among the non-communicable diseases asthma is the most common persistent lower airway disease in children both in developed and developing countries and also a major socio economic burden as well.

Childhood asthma presents challenges not seen in adults. Although many guidelines and consensus are existent but they vary in scope, methodology, focus, exclusivity in pediatric asthma. The aim is to address the various unmet needs in pediatric asthma and to highlight the key messages that are common to many of the existing guidelines, while critically analyzing and highlighting on any differences, thus providing a concise reference.

The various issues to suit our needs are: definition of pediatric asthma, classification of pediatric asthma, variability with age, phenotypes, pathophysiology, natural history, clinical evaluation, investigations, management, immunotherapy in children, control of asthma and prognosis.

13.2 DEFINITION

What is true asthma is often argued, especially in children. No doubt asthma in children is a complex and diverse entity and no guidelines proposes a differentiation between pediatric and adults asthma in regard to definition. Physiologists, pathologists, pulmonologists and allergists and internists vary in their views on various aspects and taking everything into accounts, the working definition is asthma is a chronic airway disease characterized by: (a) airway inflammation, (b) airway obstruction, (c) airway hyper-reactivity and presents with recurrent episodes of wheeze, cough, shortness of breath and chest tightness and (d) airway remodeling in uncontrolled asthma cases.

13.3 CLASSIFICATION OF PEDIATRIC ASTHMA

Age is an important factor, relevant to diagnosis and treatment. Infancy, preschool, school age and adolescents are important milestones where significant differences occur in pathophysiology and clinical features and it is reflected in the management.

Age is an important classification factor relevant to diagnosis and treatment. There is general consensus that milestone ages are around 5 and 12 years. In some documents infantile asthma (<2 or 3 years) is further distinguished. Special characteristics of adolescence are highlighted in many documents.

In respect to severity, asthma is usually classified as intermittent or persistent and persistent asthma is classified as mild, moderate and severe. These classification is currently recommended only for initial assessment and later it is replaced by the concept of 'control' which is more useful for clinicians, control is generally accepted as a dynamic classification factor, critical to guiding treatment and has categories like controlled, partly controlled, and uncontrolled. In some cases as complete control where there is no disease activity at all.

13.4 PHENOTYPES OF ASTHMA

Phenotypic classification according to apparent triggers like viral induced, exercise induced, allergen induced and unresolved should be taken into account for treatment selection. For many patients several apparent triggers may be identified which can be reflected in the future management. This can be done by asking four important questions to the parents as shown in Figure 13.1.

1. Is the child completely well between symptomatic period?
2. Colds are the most common precipitating factor?
3. Is exercise the most common or only precipitating factor?
4. Does the child have clinically relevant allergic sensitizations?

Phenotype specific biomarkers will be useful in practice, to identify the trigger factor, selection of controller medicines, prognosticate and plan preventive measures.

The ERS task force proposes viral induced wheeze or multi trigger wheeze and avoid the use of transient, late onset, and persistent wheezes in clinical practice.

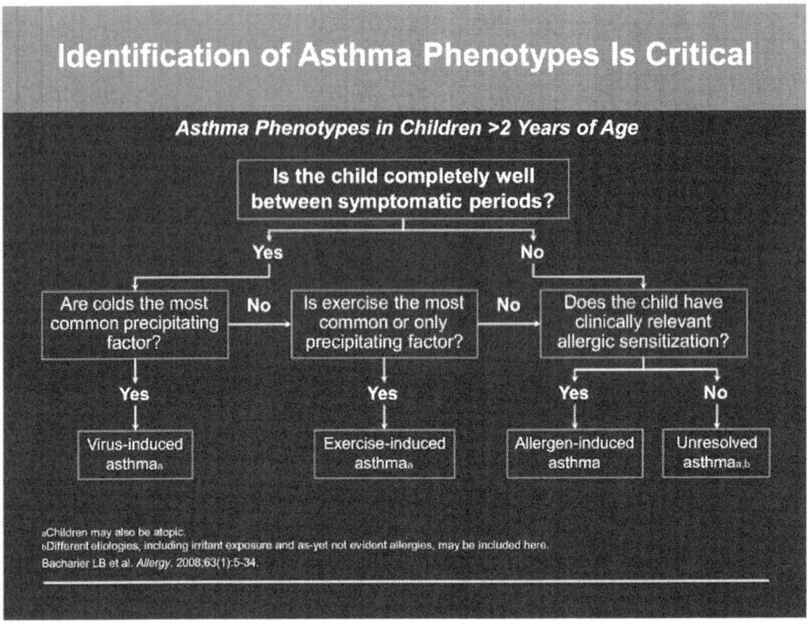

FIGURE 13.1 Identification of Asthma Phenotypes. (From ADEX Module, and Nelson Essential of Pediatrics: 1st South Asia Edition, 2016 Pg. 269. Used with permission.)

13.5 PATHOGENESIS AND PATHOPHYSIOLOGY

Studies by Yunginger et al. (1964–1992) and Paramesh (2002) have shown that asthma can begin at any age but most often has its roots in early childhood. The prevalence of asthma steadily increased in many countries, although in some studies it is leveled off. The inception of asthma depends on both interaction of genetics and environment. Modifiable environmental factors have been sought in an effort to identify targets for prevention of asthma.

Asthma is a disease of persistent inflammation, airway hyper-responsiveness and persistent structural changes has been recognized by almost all guidelines even though some focused more on diagnosis and treatment. Ever though the development of allergen specific IgE in early life for indoor pollutants is the most important risk factor for asthma more so in developing countries but not many interventional studies to give strong support. It is only the environmental tobacco smoke and its modifiable effect during pregnancy and infancy properly documented.

Persistent asthma is universally regarded as a disease of chronic airway inflammation. The interaction of epithelial cells, dendritic cells, lymphocytes, mast cells and smooth muscle cells contribute the inflammatory milieu in producing early phase reaction (EPR) and late phase reaction (LPR) as shown in Figure 13.2.

If the inflammation continues there will be structural changes of airways like increased vascularity of subepithelial tissues with deposition

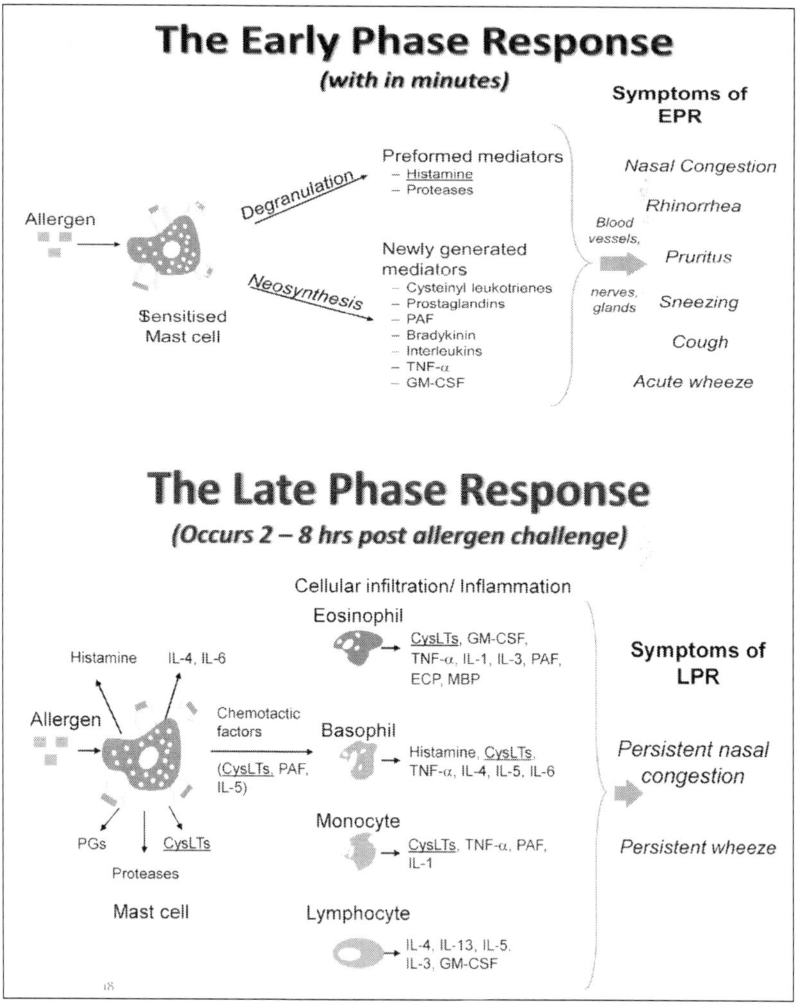

FIGURE 13.2 (a) The Early Phase-Response (with in minutes); (b) The Late Phase-Response (occurs 2–8 hrs. past allergy chemistry). (From ADEX Module. Used with permission.)

of structural proteins, thickening of basement membrane, loss of normal dispensability of airways by scarring and increased smooth muscle mass by hypertrophy what we call it as airway remodeling.

13.6 NATURAL HISTORY OF CHILDHOOD ASTHMA

Asthma may persist, remit or relapse. Natural history and prognosis are particularly important in children. Almost all patients, parents and grand parents (in our country) ask two important questions?

1. Is it asthma?
2. Is he/she going to outgrow the disease?

Even though majority of asthma 77.7% starts in childhood under 5 years we don't have specific practical, objective tests to prove.

The asthma predictive stringent index which has 2 major criteria like parental history of doctor diagnosed asthma doctor diagnosed atopic dermatitis and 3 minor criteria's like wheezing apart from cold, blood eosinophilia over 4% and doctor diagnosed allergic rhinitis. One major and two minor criterias at 3 years of age with history of recurrent wheeze are suggestive of asthma. Its sensitivity is low 14.8–27.5% only.

It is not practical in developing countries, it has more of a negative predictive value, poor evidence and extrapolation of data on future risks is difficult in clinical setting. Most of our children have more than 4% eosinophils and there is no wheeze without sneeze, over 99% of our children with asthma have allergic rhinitis, it is a major criteria for us.

Children with severe asthma in the first year of life, infants with recurrent wheeze, decrease lung function at 6 years of age in children who wheezed at less than 3 years of age, atopic asthma (high IgE levels) are the one going to have persistence course. Atopy is the strongest predictor for persistence. However both the incidence and period prevalence of wheezing decrease with increasing age.

13.7 CLINICAL EVALUATION

Clinical histories of recurrent respiratory symptoms like wheeze, cough dyspnea, and chest tightness triggered by exposure to allergens or irritants or viral infection or exercise, crying, and laughing is very important. The required rate/number of such episodes per year is generally not specified, although arbitrarily 3 or more episodes has been proposed especially these symptoms appear at night and early morning times. Personal history of atopy, eczema, allergic rhinitis, conjunctivitis and food allergy and family history of asthma strengthen the diagnosis. Other history of 'C' section, living next to heavy traffic roads, smoking in the house, ill ventilated residence, use of non commercial cooking fuel (Cow dung cakes firewood, agri-waste) may contribute in the diagnosis.

Physical examination needs to be evaluated for united airway concept from nose for allergic rhinitis rhinorrhea, sneezing, rubbing nose, nasal blockage, snoring, grinding teeth, mouth breathing and chest examination for wheeze which is a non-palpatory musical expiratory sound. Look for other atopic features of skin. Always make it a point to hear the cough to identify the location of origin of cough.

To diagnose asthma confirm the presence of episodic symptoms, reversible airway obstruction and exclude other conditions for wheeze especially in younger children.

13.8 INVESTIGATIONS

13.8.1 LUNG FUNCTION

Lung function is important for both diagnosis and monitoring. Normal lung function do not exclude the diagnosis of asthma especially for intermittent or mild cases, nevertheless it is very supportive.

Peak expiratory flow (PEF) measurements are very important for us including reversibility or variability, which help to support the suspected diagnosis. No doubt it is not a substitute for spirometry and it is more useful in monitoring.

Spirometry is recommended for children who are 5–7 years older where facilities are available. A reversibility after bronchodilators by 12%, or 10% of predicted value is taken as supportive evidence for asthma.

The newer lung function oscillometry requires less cooperation in children under 5 years of age but these tests are available only in specialized centers.

13.8.2 EVALUATION OF AIRWAY HYPER REACTIVITY (AHR)

AHR is assessed by Provocation test with inhaled methacholine, histamine, mannitol, hypertonic saline or cold air in adults either to support or to rule out the diagnosis of asthma. However accuracy in children is lacking as the inhaled dose is not adjusted for the size of the patient. Exercise can also be used to assess AHR but standardization of testing in children is difficult for differing age and limited to research than clinical practice.

13.8.3 ASSESS AIRWAY INFLAMMATION

Exhaled nitric oxide (FENO) measurement seems promising in assessing eosinophilic airway inflammation, determining the likelihood of corticosteroid responsiveness and monitoring.

Sputum eosinophils are not currently recommended for diagnosis and monitoring of childhood asthma as there is no robust supportive data.

13.8.4 EVALUATION OF ATOPY

There is general consensus that atopy be evaluated in children by skin prick test in vivo and specific IgE antibodies in vitro. This helps in diagnosis, helps in avoiding triggers and prognostic value for disease persistence.

13.8.5 CHEST X-RAY

Skiagram is needed only when there is suspicion of complication or to rule out other factors mimic like asthma. Routinely no X-ray is needed to diagnose asthma.

13.9 SPECIAL CONSIDERATION

In case of uncertainty in the diagnosis particularly in children less than 5 years of age a short course of therapeutic trial period of 3 months with inhaled corticosteroids is suggested. A considerable improvement during the trial and deterioration when it is stopped supports a diagnosis of asthma. Please note that a negative response still does not completely exclude the diagnosis.

The diversity of childhood asthma and various phenotypes or subgroups are recognized, there is little details or agreement on diagnostic requirements for particular phenotype except exercise induced asthma.

13.9.1 SEVERAL CONDITIONS THAT MIMIC ASTHMA

(a) Infections and immunological disorders; (b) Congenital anomalies; (c) Foreign body; (d) Tumor but they are rare and investigation is needed in atypical asthma case, in nonresponsive cases to therapy, persistent wheeze started in early infancy and poor growth pattern.

13.10 MANAGEMENT

Asthma management should be holistic including all the elements necessary to achieve disease control. (a) Education of the patients and parents grand parents; (b) Avoidance of triggers; (c) Pharmacotherapy with well information plan; (d) Regular monitoring; (e) Immunotherapy. All these should be adopted to the available resources as shown in Figure 13.3.

13.10.1 EDUCATION

Asthma education is a continuous process about the disease long-term therapy, environment control, and it should be tailored according to the sociocultural background of the family. Self-management is the integral part of the process. The educational intervention are complemented at school-based programme, and peer-led programme in the case of adolescents. Tailoring education according to the sociocultural level of the patients, parents and grand-parents may have important practical consequences.

13.10.2 AVOIDANCE OF TRIGGERS

The airway pathology is mediated through IgE to inhalant allergen is widely acknowledged; however, not every allergen is equally significant.

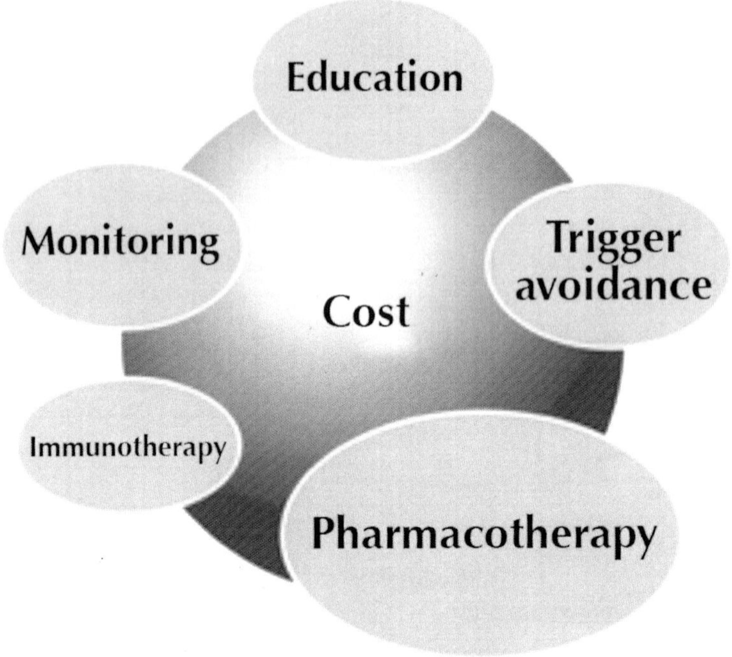

FIGURE 13.3 Asthma management. (Source: Papadopoulos, N. G., Arakawa, H., Carlsen, K. H., Custavic, A., Paramesh, H. et al. International Consensus on (ICON) Pediatric Asthma. *Allergy* 2012, 67(8), 976–997.)

Indoor and outdoor air pollution is the major trigger particularly in the developing countries. The indoor allergens (dust mite, cockroach, mold and pet allergens) are considered the main culprits and are targeted by specific interventions. Complete allergen avoidance is usually impractical or impossible and often limiting to the patients and some measures are expensive and inconvenience.

13.10.3 PHARMACOTHERAPY

The aim of asthma treatment is to control the symptoms and inflammation by using the least possible medication.

Pharmacotherapy is selected through a stepwise approach according to the level of control of the disease.

If the control is not achieved after 1–3 months stepping-up should be considered after reviewing the compliance, environmental control, and

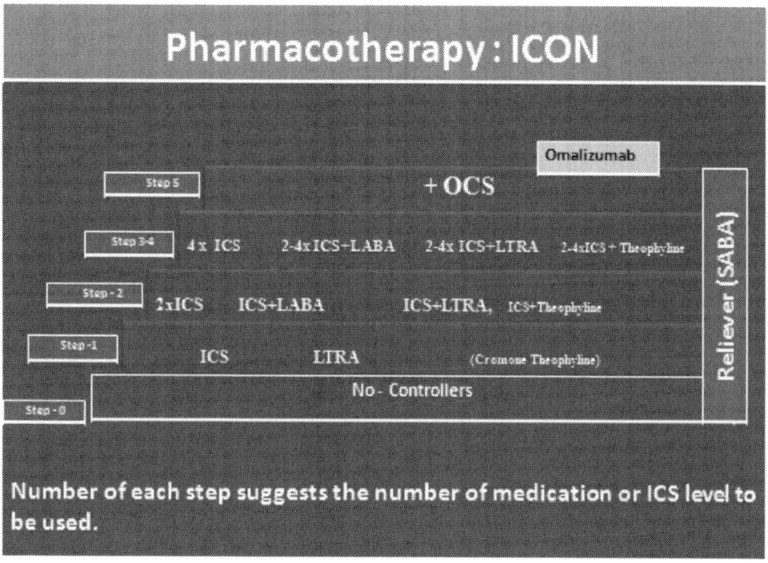

FIGURE 13.4 Pharmacotherapy (ICS = inhaled corticosteroids; LTRA = leukotriene receptor antagonist; LABA = long acting beta 2 agonist; and OCS = oral cortico steroids.) (From Papadopoulos, N. G., Arakawa, H., Carlsen, K. H., Custavic, A., Paramesh, H. et al. International Consensus on (ICON) Pediatric Asthma. Allergy 2012, 67(8), 976–997. Used with permission.)

comorbidities. When control has been achieved for at least 3 months stepping-down is considered as shown in Figure 13.4.

The dose of inhaled steroids – Beclomethasone, Budesonide, Fluticasone propionate and Mometasone is the same. Low dose is 100-microgram, medium doses is double and high dose is quadruple.

13.11 INHALED MEDICATION DELIVERY DEVICES

In children less than 5 years a static treated spacer and mask (or a mouth piece whenever child is capable of using) is used – over 5 years static treated spacer with mouthpiece, or breath activated meter dose inhalers are used. Dry powder inhalers can also be used.

Use of nebulizer is a second choice to spacer. A 500 mL plastic bottle spacer is as effective spacer in all ages. Always consider child's ability to use, preference and cost. Always rinse or gargle after inhaled corticosteroids in a dry power inhaler. Long acting B_2 against LABA should only be prescribed in combination with inhaled cortico steroids (ICS). LABA and ICS is recommended in children over 5 years of age but Japanese Guidelines (JGPA) recommends at any age.

13.12 IMMUNOTHERAPY

Immunotherapy involves in the administration of increasing doses of allergen extracts to induce persistent clinical tolerance in patients with allergen-induced symptoms.

Subcutaneous immunotherapy (SCIT) is effective in allergic asthma with sustained control of symptoms upon 6 years follow up in children. The effects are greatest with single allergen extract. It helps in disease modification and prevents allergic march. It is recommended above 3 years of age. Sublingual immunotherapy (SLIT) is most preferred and is child friendly, painless, home dosing treatment. Metaanalysis confirmed significant efficiency in children with asthma.

TABLE 13.1 Asthma Control Based on the Components

Asthma Level of Control				
Components	**Complete**	**Good**	**Partial**	**Uncontrolled**
1. Symptoms				
• Day time	None	<2/wk	>2/wk	Weekly
• Night time Disturbed Sleep	None	≤1/M	>1/M	Daily
2. Limitation of activity	None	None	Some	Extreme
3. Rescue Trt	None	≤2/wk	>2/wk	Daily
4. FEV1, PEF	>80%	≥80%	60-80%	<60%
Risks:				
5. Exacerbation / yr	0	1	2	>2
6. Side effect of Drugs	None	Variable		
* Self monitoring encouraged (Sym, PEF)				

(Adapted from Papadopoulos, N. G., Arakawa, H., Carlsen, K. H., Custavic, A., Paramesh, H. et al. International Consensus on (ICON) Pediatric Asthma. Allergy 2012, 67(8), 976–997. Used with permission.)

TABLE 13.2 Phenotypes Specific Guidelines

Phenotype-Specific Guidelines			
	Virus	**Exercise**	**Allergen**
Avoidance	In severe/persistent	NO	Intense measure with perennial allergens
Education	Hand Washing	Pre-warming	
Pharmacotherapy	Montelukast Inh.Steroids	Salbutamol PRN Montelukast Inh. Steroids	Inhaled Steroids Anti-IgE
Immunotherapy	NO	NO	YES
Monitoring	Especially after summer vacation	Follow activity	Look into allergen seasonality
Proposal by Dr. Nikos Papadapolous			

(From Unpublished suggestion of Prof. Papadopoulos.)

13.13 MONITORING

Control of asthma can be assessed at regular intervals, based on the components described in Table 13.1 only minimal symptoms are acceptable. For patients on daily controller therapy, review approximately once in 3 months is recommended, after an exacerbation, a shorter interval should be considered.

The summary of phenotypes specific guidelines as proposed by Dr. Nikos Papadopolous president of EAACI seems quite appropriate as shown in Table 13.2.

Children with viral infection triggered asthma tend to outgrow the disease by 5 years of age when the immune system attains adult levels. Some more outgrow the disease by 8 years when the airway caliber reaches adult levels, more so in boys. During adolescent period majority tend to outgrow the attacks. However, those with atopic asthma (high IgE level) and children with low lung capacities and girls have the tendency for asthma remaining for an indefinite period.

13.14 CONCLUSION

Understanding the underlying pathophysiology and improved classification of subtypes may lead a more effective personalized care local adaptation of the basic principle of management will contribute in mitigating the asthma problem.

KEYWORDS

- **childhood asthma**
- **immunotherapy**
- **pathophysiology**
- **pediatric asthma**

REFERENCES

Global Initiative for Asthma 2015. www.giasthma.org.

National Commission on Macro Economics and Health. Govt. of India: Burden of Disease in India 2005, 251–264.

Papadopoulos, N. G., Arakawa, H., Carlsen, K. H., Custavic, A., Paramesh, H. et al. International Consensus on (ICON) Pediatric Asthma. *Allergy* 2012, 67(8), 976–997.

Paramesh, H. Asthma in children: Seasonal variation. *Int J. Environ Health* 2008, 4, 410–416.

Paramesh, H. Epidemiology of Asthma in India. *Indian Journal of Pediatric*, 2002, 69, 309–312.

Paramesh, H. The unmet challenges in child health environment. *Pulmonary Clinics of India* 2014, 1(1), 217–227.

White, M. C., Etzel, R. A., Wilcox, W. D., Lloyd, C. Exacerbations of childhood asthma and ozone pollution in Atlanta, *Environmental Research,* 1994, 65, 271–290.

Yunginger, J. W., Reed, C. E., O'Connell, E. J., Melton, L. J., O'Fallon, W. M., Silverstein, M. D. A community-based study of the epidemiology of asthma. *Incidence Rates*, 1964–1992, 146, 888–894.

PART V

FOOD ALLERGY EVALUATION

CHAPTER 14

FOOD ALLERGY INSOMNIA

G. HASSAN,[1] M. ISMAIL,[1] T. MASOOD,[1] and S. SAHEER[2]

[1]*Postgraduate Department of Medicine, Government Medical College, University of Kashmir, Srinagar, Jammu and Kashmir – 190010, India, Mobile: +91-9419007335;*
E-mail: lungkashmir@rediffmail.com

[2]*Specialist Pulmonologist, International Modern Hospital, Bur Dubai, Dubai*

CONTENTS

ABSTRACT

This is a recently described disorder-involving occurrence of insomnia following exposure to certain foods among atopic individuals. The entity is well described in the International Classification of Sleep Disorders and recent texts of the sleep medicine, but the content is mainly based on hypothetical observations by previous researchers. Literature review of past century and the chapter briefly describes various aspects of this entity including most recent modalities of diagnosis and treatment.

14.1 INTRODUCTION

Food allergy insomnia is a disorder of initiating and maintaining sleep due to an allergic response to food allergens (International Classification of Sleep Disorders, 2001).

14.2 HISTORICAL OVERVIEW

The history dates back to initial published report (Schlors, 1912) that demonstrated certain forms of infantile eczema related to food protein. It was postulated that protein, in order to enter the blood stream or body tissues unaltered must be introduced through the skin (subcutaneously, intraperitoneally, intramuscularly) or intravenously, but subsequent researches postulated that a foreign protein, even when taken orally, may escape digestion and some of it can be absorbed into the blood stream in unaltered state. Similar observations were again published (Hoober, 1916), who gave the concept of allergic reactions affecting the central nervous system. Behavioral complaints in eight children that included nervousness, irritability, insomnia, decreased appetite and poor school performance were attributed to irritation of nervous system by allergic reactions (Shannon, 1922). This was clarified by marked improvement in symptoms in seven of the eight subjects upon elimination of certain foods from the diet, again suggesting food proteins as the common triggers of such allergic reactions. Observations of several patients suffering from fatigue, weakness, lack of energy, drowsiness, depression, mental confusion and body aches were reported (Row, 1930). Improvement was noted upon elimination of diets and the condition was referred to as *allergic toxemia* due to food allergy. Role of allergies in the genesis of irritability and behavioral problems in atopic children was hypothesized, that was judged after allergic problems were brought under control (Randolph, 1947). Experience of a group of patients with irritability, depression, emotional liability, difficulty in concentration, nightmares and insomnia, in a similar way as also described by the previous researchers. Other additional symptoms included twitching of muscles, unusual sensations of itching, tingling and burning, and, this entity was designated as *cerebral allergy*.

Many common foods were attributed to evoke food allergies leading to these manifestations due to involvement of central nervous system, and a review in this regard was published by him after three years (Atkins, 1986). In a similar way findings of food allergies affecting central nervous system in children leading to a variety of motor and behavioral disorders were described (Dees, 1954). Between 1954 and 1958, the condition called *allergic tension fatigue syndrome*, in atopic children with a myriad of symptoms was described (Speer, 1954, 1958). Those elements which represented exaggerated neuro-psychiatric activity were classified under the heading of *allergic tension*, and, those with depressed activity were designated as patients of *allergic fatigue*. Since both elements occurred in the same children at different times, the condition was termed as *allergic tension fatigue syndrome*. The most prominent symptoms were alternating periods of tension and excessive fatigue. Besides the usual symptoms pertaining to allergies, the more prominent mental symptoms included headaches, enuresis, depression, irritability, paranoid ideas, lack of concentration and nervous ticks, attributed mainly to food allergies capable of acting directly on the nervous system with production of characteristic behavioral abnormalities. In 1957 it was hypothesized that night waking in children could be as a result of food allergies in addition to other factors (Moore and Ukko, 1957). Another report of fifty patients referred to as *allergic toxemia* and the *allergic tension fatigue syndrome* was published subsequently (Crook et al., 1961). Foods were demonstrated as the sole cause of symptoms in 38(76%) patients. Four children improved dramatically on avoidance of certain foods from their diet. In 1976, behavioral disturbances including headaches, convulsions, learning disabilities, schizophrenia and depression occurring due to food allergies were again reviewed and eliminating diet followed by dietary rotation and avoidance of the offending agents was stressed upon (Hall, 1976).

More recently, significant research related to insomnia was contributed and report of eight infants having insomnia due to cow's milk allergy was published. On re-introduction of cow's milk the infants became severely sleepless. Once cow's milk was excluded from the diet, sleep behaviors of the study subjected normalized. The observation was again confirmed in 71 allergic infants, when sleep of the insomniac infants became normal after cow's milk was eliminated from the diet, and, again insomnia reappeared on food challenge with milk (Kahn et al., 1985, 1987). Subsequently this entity was coded and described in the International Classification of Sleep Disorders, revised by the American Academy of Sleep Medicine (International Classification of Sleep Disorders, 2001), and is also described in standard books of sleep medicine (Ferber, 2009; Lee-Chiong Jr., 2008).

To our knowledge, the present write up covering almost every aspect of the disorder, and the currently ongoing research involving pediatric as well as adult subjects being studied as per the authentic practice parameters and guidelines (yet unpublished), stand first of their kind in the world literature.

14.2.1 CLINICAL FEATURES

The sleep disturbance involves difficulty in initiating sleep accompanied by frequent arousals and awakenings leading to markedly reduced total sleep time. Other symptoms of allergy including skin irritation, rashes, respiratory difficulties with wheezing and gastrointestinal upsets may also be present. Additional symptoms include psychomotor agitation and daytime lethargy (International Classification of Sleep Disorders, 2001; Lee-Chiong Jr., 2008; Ferber, 2009). Both children and adults may suffer from this disorder, although it is more frequently encountered from infancy to 4 years of age, and, may resolve spontaneously (Ferber, 2009; International Classification of Sleep Disorders, 2001; Kahn, 1985; Kahn, 1987; Lee-Chiong Jr., 2008). A family history of food allergy may increase the risk in off-springs. Familial pattern, sex ratio and the exact pathology are not known. The exact prevalence is yet unknown, but the disorder appears to be common (International Classification of Sleep Disorders, 2001).

14.2.2 PATHOPHYSIOLOGY AND MECHANISMS

The most crucial to the pathophysiologic mechanism leading to wakefulness is the enhanced activity of histamine. Being a mediator of "wakefulness" its activity is necessary to maintain wakefulness, alertness and reaction time (Lu and Zee, 2010; Lieberman, 2009). It is evident by clinical experiences when drugs blocking histamine H1 receptors (e.g., diphenhydramine) lead to sedation and increase all the stages of sleep (Lieberman, 2009; Tasaka et al., 1989). Brain histamine localizes in both, mast cells and histamine neurons, and, the mast cells store approximately half of its levels (Yamatodani et al., 1982). The tuberomammillary nucleus in the posterior hypothalamus is the sole source of histamine in brain and it sends projections to the entire central nervous system (Figure 1). Histamine release can occur following immediate IgE-mediated allergic reactions when food antigens interact with immunocompetent cells with eventual release of antigen-specific IgE and its binding to the high affinity receptors on the surface of mast cells and even basophils. The binding of adjacent antigen-specific IgE antibodies on the surface of mast cells results in the release of granules containing histamine, prostaglandins, tumor necrosis factor alpha, and cytokines which significantly affect sleep (Chikahisa et al., 2013; Johnson and Krenger, 1992; Marshal, 2004; Yamatodani et al., 1982). In the brains of normal mammals, mast cells are located in the leptomeninges (Dropp, 1972), and are concentrated in the brain parenchyma along the blood vessels of dorsal thalamic nuclei (Goldschmidt et al., 1985). Mast cells can rapidly penetrate brain blood vessels, and this may account for the rapid increase in mast cell populations after physiological manipulations (Silverman et al., 2000). The rate of increase of mature mast cell population in the adult brain suggests the possibility that these cells translocate from extraneural sources into the central nervous system (Kitamura et al., 1993), and the mediators can alter the properties of the blood brain barrier (Zhuang et al., 1996). There is also accumulating evidence suggesting that histamine is also related to circadian rhythmicity in the body (Nowak, 1994).

The symptoms and signs of immediate allergic reactions to foods most often include gastrointestinal complaints including tingling and burning of oropharyngeal tissues, nausea, vomiting, gastrointestinal cramps and diarrhea. Findings in other organs include flushing, urticaria, eczema and respiratory tract symptoms that may also provoke sleep disturbances. *Delayed reactions* to foods occur several hours to days after ingestion of the offending food, and involve antigen-antibody complex formation with complement activation. In addition to gastrointestinal manifestations, a variety of symptoms ranging from enuresis to muscle aches and mental symptoms are known to occur with potential of disrupting normal sleep (Atkins, 1986). Chronic sleepiness or sleep fragmentation could also be related to imbalance in the metabolism of some neurotransmitters, either released excessively during the hypersensitivity state e.g. histamine, or, reduced through a depressed absorption of its precursors like serotonin (Chikahisa, 2013; Dropp, 1972; Goldschmidt, 1985; Hartmann, 1977; Johnson, 1992; Kitamura, 1993; Nowak, 1994; Silverman, 2000; Zhuang, 1996).

14.2.3 DIAGNOSIS

The appropriate evaluation of allergic patients having this disorder would need combined approach by allergist and sleep specialists, using evidence based diagnostic tools of both the elements.

14.2.3.1 Evaluation of the Food Allergy

Since there is no single diagnostic test that reliably establishes the diagnosis of food allergy, several steps are involved in the evaluation. The initial step involves a thorough medical history and physical examination, followed by the standard skin prick testing, prick-to-prick testing by using fresh foods. Atopic patch testing may improve the diagnostic accuracy in patients with delayed reactions to foods (Bock et al., 1978; Rosen et al., 1994; Spergel, 2005). *In vitro* testing using allergen-specific IgE estimation in a clinical setting may prove useful information, however, the standardized double blind, placebo controlled oral food challenge testing is the gold standard for diagnosis of food allergies (Sampson et al., 2012).

14.2.3.2 Evaluation of Insomnia

The diagnosis of insomnia is primarily based on detailed clinical evaluation of patients' subjective complaints. The detailed sleep history should include the type of complaint of insomnia, duration, course, typical sleep schedule, exacerbating and alleviating factors, perceived consequences and functional impairments and, the presence of associated medical, psychiatric or environmental factors. A complete history of medication use and consumption of alcohol, and caffeine containing food is essential. Apart from history and physical examination a variety of laboratory tests and diagnostic tools (Table 14.1) can help to identify cause of insomnia and to rule out medical causes (Consensus Statement on the Management of Insomnia: Indian Sleep Disorders Association and Indian Academy of Neurology, 2014). The use of *sleep diary* is useful not only for determining the cause of insomnia (e.g., poor sleep hygiene or circadian sleep disorders) but also in monitoring the efficacy of the treatment regimens. *Actigraphy* is the most useful tool in the evaluation of paradoxical insomnia or sleep disturbances secondary to circadian rhythm disorders. According to the American Academy of Sleep Medicine recommendations, polysomnography is indicated in the evaluation of insomnia when there is suspicion of sleep related breathing disorders, periodic limb movement disorder or when the diagnosis is uncertain (Morin and Benca, 2009; Lee-Chiong

TABLE 14.1 Evaluation of Insomnia*

1. Physical and mental examination including
    - Epworth sleepiness scale
    - Insomnia severity index
    - Pittsburg sleep quality index
    - WHO self-report questionnaire
    - Hamilton anxiety rating scale
    - Hamilton depression rating scale
    - Beck's depression inventory
    - Stait-trait anxiety inventory/Beck's anxiety scale fatigue severity scale
    - Dysfunctional beliefs and attitudes about sleep (DBAS) questionnaire
2. Sleep logs
3. Actigraphy
4. Polysomnography if indicated

*Consensus Statement on the Management of Insomnia: Indian Sleep Disorders Association and Indian Academy of Neurology, 2014.

Jr., 2008). Previously published polysomnography findings of food allergy insomnia include presence of frequent arousals and absence of electroencephalo-graphic and cardiorespiratory abnormalities (International Classification of Sleep Disorders, 2001; Lee-Chiong Jr., 2008).

14.2.4 DIAGNOSTIC CRITERIA

The recently prescribed criteria of the International Classification of Sleep Disorders need to be followed for establishing the proper diagnosis (Table 14.2).

TABLE 14.2 Diagnostic Criteria based on International Classification of Sleep Disorders*

A. The patient has complaint of insomnia.

B. The complaint is temporarily associated with the introduction of a particular food or drink.

C. Removal of the agent results in restoration of normal sleep and wakefulness, either immediately or within four weeks. Daytime behavior may improve before the sleep pattern improves.

D. Two or more of the following are present:

   a. Psychomotor agitation

   b. Day time lethargy

   c. Respiratory difficulties

   d. Skin irritation

   e. Gastrointestinal upset

E. Disturbed sleep and altered daytime behavior reoccur when the suspected allergen is reintroduced into the diet.

F. Levels of serum antibodies against the allergen are elevated.

G. Polysomnographic monitoring demonstrates frequent arousals from any sleep stage.

H. No other medical disorder accounts for the symptoms.

I. The symptoms do not meet the diagnostic criteria for any other sleep disorder producing insomnia (e.g., sleep-onset association disorder, nocturnal eating [drinking] syndrome, limit-setting disorder, etc.).

Minimal Criteria

A plus B plus C, or A plus B plus E.

Severity Criteria

Mild: Occasional arousals, crying, psychomotor agitation, and daytime lethargy; mild or no evidence of gastrointestinal upset, skin irritation or respiratory difficulties.

Moderate: Frequent arousals, crying, psychomotor agitation, and day time lethargy, moderate evidence of gastrointestinal upset, skin irritation or respiratory difficulties (in children under three years of age, physical symptoms of allergy can be absent).

Severe: Frequent and severe arousals, crying, psychomotor agitation, and daytime lethargy; severe evidence of gastrointestinal upset, skin irritation or respiratory difficulties (in children under three years of age, physical symptoms of allergy may be absent).

Duration Criteria

Acute: 7 days or less;

Subacute: more than 7 days but less than three months;

Chronic: 3 months or longer.

The ascending arousal system sends projections from the brainstem and posterior hypothalamus throughout the forebrain. Neurons of the laterodorsal tegmental nuclei (LDT) and pedunculopontine tegmental nuclei (PPT) (blue circles) send cholinergic fibers (Ach) to many forebrain targets, including the thalamus, which then regulate cortical activity. Aminergic nuclei (green circles) diffusely project throughout much of the forebrain, regulating the activity of cortical and hypothalamic targets directly. Neurons of the tuberomammillary nucleus (TMN) contain histamine (HIST), neurons of the raphe nuclei contain 5-HT and neurons of the locus coeruleus (LC) contain noradrenaline (NA). Sleep-promoting neurons of the ventrolateral preoptic nucleus (VLPO, red circle) contain GABA and galanin (Gal).

Source: Saper CB, et al. (2001).

*International Classification of Sleep Disorders (2001), with permission.

14.2.5 DIFFERENTIAL DIAGNOSIS

During the first three months of life, the disorder needs to be differentiated from infantile colic. Gastroesophageal reflux, infantile spasms and respiratory irregularities need to be excluded (International Classification of Sleep Disorders, 2001). Proper evaluation of various other causes of insomnia in adults need due consideration before attributing it solely to food allergy.

14.3 COMPLICATIONS

Allergic phenomenon in infants and children can lead to progression of other allergic disorders as part of atopic march (Juan, 2014). Stress is usually limited to the caretakers, and the sedative medications may lead to adverse effects (International Classification of Sleep Disorders, 2001). In older children and adults, consequences of insomnia include impaired performance, fatigue, sleepiness, accidents and mood changes with eventual decline in quality of life (Lee Chiong Jr., 2008).

14.4 PREVENTION AND TREATMENT

The basic principle of food allergy treatment is to avoid the identified foods leading to allergy reactions. Allergen immunotherapy for food allergy is not yet approved by the United States Food and Drug Administration, however several trials are going on across the globe. As per published reports oral immunotherapy appears to be effective in inducing desensitization as well as oral tolerance in patients with food allergy (Zukiewicz et al., 2013; Scurlock and Jones, 2010). Prompt diagnosis is necessary, as sleep normalizes following removal of the inciting food allergens. Management of chronic insomnia in adults includes adaptation of sleep hygiene measures, cognitive behavioral therapy in addition to proper treatment of the other associated sleep disorders (Consensus Statement on the Management of Insomnia: Indian Sleep Disorders Association and Indian Academy of Neurology, 2014; Morin, 2009; Lee-Chiong Jr., 2008).

14.5 FUTURE PERSPECTIVES

In view of the increasing burden of allergies globally, the prevalence of food allergy insomnia is also expected to rise. The increase in incidence of the disease, which underlies the phenomenon associated with hypersensitivity to foods, and the knowledge in new fields like immunology, molecular biology and genetics over the last years has lead to an unprecedented increase in the interest in the field of allergy (Zukiewicz et al., 2013). We hope that this knowledge in future will be further expanded. Large sample studies using evidence-based scientific tools for prompt diagnosis and early treatment are recommended.

KEYWORDS

- **central nervous system**
- **food allergy**
- **histamine**
- **insomnia**
- **mast cells**
- **sleep disorders**

REFERENCES

Atkins, F. M. Food allergy and behavior, definitions, mechanisms and review of literature. *Nutrition Rev* 1986, Suppl, 104–112.

Bock, S., et al. Proper use of skin tests with food extracts in diagnosis of food hypersensitivity. *Clin Allergy* 1978, 8, 559–564.

Chikahisa, S., et al. Histamine from brain resident mast cells promotes wakefulness. PLoSONE 2013, 8(10), e78434. doi: 10.1371/journal.pone.0078434.

Consensus Statement on the Management of Insomnia, *Indian Sleep Disorders Association and Indian Academy of Neurology*, 2014, Elsevier, New Delhi.

Crook, W. G., et al. Systemic manifestations due to allergy. *Pediatrics* 1961, 27, 790–799.

Dees, S. C. Neurologic allergy in childhood. *Pediatric Clin North Am* 1954, 5, 1017–1025.

Dropp, J. J. Mast cells in the central nervous system of several rodents. *Anat Rec* 1972, 174, 227–238.

Ferber, R. Sleep disorders of childhood. In: Chokroverty, S., ed., *Sleep Disorders Medicine, Basic Science, Technical Considerations and Clinical Aspects.* 3rd ed. Saunders-Elsevier, USA 2009, 621–629.

Goldschmidt, R. C., et al. Rat brain mast cells, contribution to brain histamine levels. *J Neurochem* 1985, 44, 1943–1947.

Hall, K. Allergy of the nervous system, a review. *Ann Allergy* 1976, 36(1), 49–64.

Hartmann, E. L. Tryptophan, a rational hypnotic with clinical potential. *Am J Psychiatry* 1977, 134, 366–370.

Hoobler, B. R. Some early symptoms suggesting protein sensitization in infancy. *Am J Dis Child* 1916, 12, 129–135.

Insomnia. In: Lee-Chiong Jr. T. (ed.). *Sleep Medicine. Essentials and Review. Oxford*, USA 2008, 73–131.

Johnson, D., Krenger, W. Interaction of mast cells with the nervous system, recent advances. *Neurochem Res* 1992, 17, 939–951.

Juan, F., Salazar-Espinosa. The Atopic March. A Literature Review. *Int J Med Students* 2014, 2(3), 119–124. Kahn, A., et al., Insomnia and cows' milk allergy in infants. *Pediatrics* 1985, 76(6), 880–884.

Kahn, A., et al. Difficulty in initiating and maintaining sleep associated with cows' milk allergy in infants. *Sleep* 1987, 10(2), 116–121.

Kitamura, Y., et al. Development of mast cells and basophils, processes and regulation mechanisms. *Am J Med Sci* 1993, 306, 185–191.

Lee-Chiong T. Jr. Insomnia. In: Lee Chiuong T., Jr. (Ed). *Sleep Medicine, Essentials and Review*. Oxford, New York, 2008, 73–131.

Lieberman. Histamine, antihistamines and the central nervous system. *Allergy Asthma Proc* 2009, 30(5), 482–486.

Lu, B. S., Zee, P. S. Neurobiology of sleep. *Clin Chest Med* 2010, 31(2), 309–318.

Marshal, J. S. Mast cell responses to pathogens. *Nat Rev Immunol* 2004, 4, 787–799.

Moore, T., Ucko, L. E. Night walking in early infancy, Part I. *Arch Dis Child* 1957, 32, 333–342.

Morin, C. M., Benca, R. M. Nature and treatment of insomnia. In: Chokroverty, S. (ed.). *Sleep Disorders Medicine, Basic Science, Technical Considerations and Clinical Aspects*, 3rd ed., Saunders-Elsevier, USA 2009, 361–376.

Nowak, J. Z. Histamine in the central nervous system, its role in circadian rhythmicity. *Acta Neurol Exp* 1994, 54(Suppl.), 65–82.

Randolph, T. G. Allergy as a causative factor of fatigue, irritability and behavioral problems of children. *J Pediatr* 1947, 31(5), 560–572.

Rosen , J., et al. Skin testing with natural foods in patients suspected of having food allergies – is it necessary? *J Allergy Clin Immunol* 1994, 93, 1068–1070.

Row, A. H. Allergic toxemia and migraine due to food allergy, California and West 1930, 33, 785–793.

Sampson, H. A., et al. Standardizing double-blind, placebo-controlled oral food challenges, American Academy of Allergy, Asthma and Immunology – European Academy of Allergy and Clinical Immunology PRACTALL Consensus Report. *J Allergy Clin Immunol* 2012, 130(6), 1260–1274.

Saper, C. B., et al. The sleep switch, hypothalamic control of sleep and wakefulness. *Trends Neurosci* 2001, 24(12), 726–731.

Schloss, O. M. A case of allergy to common foods. *Am J Dis Child* 1912, III, 341–362.

Scurlock, A. M., Jones, S. M. An update on immunotherapy for food allergy. Curr Opin Allergy Clin Immunol 2010, 10, 587–593.

Shannon, W. R. Neuropathic manifestations in infants and children as a result of anaphylactic reaction to foods container in their diet. *Am J Dis Child* 1922, 24, 89–94.

Silverman, A. J., et al. Mast cells migrate from blood to brain. *J Neurosci* 2000, 20(1), 401–408.

Speer, F. The allergic tension fatigue syndrome in children. *Int Arch Allergy* 1958, 12, 207–214.

Speer, F. The allergic tension fatigue syndrome. *Pediatr Clin North Am* 1954, 1, 1029–1037.

Spergel, J. M., et al. The use of patch testing in the diagnosis of food allergy. *Curr Allergy Asthma Rep* 2005, 5, 86–90.

Tasaka, K., et al. Excitatory effect of histamine on the arousal system and its inhibition by H1 blockers. *Brain Res Bull* 1989, 22, 271–275.

The International Classification of Sleep Disorders, Revised, Diagnostic and Coding Manual 2001, 98–100.

Yamatodani, A., et al. Tissue distribution of histamine in a mutant mouse deficient in mast cells, clear evidence for the presence of non-mast cell histamine. *Biochem Pharmacol* 1982, 31, 305–309.

Zhuang, X., et al. Brain mast cell degranulation regulates the blood brain barrier. *J Neurobiol* 1996, 31, 393–403.

Zukiewicz-Sobczak, W. A., et al. Causes, symptoms and prevention of food allergy. *Postep Derm Alergol* 2013, 2, 113–116.

CHAPTER 15

SCIENCE BASED EVALUATION OF POTENTIAL RISKS OF FOOD ALLERGY FROM GENETICALLY ENGINEERED CROPS

R. E. GOODMAN

Food Allergy Research and Resource Program, Deptartment of Food Science and Technology, University of Nebraska-Lincoln, 1901 North 21st Street, P.O. Box 886207, Lincoln, NE, 68588-6207, USA

CONTENTS

ABSTRACT

India developed a safety assessment process to evaluate food safety of genetically engineered (GE) crops around the same time as the Food and Drug Administration was developing a process for the US. The Indian guideline for allergenicity adopted in 1989 was based on the toxicity assessment for chemical pesticides rather than risks of allergy from dietary proteins. Under the 1989 Indian guidelines the only GE crops approved for cultivation in India were two varieties of cotton containing genes from *Bacillus thuringiensis* (*Bt*) that encode specific crystal proteins that are toxic to caterpillars that consume the GE cotton plants in 2002 and 2005. While a number of scientists in India have worked on development of GE crops (brinjal, cauliflower, cotton, mustard, peanuts, potatoes, rice and wheat) to improve crop production or improve safety, none have been approved for commercial production or human consumption. Regulatory and public opinion hurdles in India in addition to a less developed commercial seed industry have blocked progress. However, recent increased demand for Indian agricultural products and the need to reduce dependence on chemical pesticides along with increasingly unstable environmental conditions brings pressure for change. The safety assessment of genetically engineered (GE) food crops was outlined by the Codex Alimentarius Commission, a body of the World Health Organization (WHO) and the Food and Agricultural Organization (FAO) of the United Nations adopted a comprehensive guideline in 2003, reaffirmed in 2009, includes evaluating potential risks of food allergy and toxicity of GE crops based on extensive scientific knowledge of allergies and allergens as well as the toxicity of proteins and specific metabolites. The assessment also considers the nutritional properties of complex foods. The Indian Council of Medical Research adopted a similar guideline for the safety assessment of GE crops in 2008. The primary concern for food allergy is whether the newly transferred protein is known to cause any type of IgE mediated allergy (food, contact or inhalation), or whether the protein is sufficiently similar to any known allergen to suspect potential IgE cross-reactivity. The goal is to prevent the transfer of a protein that would cause immediate reactions in those who are already allergic as they must avoid the proteins that cause their allergies to remain symptom free. The guidelines also recommend steps intended to identify proteins that may have a higher probability of becoming allergens based on stability of the protein in pepsin at low pH, and the abundance of the protein in the food since many important food allergens are stable and abundant in the food source. They also recommend evaluating potential changes in endogenous allergen expression for commonly allergenic crops that are modified (e.g., soybeans, wheat, peanuts). The safety assessment is intended to ensure the GE crops are as safe as conventional counterparts as discussed here for allergenicity.

15.1 INTRODUCTION

The food safety assessment of genetically engineered (GE) crops, also referred to as genetically modified (GM) crops, is based on a scientific understanding of the complexity of plant genetics and composition as well as risks of food allergy, toxicity and nutritional properties posed by "conventional" food crops. Generation of the first GE plants occurred in the early-1980s although no GE crop was allowed to be commercially produced and used until 1996 when two separate GE tomato events that delayed ripening were approved for food use in the US (1994) were sold in the United Kingdom (http://isaaa.org/resources/publications/pocketk/12/default.asp; http://www.ncbe.reading.ac.uk/NCBE/GMFOOD/tomato.html). Current GE crops are produced by inserting one or a few genes (segments of DNA encoding a protein, a regulatory element or an antisense RNA) into the mixture of naturally occurring genes in the plant. Different "conventional" varieties of these species (maize, soybean, cotton, wheat and rice) are highly genetically diverse (Choudhury et al., 2014; Faris et al., 2014; Lin et al, 2010; Springer and Stupar, 2007; Stupar, 2010). Natural crop species like soybeans (*Glycine max*), corn (*Zea mays*) or wheat (*Triticum aestivum*) have from 20,000 to 40,000 genes, or genetic units, which include regulatory sequences and protein coding regions that are transcribed into RNA, which is then translated to proteins or serve as regulators of gene expression. Natural genetic changes that occur in these species include point mutations leading to loss or change of function, gene duplication or gene deletion. Those changes occur during natural reproduction (mitosis and meiosis). Most of the parental plant species (the gene recipient) have been grown for food or fiber production for centuries or millennia. Few plants, except those that self-pollinate, have identical copies of the genes at nearly every genetic locus. Self-pollinating species are still changed through random mutations that may be passed on to the next generation. Survival of the plants in different environments and with different pest and physical pressures depends on genetic diversity to provide adaptability to change. The genetic changes introduced through the process of transgenesis (genetic engineering) are quite minor compared to the natural genetic variation of the individual agricultural species.

New GE varieties have been produced in ways that introduce small changes in their DNA, by the introduction of one or more specific genes from another species using transformation techniques of modern biotechnology. Typically that is through the use of biolistics (DNA coated particles "shot" into cells), or through "infection" with a recombinant Agrobacterium vector. *Agrobacterium tumefaciens* is a natural plant pathogenic bacterium that carries a plasmid (DNA) element capable of transferring into cells of a number of plants and integrating genetic material into the chromosome of the host plant. The natural plant genetic engineering system has been modified by scientists to allow controlled transfer and integration of very specific traits into agricultural plants that cannot be achieved by other methods, certainly not by conventional plant breeding (Harlander, 2002; Delmer, 2014; Newell-McGloughlin, 2014). Some GE plants have been made resistant to specific insect pests such as corn-borer resistant MON810 from Monsanto, by introduction of one gene from *Bacillus thuringiensis*, a bacterium with ~5,000 genes, which is used as an organic pesticide (Walker et al., 2000). Papaya has been made resistant to pathogenic ringspot virus (PRSV) by insertion of a chimeric gene from the virus, which does not express a protein (Chiang et al., 2001). Some GE crops are transformed with genes expressing proteins that provide protection from herbicides in order to facilitate post-emergent weed control (Padgette et al., 1995). The fatty acid profile of soybeans has been altered to improve cooking oil stability by silencing the expression of a soybean desaturase gene to produce high oleic, low linolenic acid oil by insertion of DNA with a partial soybean fatty acid desaturase (Delaney et al., 2008). These genetic changes are quite small compared to the genetic diversity introduced through crosses with wild plant relatives by traditional plant breeding or by the unknown mutations achieved with radiation or specific chemicals to induce random mutations (Wu et al., 2015). While wide-crosses and mutagenesis have produced many important new traits in crop plants, the primary focus of evaluating the altered plants is simply productivity under specific environmental conditions.

Transgenesis introduces specific new DNA constructs that are detectable, are characterized and checked for safety and performance. Currently there are well over 100 GE crop varieties that have been approved for plant production in the US between 1995 and 2015 (http://www.cera-gmc.org/GmCropDatabase; http://www.isaaa.org/gmapprovaldatabase). Some approved GE events are not used in commerce today because they were not economically viable or were not accepted by growers or commercial markets. However, many other useful events are grown commercially. The US Department of Agriculture estimated 93% of soybeans, 90% of corn and 90% of cotton grown in the US in 2012 (Fernandez-Cornejo et al., 2014). India has become the leading cotton producing country in the world, partly because of adoption of insect protected GE cotton, which was grown on 93% of cotton fields in 2013 (James, 2014). Adopting insect resistant, *Bt* cotton has allowed Indian farmers to reduce the application of chemical pesticides for certain insect pests by up to 90% Scientists in India have produced a number of potentially useful GE varieties of a number of crops. Some, like those incorporating the *Cry 1* genes of *B. thuringiensis* would likely present no significant risks to consumers as they express similar low levels of the *Bt* proteins that are already approved in the U.S. or elsewhere. Yet the regulatory and political challenges facing GE crops in India have prevented the introduction of insect resistant brinjal or other important GE crops (Choudhury et al., 2014; Herring, 2014). A number of *Bt* cotton hybrids have been approved for commercial use in India, but only five new GE crop events (corn and cotton) are currently undergoing field trials (http://igmoris.nic.in/status_gmo_products.asp). At the same time, 20 GE pharmaceutical products are approved for use in India, including human insulin, erythropoietin, hepatitis B vaccine and a number of cytokines (http://igmoris.nic.in/ status_gmo_products.asp).

A high protein potato developed by Chakraborty et al. (2000) was partly analyzed by the developers (Chakraborty et al., 2000). A number of other potentially beneficial GE crops have been or are under development in India, for use in India including mustard, peanuts and rice (Jagannath et al., 2001; Jagannath et al., 2002; Krishna et al., 2015). Some events help agronomists in producing better seeds or in production by reducing crop losses to insects (e.g., *Bt* brinjal), plant fungal pests or plant viruses (Cletus et al., 2013; Giri and Vijaya Laxmi, 2000; Jagannath et al., 2002; Kumar et all, 2011; Reddy et al., 2009; Seetharam, 2010; Vasavirama and Kirti, 2012). From my observations, there are many articles in the public media decrying the safety, testing, economics and performance of the GE crops in India that do not provide substantiation with facts. There are a number of peer-reviewed publications that make similar adverse claims of risks or ethical issues to consider, without facts and with inaccurate description (Bawa and Anilakumar, 2013; Reddy et al., 2009). Most use subjective inference that the process of transgenesis is against nature and that GE crops would somehow replicate exponentially, displacing local crop genetic pools or that long-term human food safety trials are needed to prove safety (Bawa and Anilakumar, 2013). Yet those familiar with plant genetics, agronomy, historical development of agriculture and food science should see many flaws in those arguments. Minor changes to food crops that have been historically consumed without evidence of harm to consumers should require straight forward evaluation of the specific changes, not long term feeding trials. Food safety experts who attempt to undertake evaluation of potential human health effects from the consumption of foods or specific ingredients understand the remarkable challenge of gathering valid information about intake (exposure), enumeration of differences in consumption or other factors that may impact health outcomes and the cost and complexity of measuring individual health parameters that are not hypothesis driven (Hepburn et al., 2008; Goldstein, 2014). Therefore the focus of the allergenicity assessment of GM crops centers on understanding the specific modification of the event and evaluating the potential allergenicity of the introduced protein (Delaney et al., 2008a; Goodman et al., 2008; Goodman, 2014).

15.2 RISKS OF FOOD ALLERGY

The allergenicity assessment of GE crops must take into account the natural risks presented in currently consumed foods, knowledge of allergenic proteins and relative risks of reactions. Food allergens do not all share a common characteristic. Thus we are not able at this time to accurately predict the allergenicity of proteins without having a history of exposure. However, the risks of de novo sensitization are much lower than risks associated with exposure for those already allergic to a protein. The prevalence of allergies to a number of foods has been reportedly rising during the past 20 in industrialized countries (Prescott et al., 2013; Sicherer and Sampson, 2014).

15.3 ALLERGENIC FOODS

Although the most prominent allergenic food sources are similar in 2014 to those reported in the 1990's, estimates of the prevalence have gone up from 1 to 2% of adults having allergies to 4–6% or more in the U.S. (Sicherer and Sampson, 2014). In the late 1990's pediatric allergists were recommending that parents of infants at high risk of developing food allergy to peanuts and other commonly allergenic foods delay feeding infants those foods for the first 2 to 4 years of age (Sampson, 1997). However, a new randomized food trial in the United Kingdom (UK) with peanut, one of the most common and serious foods for the US and UK demonstrate that avoiding consumption of peanut in early infancy actually increases the prevalence of food allergy to peanuts in those at higher risk of developing food allergy (Du Toit et al., 2015). Clinicians from the major international allergy organizations including the American Academy of Allergy Asthma and Immunology (AAAAI) and the European Academy of Allergy and Clinical Immunology (EAACI) just published a new consensus document changing their recommendations to reflect the new evidence based observation that avoidance has increased food allergy and that early introduction leads to tolerance in the majority of children (Fleischer et al., 2015).

In other industrialized countries the prevalence reports are fairly similar to the experience in the US although there are some differences in the identity of the most common causes of allergy due to differences in diets. Clearly it is difficult to obtain accurate estimates of food allergy prevalence as allergy to many foods is relatively rare and there are few medical health systems that have requirements for reporting food allergy. In addition, the availability and sensitivity of diagnostic tests and criteria have changed. While there is general agreement that prevalence of food allergy has increased, statements suggesting doubling of food allergy prevalence in five or even ten years may not be accurate. The EuroPrevall study was funded by the European Commission in an attempt to obtain better prevalence data across Europe (Kummeling et al., 2009). A population based study in Mysore and Bangalore, India of randomly selected households used questionnaires to select subjects for skin prick tests with foods common to India and to sample blood for IgE measurements to evaluate prevalence (Wong et al., 2010). The results demonstrated that many more subjects think they or family members are food allergic than is supported by SPT and specific IgE, and that those tests also over-estimate evidence based food allergy (Janse et al., 2014). A significant amount of useful data has been coming out of population studies, but much of it demonstrates heterogeneity of sensitivities (or at least detection and reporting) and results suggest there are a number of potentially factors across geographies that influence sensitization (Cerecedo et al., 2014; Fernandez-Rivas et al., 2015). A few countries in the European Union report mustard seed, celery root (celeriac), sesame seed and lupine as common sources of allergy, but in many countries allergy to those sources seem rare (Pauli et al., 1988; Taylor et al., 2014; Vejvar et al., 2013). Some allergenic foods, especially fruits and vegetables are common in causing allergies, although often reactions are generally relatively mild and rarely severe. A few foods, such as peanut, a few tree nuts and crustacean shellfish cause more fatal reactions than other foods (Bock et al., 2007; Xu et al., 2014; Turner et al., 2014).

15.4 ALLERGENS (PROTEINS)

Although many physicians and most patients think of the whole food as the allergen, specific proteins within the food are the allergen, the molecules that elicit reactions. These proteins are bound specifically by protein-specific

IgE antibodies in allergic subjects, which cross-link FcβRI receptors on the surface of mast cells and basophils, inducing release of histamine and leukotriene mediators that drive the reactions. Some allergenic proteins are extremely effective at causing reactions as they have multiple epitopes, or IgE binding sites. Others have fewer epitopes, although at least two epitopes are required to cross-link receptors or the proteins themselves must be cross-linked. Other proteins are bound weakly and are thus ineffective as antigenic targets. Most epitopes are comprised of amino acids in a specific structural conformation (peptides), specific to the individual allergic subject and antibody. Some epitopes are specific structures (α-1,3 fucose or β-1,2 xylose) on the stem structure of a few asparagine-linked complex carbohydrates common to many proteins and sources and they are typically not effectively bound by IgE or inducing reactions (van Ree, 2000; Mari et al., 2008). The peptide epitopes may be contiguous (sequential) or discontinuous (conformational). There are typically 3–5 key amino acid residues that are essential for determining specificity based on spatial arrangement, charge or polarity, with some allowed substitutions in adjacent amino acid residue types. However, the structures presented by epitopes are strongly influenced by surrounding amino acids that influence protein folding. In many cases homologous proteins from closely related sources can share some similar or nearly identical epitopes that act as cross-reactive epitopes for some antigen-specific IgE antibodies, with varying degrees of efficacy in binding. For peanut (*Arachis hypogaea*), one of the most potent allergenic foods, there are 13 or more proteins within the seeds that bind IgE from sera of peanut allergic subjects. Not all IgE binding peanut proteins are thought to elicit allergic reactions. The relatively abundant 2S albumins, known as Ara h 2 and Ara h 6, are thought to be the most potent and common of the biologically important allergens (Zhuang and Dreskin, 2013). The very abundant major seed storage proteins, Ara h 1 (vicilin) and Ara h 3 (conglycinin or legumin), are also relatively potent allergens, although in vivo reactivity may require considerably higher concentrations of these proteins than for the 2S albumins (Peeters et al., 2007). Some lower abundance, small molecular weight proteins that are stable to pepsin and thermal treatment as are the 2S albumins, may or may not be important allergens in peanuts. Those include oleosins (Ara h 10 and 11) and lipid transfer protein (Ara h 9). Other proteins that bind IgE from a few allergic subjects are not likely to be important allergens due to small molecular weight, low abundance and rapid digestion by pepsin and those include profilin (Ara h 5) and pathogenesis related PR-10 (Ara h 8) proteins. Some others including peanut agglutinin bind to carbohydrates on IgE or have cross-reactive carbohydrate binding (CCD) specificities that bind CCD on many plant proteins, but do not seem to cause allergy.

Although taxonomically not closely related to peanut (a legume), tree nuts such as almond, walnut and pecan, pistachio and cashews have similar homologous seed storage proteins that are the dominant allergens (2S albumins, vicilins or legumins). Those nuts cause severe allergic reactions in some consumers and the key allergens are likely to be the abundant seed storage proteins. While the corresponding homologous sequences between these nuts share 30–45% identity, there is limited IgE cross-reactivity for some subjects, but co-reactivity is rare except to highly identical, closely related homologues (e.g., walnut and pecan). The binding affinities are thought to be weak across these distant homologues. A number of plant proteins that are homologous to PR-5 (thaumatin like proteins) and PR-10 (Bet v 1, Mal d 1 like proteins), from diverse plant taxa are more likely to bind IgE from many subjects who have either mild airway or oral mucosal itch or mild angioedema if they are symptomatic. Generally they elicit mild symptoms. Allergy to crustacean shellfish is common and cross-reactive in adults, often causing severe symptoms following high dose exposure. Typically the primary IgE binding target in crustacean shellfish is tropomyosin, a double alpha-helical protein that forms stable coiled coils and is involved in regulation of muscle contraction. Tropomyosins of crustaceans and arthropods typically share >50% identity and cross-reactive IgE binding is common. Tropomyosin is an abundant protein and with repeated domains is likely to include multiple epitopes per molecule, allowing for efficient cross-linking of IgE bound to FcåRI to signal activation and activator release from mast cells and basophils.

Recently some additional proteins have been identified as probable allergens from crustaceans: arginine kinase, sarcoplasmic calcium-binding protein, myosin and triosephosphate isomerase (*see* IUIS, www.allergen.org). However, the abundance of these proteins in edible portions of various crustaceans and eliciting strength of each is not yet clear. The prevalence of food allergy to fresh water and salt-water boney fish is moderately high (~0.4% by some estimates), and the primary allergenic protein is parvalbumin (Lim et al., 2008; Sicherer, 2011; Van Do et al., 2005). Cross-reactivity is relatively high if measured by IgE binding and less if individuals are tested by food challenge (Sharp et al., 2015; Schulkes et al., 2014). Other important allergenic foods and allergens (proteins) include chicken egg (ovomucoid, ovalbumin and less important, lysozyme and ovotransferrin); cow's milk (beta-lactoglobulin, caseins and less commonly alpha-lactalbumin, albumin and lipocalin); soybean (beta-conglycinins with three subunits and glycinins with five subunits and to a lesser degree six or seven other proteins including a 2S albumin and a lipid transfer protein) and wheat (omega-5 gliadin for exercise induced anaphylaxis and a number of other less important IgE binding 'proteins as well as celiac eliciting glutens), (*see* www.allergenonline.org for additional references).

15.5 GLUTENS AND CELIAC DISEASE

Celiac disease affects approximately 1–1.5% of consumers in most geographical regions. Celiac disease (CD) is an autoimmune disease that is restricted to a subset of consumers who have the class II major histocompatibility antigen restrictions of either MHC DQ 2.5 or MHC DQ 8 or some variations of those (Tjon et al., 2010). However, while ~30% of many populations do have one or both alleles of the correct type that is associated with CD, less than 2% of the whole population has symptoms and pathology consistent with the disease (Rubio-Tapia and Murray, 2010). Symptoms occur following ingestion of gluten proteins from wheat, barley, rye grains or for some oats. Different wheat family members carry different glutinin and gliadin genes that are associated with the disease but it is the specific peptides from those proteins that are bound by the correct form of antigen presentation (MHC II, DQ 2.5 or DQ 8) that are able to stimulate T cells to elicit CD specific autoimmune pathology (Sollid et al., 2012). Today the concept of non-CD gluten sensitivity has become a fad for many, but true CD diagnosis is set by some fairly strict criteria (Ludvigsson et al.,

2014). A highly predictive diagnosis usually involves serology (anti-tissue transglutaminase antibody measurement) and duodenal biopsy, which is more predictive if performed with the patient on a normal (gluten containing) and with a gluten-free diet. Intestinal villous atrophy is a normal significant finding, or if little atrophy, then greater than 25 interepithlial lymphocytes per high-power field with IgA-anti-endomesial antibodies, anti-tissue transglutaminase antibodies and an appropriate HLA genotype.

Other histological markers are important. One important concept is that it often takes from four to six sites of biopsy to confirm the diagnosis as local regions of normal or abnormal structure are common (Rostom et al., 2006). Recovery and normal histology on a carefully restricted gluten-free diet (GFD) provides the demonstration of probable celiac disease although some clinicians would recommend re-challenge following many weeks of recovery for absolute proof of causality (Rostom et al., 2006). Maintaining an absolutely GFD is almost impossible without occasional instances of exposure as traces of wheat are common in oats and other agricultural products that are grown in the same geographical areas due to shared farm equipment. And processing foods in factories that also process any wheat fractions can lead to accidental and incidental minor contamination in many packaged foods, salad dressings and other foods. Glutens (gliadins and glutenins) are major grain seed storage proteins that are responsible for the elasticity of bread dough. Bread wheat flour is approximately 13% protein, with nearly 80% of that being a combination of various gluten and gliadin proteins. Glutens are relatively insoluble in water and saline at neutral pH, but soluble in alcohol. Grain from grass family members outside of Pooideae do not cause CD as affected individuals can consume rice, maize, pearl millet and seeds from other monocotyledonous plants outside of the family with no apparent disease. The homologous proteins are up to 45% identical to other gluten proteins that do cause celiac disease and the selective mechanism is the specificity of binding of gluten derived peptides by MHC Class II binding (DQ 2.5 and DQ 8) and the T-cell receptors specific to gluten peptides (manuscript in preparation, Goodman and Amnuaycheewa, 2015).

15.6 POTENTIAL RISKS OF GMOS: ALLERGENICITY AND CELIAC DISEASE

The primary risks of food allergy or celiac disease that can occur from new proteins expressed following insertion of a new gene into a food crop through genetic engineering are due to the characteristics of the gene and protein. If the gene is from an allergenic source or a grain related to wheat, there is a chance that the gene encodes an allergen or gluten and that there are already consumers who are sensitive to the protein. Then the first time the consumer with the specific allergy or CD consumes food produced using the new GE crop products, they could suffer a reaction. In addition, if the protein is nearly identical to an allergen, the protein might elicit a cross-reaction of equal severity. The risks are the same as having processed foods that are not labeled as being made from the allergenic or celiac eliciting source. The affected consumers would not know to avoid the foods that would present risk. Other unaffected consumers (>99% of all consumers for most allergens) are likely to be able to consume the food without any adverse effect. In the late 1980's scientists and regulators recognized those potential risks. Regulators, industry scientists and independent academic scientists discussed the issues and possible ways to evaluate those risks years before the first GE food crops were approved and grown commercially as reviewed by Goodman (2014).

The US FDA posted their first official guideline in the Federal Register in 1992 (FDA, 1992). The recommendations in the guideline provided the model for the scheme for evaluating potential food allergenicity as describe in a 1996 publication by the International Life Sciences and International Food Biotechnology Council (Metcalfe et al., 1996). The document summarizes the primary concerns and a decision tree evaluation process to regarding science-based evaluation process to minimize the risk of transferring an allergen from one organism into the GE food source. However, the description in the text did not completely match the suggestions by their decision tree diagram in that publication (Metcalfe et al., 1996). Therefore I modified the decision tree based on my interpretation of the whole document in 2014 and present as figure 1 in an open access journal article (Goodman, 2014). The allergenicity assessment as it is outlined in the Codex Alimentarius Commission guidelines (Codex,

2003, 2009) are quite similar to the overall process outlined by Metcalfe et al. (1996). Although the Codex intentionally did not use a decision tree as they focused establishing an integrated "weight of evidence" approach. An illustrated interpretation of Codex is provided in a review (Goodman et al., 2008). The Codex guideline is intended as an international treat-backed recommendation intended to help harmonize food safety regulations to improve international safety and international trade. Both ask similar questions with the order of importance outlined as follows:

1. Is the protein already known to be an important ingestion, inhalation or contact allergen?
2. Does the protein share sufficiently high sequence identity with a known allergen so that there is a possibility of cross-reactivity?
3. Does the protein have characteristics similar to many food allergens in being resistant to digestion by pepsin at pH 1.2, being abundant and resistant to unfolding by heating, which might predict sensitization or elicitation?
4. Did insertion of the DNA significantly increase the expression of endogenous allergens if the recipient plant is a commonly allergenic food source?
5. If the gene is transferred from wheat or a near-wheat relative, evaluate the protein for possible elicitation of Celiac Disease?

The first two questions are the most critical as the transfer of a gene encoding a protein that already known to cause allergy in a number of potential consumers into a different food source (e.g., from peanut into rice), would put those who are already allergic at an immediate risk. Food allergic consumers know to avoid consuming the source that causes their allergies. That is why most countries have strict laws requiring clear labeling of allergenic ingredients and glutens in processed foods (Taylor and Baumert, 2015). Without knowledge of ingredients, allergic consumers are vulnerable to exposure and for some, anaphylactic reactions.

15.7 LITERATURE REVIEW WITH GENE SOURCE FOR INFORMATION ON ALLERGENICITY OR CELIAC DISEASE

Question one should be addressed first by considering the source of the gene that was transferred. A literature search should be performed using

PubMed (US National Library of Medicine, National Institutes of Health, searchable database www.ncbi.nlm.nih.gov/pubmed) with the scientific and common names of the source of the gene and keywords "allergy" and "allergen." Additional searches of internet resources may be performed using web-browsers. This question is intimately tied to the concept of proteins having a "history of safe use." In the U.S., ingredients from foods that have an established record of being consumed safely are often recognized as being safe for human consumption if the history of the safe use/consumption can be documented. If however, the source is a common source of allergy, then a study would likely be required (and would be possible) using sera from subjects allergic to the source to evaluate possible IgE binding to the protein of expressed by the transferred gene. In addition, if the source of the gene is a member of the Pooideae subfamily of grasses that includes wheat, barley, rye and oats, the protein should be evaluated as a potential elicitor of celiac disease. The AllergenOnline.org database includes a link to our Celiac Database (http://www.allergenonline.org/celiachome.shtml) that provides bioinformatics tools of exact peptide matches to peptides known to stimulate T cells from some subjects with celiac disease. It also provides a FASTA comparison to proteins containing known celiac inducing peptide as a secondary risk assessment tool.

15.8 BIOINFORMATICS SEARCHES FOR MATCHES TO ALLERGENS

Question two should be addressed using bioinformatics approaches to compare the amino acid sequence of the expressed protein (if any) with those of known allergens. The source of the search should be a well-recognized public allergen database (Goodman, 2006). The AllergenOnline.org database (http://www.allergenonline.org) is widely used by developers of biotechnology companies. It is updated annually and entries are reviewed by a panel of allergy experts to ensure there is published scientific information to support inclusion of specific protein sequences in the database using criteria for source, characterization of the protein, serum IgE binding for appropriately allergic subjects. Optimum published criteria include

IgE binding with appropriate methods and controls and additional demonstration of biological relevance either by basophil activation, by skin prick tests or in vivo (human) allergen challenges. The AllergenOnline.org database, also referred to as the FARRP database (Food Allergy Research and Resource Program) is maintained at the University of Nebraska-Lincoln. References are provided for inclusion of the individual allergenic protein groups as well as an explanation of the review process and sequence comparison methods and criteria. There are other searchable allergen databases that some investigators use including SDAP (http://fermi.utmb.edu/ and Allermatch (http://www.allermatch.org/database.html) as well as informational databases including the WHO/IUIS database (http://www.allergen.org) and allergome (http://www.allergome.org/). The NCBI Protein database (http://www.ncbi.nlm.nih.gov/protein/) is an all-protein inclusive database that can be searched by keywords (e.g., allergen) and sequences can be searched using BLAST local alignment tool with key word limits.

As described previously, the most meaningful searches are accomplished using the full-length amino acid sequence of the introduced protein and either a FASTA or BLAST algorithm to perform local alignment comparisons against the allergen database (Goodman, 2008). If there is an identity match to a known allergen of >50% over nearly the full-length, there would be a relatively high risk of cross-reactivity (Aalberse, 2000). Matches in such cases should be evaluated closely by reviewing the primary literature and finding the at-risk population of allergic subjects. Allergists likely to have patients allergic to the source of the matched allergen should be contacted to recruit study subjects and sera from willing donors with appropriate confirmed allergies should be used to test specific IgE binding (Goodman, 2008). In addition the Codex guideline (2003) and the ICMR guideline (2008) ask for the identification of matches to allergens of any 80 amino acid segment that has 35% identity or more to any known allergen. If such matches are identified, similar evaluation is done. In addition, the Codex guideline suggests looking for identity matches of 6 to 8 amino acids, but since anything less than 8 amino acids identifies far more false positives than true positive matches, an 8 amino acid match would be the minimum size recommended for this evaluation. The question of false positive matches has been demonstrated by a number of publications demonstrating the lack of predictive value of such alignments (Goodman et al., 2008; Hileman et al., 2002; Stadler and Stadler, 2003; Silvanovich, 2006).

15.9 EXAMPLE EVALUATION OF AMARANTIN FOR ALLERGENICITY

The 11S globulin gene encoding Amarantin, was transferred from *Amaranthus hypochondriacus* to maize to provide a higher protein content in the grain of maize (Rascon-Cruz et al, 2004). Grain from *Amaranthus sp.* has been consumed for centuries in Africa and Mexico (Wikipedia). PubMed shows 487 references when searched with "food" and "Amaranthus." When searching PubMed with keywords "Amaranthus" and "allergy" four references were retrived. One reported on a partial food safety evaluation of the 11S globulin produced by this particular GE maize (Sinagawa-Garcia et al., 2004). The other three references were about pollen allergens and not seed proteins and specifically related to the 11S albumin. A search with the terms "Amaranthus" and "allergy" identified 34 references. One related to ingestion of flour from a different species, *Amaranthus paniculatus* (Kasera et al., 2013). The immunoblot is not clear, as there were multiple bands that seem to have been marked by the patient's IgE although no proteins were identified. Other control extracts and proteins were not included, thus it is not possible to conclude whether 11S globulin was bound by IgE or not. A bioinformatics comparison of the sequence of the protein (locus CAA57633, 501 amino acids from Barba de la Rosa et al., 1996) was searched against AllergenOnline.org using a Full-length FASTA (Goodman, 2015). The results show highly significant *E* scores of 1e-60 or smaller to seven 11S globulins of seeds from buckwheat, mustard, pistachio, Brazil nut, mustard, cashew and sesame with 40 to 51% identity over alignments of 450 to 508 amino acids. That result suggests a moderately high probability of cross reactivity for those allergic to one or more of those seeds or nuts. A search of AllergenOnline.org using the 80 mere sliding window search identified matches as high as 71% to pistachio 11S globulin, 70% to hazelnut, 66% to pecan and walnut, 63% to Brazil nut and slightly less to a number of 11S globulin proteins that are known to be allergens. There were a number of allergenic proteins that were found to have a match of 8 or more contiguous amino acids to the Amarantin protein. These results demonstrate that the GE maize (corn) produced by transforming the 11S gene from *Amaranthus hypochondriacus* has a high probability of having shared IgE binding with a number of allergenic seed storage proteins. In order to allow such a product on the market, regulatory agencies would likely require serum IgE tests to many seed/nut allergic subjects to evaluate potential risks for those with existing allergies to various 11S globulins. As discussed below, the serum IgE binding tests need to be well designed with samples of serum from relevant subjects in order to have validity.

Serum IgE tests would require at least eight qualified, specifically-allergic sera would be tested along with sera from a few subjects not allergic to the protein or source of interest, but allergic to some other organisms and one or more non-atopic donors (Metcalfe et al., 1996). While there has been discussion suggesting a need to use high numbers of serum donors for statistically significant power evaluations, it is extremely difficult to identify more than eight to ten subjects sensitized to any allergen and especially for sources that are not common allergenic sources. It is important that all serum IgE tests that are performed use highly specific secondary antibodies and detection methods (Goodman and Leach, 2004; Satinover et al., 2005). The specific antigen controls must also be included to demonstrate positive detection of IgE binding to a source that the allergic donor is sensitized to in order to demonstrate true positive. In almost every case the sensitivity of the assay can be pushed to the point that non-specific signals occur. Appropriate blocking solutions, controls and highly specific anti-IgE and standards of pure IgE are required to demonstrate specificity (Goodman and Leach, 2004; Holzhauser et al., 2009). Test materials must be well characterized to demonstrate that binding is to the protein(s) of interest and that the intended full-length or partial protein is used as the binding target. In addition we must recognize that the correlation between soluble serum IgE and clinical symptoms is not perfect, so a positive detection will not perfectly predict clinical allergic responses (Purohit et al., 2005). In some cases serum IgE tests may not sufficiently resolve the question of whether there is likely important IgE binding to the protein of interest. There are times when either skin prick tests (SPT), basophil activation or basophil histamine release (BHR) or food challenge might be needed to confirm either a lack of response or the relevance of a weak positive IgE binding response (Bolhaar et al., 2005). Since many subjects have IgE that binds to cross-reactive carbohydrate determinants (CCD) on plant proteins, but without clinical reactivity, it is essential that the transgenic protein be characterized to understand whether it contains CCD (Goodman et al., 2008; van Ree et al., 2000). Sufficient positive and negative allergen and serum controls must be included to ensure the validity of results (Hoff et al., 2007). Finally, if serum test results are equivocal or weak, tests designed to evaluate the biological relevance of IgE binding should be undertaken to demonstrate the binding involves more than one IgE epitope and is able to effectively cross-link FcåRI on basophils and mast cells.

15.10 STABILITY OF THE PROTEIN IN PEPSIN AND ABUNDANCE

The FAO/WHO consultation (2001) recommended testing stability of the protein in pepsin at two pH's (1.2 and 2.0) rather just pH 1.2 recommended by Metcalfe et al., (1996). We tested digestion of a number of proteins and found very little difference in digestion results between pH 1.2 and 2.0 for a number of proteins using similar conditions (Ofori-Anti et al., 2008). A laboratory ring-test was performed and reported in 2004 demonstrating only minor differences in the time of disappearance of purified proteins using the standard method of digestion used by developers at that time (Thomas et al., 2004). Additional tests have been performed to establish a limit of measuring digestion in a standard way following evaluation of the pepsin activity and protein detection using a 10% residual sample of test protein as the limit of detection (Ofori-Anti et al., 2008). Other methods of measuring the digestion of test proteins by pepsin have also been reported for evaluating potential risks Herman et al., 2005). Some risk assessments have used a sequential digestion method of pepsin followed by trypsin to evaluate protein stability (Liu et al., 2011). While there seems to be some positive predictive value in assessing stability of a protein in pepsin relative to probability of that protein being a food allergen, abundance and heat stability along with stability in pepsin may be related to food allergy risk due to higher likelihood of eliciting a reaction if a person is sensitized. The addition of simulated intestinal digestion (pancreatin or trypsin-chymotrypsin digestion) does not seem to increase the predictive power of the assessment.

It is important to note that regulatory safety guidelines for assessing potential allergenicity of proteins do not outline abundance as an important factor. Yet it is clear that on an individual basis, the amount of allergen present in food is an important determinant regarding likely clinical reactivity (Ballmer-Weber et al., 2015). However, there are large differences in thresholds between individuals and there is little agreement in establishing thresholds (Taylor et al., 2015). A number of transgenic proteins, such as Cry 1 in maize, cotton and brinjal are expressed at very low levels and are unlikely to be above food allergy thresholds even if someone developed specific IgE to the protein.

15.11 EVALUATING POTENTIAL CHANGES IN ENDOGENOUS ALLERGENS

Evaluating potential changes in the abundance of endogenous allergens due to insertion of the transgene, has been suggested as an important part of assessing potential risks for those host plants that are common allergens (peanut, soybeans, wheat). That is part of the substantial equivalence evaluation described in the Codex 2003 document, and was recommended by Metcalfe et al. (1996). Studies have been performed to evaluate potential changes for each of the approved GE soybean events, beginning with glyphosate (Roundup®) tolerant soybeans (Fuchs and Burks, 1995). My laboratory performed comparative serum IgE tests for five events, and published some results, although most data was only presented in regulatory dossiers (Goodman et al., 2013; Panda et al., 2013, 2013). Other investigators have used 2D-gel separation followed by LC-MSMS to identify and estimate quantities of many proteins, or gel-free LC-MSMS (Hajduch et al., 2005; Houston, 2011). Both methods have advantages and drawbacks. Both are expensive, time consuming and in the end the evaluation is not complete. So far the results demonstrate that there are variations between soybean lines and that environmental factors influence expression of proteins that are thought to be allergens. However, there is no context for food safety in terms of the levels of difference, or the protein identities that lead to higher or lower risks of food allergy (Goodman et al., 2013).

15.12 EVALUATING GENES AND PROTEINS FOR RISKS OF ELICITING CELIAC DISEASE

We have collected many gluten peptides that have been implicated as causal agents of CD in our http://www.allergenonline.org/celiacfasta.shtml database that includes peptides that have been demonstrated in peer-reviewed publications to stimulate T cell proliferation or activation from CD subjects when exposed to the peptides, or have been demonstrated to be toxic for intestinal epithelial tissues of CD subjects. We have included both an exact peptide match and a high-identity FASTA protocol for screening and presumptive positive proteins. We have also included a FASTA search routine compared to a limited number of glutens with high identity matches as presumptive criteria that can be used to evaluate dietary proteins from wheat and near wheat relatives (members of the Pooideae subfamily). If a developer used a gene from the Pooidaea family and had a positive peptide identity match or high scoring FASTA alignment, the protein should be evaluated by in vitro T-cell activity or in vivo challenge using well characterized subjects with celiac disease.

15.13 GENETICALLY ENGINEERED CROPS IN INDIA

Scientists in India have developed a number of promising GE crops, both from the public and the private sector. The Bt brinjal that has been rejected by the Ministry of the Environment in India expresses the same Cry 1 Ac protein that is present in Bollgard® and Bollgard II® cotton, which was approved in 2002 and 2005 respectively. Insecticide applications on cotton have been reduced dramatically due to the expression of the Cry 1 Ac protein, which specifically affects caterpillars that consume the crop, but not mammals. Chakraborty et al. (2000) expressed a transgenic protein from *Amaranthus hypochondriacus* (AmA1, GI#20067185) in potato to improve the protein content of potatoes (Chakraborty et al., 2000). That product has not been advanced. A bioinformatics search (unpublished by Goodman, 4 Sept, 2015) using Allergen Online.org database to evaluate GI#20067185 shows very low identity matches to any allergen, at only 35.8% identity to a latex allergen (Hev b 7.0201, GI#41581137). That is unlikely to be cross-reactive as the identity is low and the *E* score is very large at 0.37. Some regulators might assume that the product would require serum IgE tests using samples from latex allergic subjects, but the match is very weak and it is unlikely to cause cross-reactions for those with allergy to latex based on information from studies on latex allergens (Sowak et al., 1999; Wagner and Breiteneder, 2005). A potentially useful GE mustard hybrid breeding system was developed at Delhi University (Jagannath et al., 2001, 2002). The GE mustard plants await safety and environmental evaluation under by regulators in the government of India. A bioinformatics evaluation of the two transgenic lines was recently published and shows no reason to be concerned related to potential allergenicity (Siruguri et al., 2015). Many scientists are developing tools to advance crop production in India, such as demonstration of the value of the 2S albumin promoter from sesame as a potential regulatory element for a number of oilseed crops (Bhunia et al., 2014). These potential products must be evaluated for food safety based on current scientific knowledge. The mechanisms for evaluation are in place, but the regulatory process in India is stalled, having failed to approve any genetically engineered crop except certain cotton traits.

15.14 DISCUSSION

The risk assessment process established with the U.S. FDA Federal Register guidance in 1992 worked well in outlining a process that led to the identification of the only potential GE product that would have represented a significant risk of food allergy to date, the transfer of a 2S albumin from Brazil nut into soybean. The product was under development by Pioneer. Due to the 1992 guideline, Pioneer worked with Steve Taylor, Professor at the University of Nebraska, to test potential IgE binding using sera from Brazil nut allergic subjects. At that time no one know what proteins in Brazil nut caused food allergy, but since the gene was from an allergenic source, Brazil nut allergic subjects were identified and serum IgE immunoblots and RAST Inhibition studies were used to evaluate possible binding (Nordlee et al., 1996). Results demonstrated clear IgE binding to the introduced protein and positive skin prick test (SPT) results, thus the potential product was stopped by the developer.

The primary risk management step is to avoid is the transfer of a gene encoding an important allergen into a new food source. In 2015 we have significantly more knowledge of the allergenic food sources and most of the important allergenic proteins. To date no new GE crop that has been approved for commercial use in the U.S. or elsewhere that has any caused any documented case of food allergy. The assessment has worked extremely well when it is used. In the U.S. there are more than 100 approved GE events. In India there are still only two approved events for growing. And import approval has only been for highly refined oil from GE soybean. There are many potential beneficial GE products that have been developed in India and many others developed outside of India that has not been evaluated. Approvals have been blocked by political and philosophical argument and not because of a lack of sufficient safety information. As the population grows in India and environmental changes make food production more difficult, it is important that a science based evaluation process becomes the primary determinant regarding the future of GE crop approvals rather than political decisions driven by unfounded and unsubstantiated claims of harm by individuals and a few Non-Governmental Organizations.

KEYWORDS

- **allergens**
- **food allergy**
- **genetically engineered**
- **genetically modified**
- **IgE**
- **risk assessment**

REFERENCES

Aalberse, R. C. Structural biology of allergens. *J. Allergy Clin. Immunol.* 2000, 106, 228–238.

Ballmer-Weber, B. K., Fernandez-Rivas, M., Beyer, K., Defernez, M., Sperrin, M., Mackie, A. R., Salt, L. J., Hourihane, J. O., Asero, R., Belohlavkova, S., Kowalski, M., de Blay, F., Papadopoulos, N. G., Clausen, M., Knulst, A. C., Roberts, G., Popov, T., Sprikkelman, A. B., Dubakiene, R., Vieths, S., van Ree, R., Crevel, R., Mills, E. N. C. How much is too much? Threshold dose distributions for 5 food allergens. *J. Allergy Clin. Immunol.* 2015, 135(4), 964–971.

Barba de la Rosa, A. P., Herrera-Estrella, A., Utsumi, S., Paredes-Lopez, O. Molecular characterization, cloning and structural analysis of a cDNA encoding an amaranth globulin. *J. Plant Physiol.* 1996, 149, 527–532.

Bawa, A. S., Anilakumar, K. R. Genetically modified foods, safety, risks and public concerns—a review. *J. Food Sci. Technol.*, 2013, 50, 1035–1046.

Bhunia, R. K., Chakraborty, A., Kaur, R., Gayatri, T., Bhattacharyya, J., Basu, A., Maiti, M. K., Sen, S. K. Seed-specific increased expression of 2S albumin promoter of sesame qualifies it as a useful genetic tool for fatty acid metabolic engineering and related transgenic intervention in sesame and other oil seed crops. *Plant Mol. Biol.*, 2014, 86, 351–365.

Bock, S. A., Munoz-Furlong, A., Sampson, H. A. Further fatalities caused by anaphylactic reactions to food, 2001–2006. *J. Allergy Clin. Immunol*, 2007, 119(4), 1016–1018.

Bolhaar, S. T., Zuidmeer, L., Ma, Y., Ferreira, F., Bruijzeel-Koomen, C. A., Hoffmann-Sommergruber, K., van Ree, R., Knulst, A. C. A mutant of the major apple allergen, Mal d 1, demonstrating hypo-allergenicity in the target organ by double-blind placebo-controlled food challenge. *Clin. Exp. Allergy*, 2005, 35(12), 1638–1644.

Burks, A. W., Fuchs, R. L. Assessment of the endogenous allergens in glyphosate-tolerant commercial soybean varieties. *J. Allergy Clin. Immunol.*, 1995, 96(6 Pt. 1), 1008–1010.

Cerecedo, I., Zamora, J., Fox, M., Voordouw, J., Plana, N., Rokicka, E., Fernandez-Revas, M., Vazquez, C. S., Reche, M., Fiandor, A., Kowalski, M., Antonides, G., Mugford, M., Frewer, L. J., De la Hoz., B. The impact of double-blind placebo-controlled food challenge (DBPCFC) on the socioeconomic cost of food allergy in Europe. *J. Inv. Allergol. Clin. Immunol.*, 2014, 24(6), 418–424.

Chakraborty, S., Chakraborty, N., Datta, A. Increased nutritive value of transgenic potato by expressing a non-allergenic albumin gene from *Amaranthus hypochondriacus*. *Proc. Natl. Acad. Sci.*, USA, 2000, 97(7), 3724–3729.

Chiang, C. H., Wang, J. J., Jan, F. J., Yeh, S. D., Gonsalves, D. Comparative reactions of recombinant papaya ringspot viruses with chimeric coat protein (CP) genes and wild-type viruses on CP-transgenic papaya. *J. Gen. Virol.*, 2001, 82(Pt 11), 2827–2836.

Choudhury, B. I., Khan, M. L., Dayanandan, S. Genetic relatedness among indigenous rice varieties in the Eastern Himalayan region based on nucleotide sequences of the *Waxy* gene. *BMC Research Notes*, 2014, 7, 953.

Choudhury, B., Gheysen, G., Buysee, J., van der Meer, P., Burssens, S. Regulatory options for genetically modified crops in India. *Plant Biotechnol. J.*, 2014, 12,135–146.

Cletus, J., Balasubramanian, V., Vashisht, D., Sakthivel, N. Transgenic expression of plant chitinases to enhance disease resistance. *Biotechnol. Lett.*, 2013, 35,1719–1732.

Codex Alimentarius Commission Guidelines. Alinorm 03/34, Joint FAO/WHO Food Standard Programme, Codex Alimentarius Commission, Twenty-Fifth Session, Rome, 30 June–5 July, 2003. Appendix III, Guideline for the conduct of food safety assessment of foods derived from recombinant-DNA plants and Appendix IV, Annex on the assessment of possible allergenicity, 2003, pp. 47–60.

Delaney, B., Appenzeller, L. M., Munley, S. M., Hoban, D., Sykes, G. P., Malley, L. A., Sanders, C. Subchronic feeding study of high oleic acid soybeans (Event DP-305423–1) in Sprague-Dawley rats. *Food Chem. Toxicol.*, 2008 46(12), 3808–3817.

Delaney, B., Astwood, J. D., Cunny, H., Conn, R. E., Herouet-Guicheney, C., MacIntosh, S., Meyer, L. S., Privalle, L, Gao, Y., Mattsson, J., Levine, M. Evaluation of protein safety in the context of agricultural biotechnology. *Food Chem. Toxicol.*, 2008, 46, S71–S97.

Delmer, D. GM crops and food security. *J. Huazhong Agr. Univ.*, 2014, 33(6), 1–10. (Chinese and English), http,//hnxbl.cnjournals.net/hznydxzr/ch/reader/create_pdf.aspx?file_no=20140601&year_ id=2014&quarter_ id=06&falg=1.

Du Toit, G., Roberts, G., Sayre, P. H., Bahnson, H. T., Radulovic, S., Santos, A. F., Brough, H. A., Phippard, D., Basting, M., Feeney, M., Turcanu, V., Sever, M. L., Gomez Lorenzo, M., Plaut, M., Lack, G. Randomized trial of peanut consumption in infants at risk for peanut allergy. *N. Engl. J. Med., 2015,* 372(9), 803–813.

FAO/WHO. Evaluation of allergenicity of genetically modified foods. Report of a Joint FAO/WHO expert panel consultation on allergenicity of foods derived from Biotechnology. Rome, Italy, 21–25 January, 2001.

Faris, J. D., Zhang, Q., Chao, S., Zhang, Z., Xu, S. S. Analysis of agronomic and domestication traits in a durum x cultivated emmer wheat population using a high-density single nucleotide polymorphism-based linkage map. *Theor. Appl. Gen.*, 2014, 127, 2333–2348.

FDA. Policy statement on the safety and evaluation process for foods derived from new plant varieties including those derived from recombinant DNA techniques under the Federal Food, Drug and Cosmetic act. Federal Register vol. 57, No. 104, docket No. 92N-0139, 1992.

Fernandez-Cornejo, J., Wechsler, S., Livingston, M., Mitchell, L. Genetically engineered crops in the United States. Econ. Res. Report number 162, February, 2014. http://www.ers.usda.gov/media/1282246/err162.pdf.

Fernandez-Rivas, M., Barreales, L., Mackie, A. R., Fritsche, P., Vazquez-Cortes, S., Jedrzejczak-Czechowicz, M., Kowalski, M. L., Clausen, M., Gislason, D., Sinaniotis, A., Kompoli, L, Le, T. M., Knulst, A. C., Porohit, A., de Blay, F., Kralimarkova, T., Popov, T., Asero, R., Belohlavkova, S., Seneviratne, S. L., Dubakiene, R., Lidholm, J., Hoffmann-Sommergruber, K., Burney, P., Crevel, R., Brill, M., Fernandez-Perez, C., Vieths, S., Mills, E. N. C., van Ree, R., Ballmer-Weber, B. K., The EuroPrevall outpatient clinical study on food allergy, background and methodology. *Allergy,* 2015, doi, 10.1111/all.12585 [Epub ahead of print].

Fleischer, D. M., Sicherer, S., Greenhawt, M., Campbell, D., Chan, E., Muraro, A., Halken, S., Katz, Y., Ebisawa, M., Echenfield, L., Sampson, H. A. Consensus communication on early peanut introduction and the prevention of peanut allergy in high-risk infants. *Allergy*, 2015, E-Pub ahead of print, doi 10.1111/all.12687, July 5, 2015.

Giri, C. C., Vijaya Laxmi, G. 2000. Production of transgenic rice with agronomically useful genes, an assessment. *Biotech. Adv.*, 2000, 18, 653–683.

Goldstein, D. A. Tempest in a tea pot, how did the public conversation on genetically modified crops drift so far from the facts? *J. Med. Toxicol.* 2014, 10, 194–201.

Goodman, R. E. Biosafety, evaluation and regulation of genetically modified (GM) crops in the United States. *J. Huazhong Agr. Univ.*, 2014, 33(6), 93–114. (Chinese and English), http,//hnxbl.cnjournals.net/hznydxzr/ch/reader/create_pdf.aspx?file_no=20140611&year_id=2014&quarter_id=06&falg=1.

Goodman, R. E. Performing IgE serum testing due to bioinformatics matches in the allergenicity assessment of GM crops. *Food Chem. Toxicol.*, 2008, 46, S24–S34.

Goodman, R. E. Practical and predictive bioinformatics methods for the identification of potentially cross-reactive protein matches. *Mol., Nutri., Food Res.* 2006, 655–660.

Goodman, R. E., Leach, J. N. Assessing the allergenicity of proteins introduced into genetically modified crops using specific human IgE assays. *J. AOAC Int.*, 2004, 87(6), 1423–1432.

Goodman, R. E., Panda, R., Ariyarathna, H. Evaluation of endogenous allergens of the safety evaluation of genetically engineered food crops, review of potential risks, test methods, examples and relevance. *J. Agr. Food Chem.*, 2013, 61(35), 8317–8332.

Goodman, R. E., Vieths, S., Sampson, H. A., Hill, D., Ebisawa, M., Taylor, S. L., van Ree, R. Allergenicity assessment of genetically modified crops—what makes sense? *Nat. Biotechnol.*, 2008, 26, 73–8168.

Hajduch, M., Ganapathy, A., Stein, J. W., Thelen, J. J. A systematic proteomic study of seed filling in soybean. Establishment of high-resolution 2-dimensional reference maps, expression profiles and an interactive proteome database. *Plant Physiol.*, 2005, 137(4), 1397–1419.

Harlander, S. K. The evolution of modern agriculture and its future with biotechnology. *J. Amer. Coll. Nutr.*, 21(3), 161S-165S.

Hepburn, P., Howlett, J., Boeing, H., Cockburn, A., Constable, A., Davi, A., de Jong, N., Moseley, B., Oberdorfer, R., Robertson, C., Wal, J. M., Samuels, F. The application of post-market monitoring to novel foods. *Food Chem. Tox.*, 2008, 46,9–33.

Herman, R. A., Korjagin, V. A., Schafer, B. W. Quantitative measurement of protein digestion in simulated gastric fluid. *Reg. Toxicol. Pharmacol.*, 2005, 41(3), 175–184.

Herring, R. J. On risk and regulation, Bt crops in India. *GM Crops & Food*, 2014, 5(3), 204–209.

Hileman, R. E., Silvanovich, A., Goodman, R. E., Rice, E. A., Holleschak, G., Astwood, J. D., Hefle, S. L. Bioinformatic methods for allergenicity assessment using a comprehensive allergen database. *Int. Arch. Allergy Immunol.* 2002, 128(4), 280–291.

Hoff, M., Son, D. Y., Gubesch, M., Ahn, K., Lee, S. I., Vieths, S., Goodman, R. E., Ballmer-Weber, B. K., Bannon, G. A. Serum testing of genetically modified soybeans with special emphasis on potential allergenicity of the heterologous proteins CP4 EPSPS. *Mol. Nutr. Food Res.* 2007, 51, 946–955.

Holzhauser, T., Wackermann, O., Ballmer-Weber, B. K., Bindslev-Jensen, C., Scibilia, J., Perono-Garoffo, L., Utsumi, S., Poulsen, L. K., Vieths, S. Soybean (*Glycine max*) allergy in Europe, Gly m 5 (β-conglycinin) and Gly m 6 (glycinin) are potential diagnostic markers for severe allergic reactions to soy. *J. Allergy and Clin. Immunol.* 2009, 123, 452–458.

Houston, N. L., Lee, D. G., Stevenson, S. E., Ladics, G. S., Bannon, G. A., McClain, S., Privalle, L., Stagg, N., Herouet-Guicheney, C., MacIntosh, S. C., Thelen, J. J. Quantitation of soybean allergens using tandem mass spectrometry. *J. Prot. Res.,* 2011, 10(2), 763–773.

Jagannath, A., Arumugam, N., Gupta, V., Pradhan, A., Burma, P. K., Pental, D. Development of transgenic barstar lines and identification of a male sterile (barnase)/restorer (barstar) combination for heterosis breeding in Indian oilseed mustard (*Brassica juncea*). *Curr. Sci., 2002,* 82, 46–52.

Jagannath, A., Bandyopadhyay, P., Arumugam, N., Gupta, V., Burma, P. K., Pental, D. The use of a Spacer DNA fragment insulates the tissue-specific expression of a cytotoxic gene (barnase) and allows high-frequency generation of transgenic male sterile lines in *Brassica juncea* L. *Mol. Breeding,* 2001, 8, 11–23.

James, C. Global status of commercialized biotech/GM crops. *ISAAA brief No. 49.* ISAAA, Ithaca, New York, 2014.

Janse, J. J., Wong, G. W., Potts, J., Ogorodova, L. M., Fedorova, O. S., Mahesh, P. A., Sakellariou, A., Papadopoulos, N. G., Knulst, A. C., Versteeg, S. A., Kroes, A. C., Vossen, A. C., Campos Ponce, M., Kummeling, I., Burney, P., van Ree, R., Yazdanbakhsh, M. The association between foodborne and orofecal pathogens and allergic sensitization—EuroPrevall study. *Pediatr. Allergy Immunol.*, 2014, 25(3), 250–256.

Kasera, R., Niphadkar, P. V., Saran, A., Mathur, C., Singh, A. B. First case report of anaphylaxis caused by Rajgira seed flour (Amaranthus paniculatus) from India, A clinic-immunologic evaluation. *Asian Pac. J. Allergy Immunol.* 2013, 31, 79–83.

Krishna, G., Singh, B. K., Kim, E.-K., Morya, V. K., Ramteke, P. W. Progress in genetic engineering of peanut (*Arachis hypogaea* L.)—A review. *Plant Biotech. J.*, 2015, 13, 147–162.

Kumar, S., Misra, A., Verma, A. K., Roy, R., Tripathi, A., Ansari, K. M., Das, M., Dwivedi, P. D. *Bt* brinjal in India, a long way to go. *GM Crops*, 2011, 2, 92–98.

Kummeling, I., Mills, E. N., Clausen, M., Dubakiene, R., Perez, C. F., Fernandez-Rivas, M., Knulst, A. C., Kowalski, M. L., Lidholm, J., Le, T. M., Metzler, C., Mustakov, T., Popov, T., Potts, J,. van Ree, R., Sakellariou, A., Tondury, B., Tzannis, K., Burney, P. The EuroPrevall surveys on the prevalence of food allergies in children and adults, background and study methodology. *Allergy, 2009,* 64(10), 1493–1497.

Lim, D. L.-C., Neo, K. H., Yi, F. C., Chua, K. Y., Goh, D. L.-M., Shek, Giam, Y. C., Van Bever, H. P. S., Lee, B. W. Parvalbumin-the major tropical fish allergen. *Ped. Allergy and Immunol., 2008,* 19, 399–407.

Lin, J.-Y., Stupar, R. M., Hans, C., Hyten, D. L, Jackson, S. A. Structural and functional divergence of a 1-Mb duplicated region in the soybean (*Glycine max*) genome and comparison to an orthologous region from *Phaseolus vulgaris. The Plant Cell* 2010, 22, 2545–2561.

Liu, G. M., Huang, Y. Y., Cai, Q. F., Weng, W. Y., Su, W. J., Cao, M. J. Comparative study of in vitro digestion of major allergen, tropomyosin, and other proteins between Grass prawn (*Penaeus monodon*) and Pacific white shrimp (*Litopenaeus vannamei*). *J. Sci. Food Agric.*, 2010, 91(1), 163–170.

Ludvigsson, J. F., Bai, J. C., Biagi, F., Card, T. R., Ciacci, C., Ciclitira, P. J., Green, P. H. R., Hadjivassilou, M., Holdoway, A., van Heel, D. A., Kaukinen, K., Leffler, D. A., Leonard, J. N., Lundin, K. E. A., McGough, N., Davidson, M.l, Murray, J. A., Swift, G. L., Walker, M. M., Zongone, F., Sanders, D. S., Diagnosis and management of adult celiac disease, guidelines from the *Br. Soc. Gastro. Gut*, GID, 2014, 63, 1210–1228.

Mari, A., Ooievaar-de Heer, P., Scala, E., Giani, M., Pirrotta, L., Zuidmeer, L., Bethell, D., van Ree, R. Evaluation by double-blind placebo-controlled oral challenge of the clinical relevance of IgE antibodies against plant glycans. *Allergy,* 2008, 63, 891–896.

Metcalfe, D. D., Astwood, J. D., Townsend, R., Sampson, H. A., Taylor, S. L., Fuchs, R. L. Assessment of the allergenic potential of foods derived from genetically engineered crop plants. *Crit Rev. Food Sci Nutr, 1996,* 36 (Suppl), S165–S186.

Newell-McGloughlin, M. Future directions, development and application of GM crops in the USA. *J. Huazhong Agr. Univ,* 2014, 33(6), 33–39. http,//hnxbl.cnjournals.net/hznydxzr/ch/reader/create_pdf.aspx?file_no=20140605&year_id=2014&quarter_id=06&falg=1.

Nordlee, J. A., Taylor, S. L., Townsend, J. A., Thomas, L. A., Bush, R. K. Identification of a Brazil-nut allergen in transgenic soybeans. *N. Engl. J. Med.* 1996, 334(11), 688–692.

Ofori-Anti, A. O, Ariyarathna, H., Chen, L., Lee, H. L., Pramod, S. N., Goodman, R. E. Establishing objective detection limits for the pepsin digestion assay used in assessment of genetically modified foods. *Reg. Tox. Pharma.* See Huazhong Medical, India, 2014, 52(2), 94–103.

Padgette, S. R., Taylor, N. B., Nida, D. L., Bailey, M. R., MacDonald, J., Holden, L. R., Fuchs, R. L. The composition of glyphosate-tolerant soybean seeds is equivalent to that of conventional soybeans. *J. Nutr.* 1995, 126(3), 702–716.

Panda, R., Ariyarathna, H., Amnuaycheewa, P., Tetteh, A., Pramod, S. N., Taylor, S. L., Ballmer-Weber, B. K, Goodman, R. E. Challenges in testing genetically modified crops for potential increases in endogenous allergen expression for safety. *Allergy,* 68(2), 142–151.

Pauli, G., Bessot, J. C., Braun, P. A., Dietemann-Molard, A., Kopferschmitt-Kubler, M. C., Theirry, R., Celery allergy, clinical and biological study of 20 cases. *Ann. Allergy,* prime suspect 1888, 60(3), 243–246.

Peeters, K. A., Koppelman, S. J., van Hoffen, E., van der Tas, C. W., den Hartog Jager, C. F., Penninks, A. H., Hefle, S. L., Bruijnzeel-Koomen, C. Al, Knol, E. F., Knulst, A. C. Does skin prick test reactivity to purified allergens correlate with clinical severity of peanut allergy? *Clinical and Experimental Allergy* 2007, 37(1), 108–115.

Prescott, S. L., Pawankar, R., Allen, K. J., Campbell, D. E., Sinn, J. K. H., Fiocchi, A., Ebisawa, M., Sampson, H. A., Beyer, K., Lee, B.-W. A global survey of changing patterns of food allergy burden in children. *WAO J.*, 2013, 6, 21–33.

Purohit, A., Laffer, S., Metz-Favre, C., Verot, A., Kricek, F., Valenta, R., Pauli, G. Poor association between allergen-specific serum immunoglobulin E levels, skin sensitivity and basophil degranulation, a study with recombinant birch pollen allergen Bet v 1 and an immunoglobulin E detection system measuring immunoglobulin E capable of binding to FcåRI. *Clin. Exp. Allergy*, 2005, 35, 186–192.

Rascon-Cruz, Q., Sinagawa-Garcia, S., Osuna-Castro, J. A., Bohorova, N., Parades-Lopez, O. Accumulation, assembly, and digestibility of amarantin expressed in transgenic tropical maize. *Theor. Appl. Genet.* 2004, 108, 335–342.

Reddy, D. V., Sudarshana, M. R., Fuchs, M., Rao, N. C., Thottappilly, G. Genetically engineered virus-resistant plants in developing countries, current status and future prospects. *Adv. Virus Res.* 2009, 75,185–220.26. Vasavirama, K., Kirti, P. B. Increased resistance to late leaf spot disease in transgenic peanut using a combination of PR genes. *Funct. Integr. Genomics*, 2012, 12,625–634.

Rostom, A., Murray, J. A., Kagnoff, M. F. American Gastroenterological Association (AGA) Institute technical review on the diagnosis and management of Celiac Disease. *Gastroenterol.* 2006, 131, 1981–2002.

Rubio-Tapia, A., Murray, J. A. Celiac Disease. *Current Opinions in Gastroenterology*. 2010, 26(2), 116–122.

Sampson, H. A. Food allergy. *JAMA*, 1997, 278(22), 1888–1894.

Satinover, S. M., Reefer, A. J., Pomes, A., Chapman, M. D., Platts-Mills, T. A., Woodfolk, J. A. Specific IgE and IgG antibody-binding patterns to recombinant cockroach allergens. *J. Allergy Clin. Immunol.*, 2005, 15(4), 803–809.

Schulkes, K. J., Klemans, R. J., Knigge, L., de Bruin-Weller, M., Bruijnzeel-Koomen, C. A., Marknell deWitt, A., Lidholm, J., Knulst, A. C., 2014. Specific IgE to fish extracts does not predict allergy to specific species within an adult fish allergic population. *Clin. Trans. Allergy* 4, 27. doi 10.1186/2045-7022-4-27.

Seetharam, S. Should the *Bt* brinjal controversy concern healthcare professionals and bioethicists? *Indian J. Med. Ethics* 2010, 7(1), 9–12.

Sharp, M. F., Stephen, J. N., Kraft, L., Weiss, T., Kamath, S. D., Lopata, A. L. Immunological cross-reactivity between four distant parvalbumins-impact on allergen detection and diagnostics. *Mol. Immunol.*, 2015, 63(2), 437–448.

Sicherer, S. H. Epidemiology of food allergy. *J. Allergy Clin. Immunol.* 2011, 127, 594–602.

Sicherer, S. H., Sampson, H. A. Food allergy, Epidemiology, pathogenesis, diagnosis, and treatment. *J. Allergy Clin. Immunol.* 2014, 133, 291–307.

Silvanovich, A., Nemeth, M. A., Song, P., Herman, R., Tagliani, L., Bannon, G. A. The value of short amino acid sequence matches for prediction of protein allergenicity. *Toxicol. Sci.*, 2006, 90(10), 252–258.

Sinagawa-Garcia, S. R., Rascon-Cruz, Q., Valdez-Ortiz, A., Medina-Godoy, S., Escobar-Gutierrez, A., Paredes-Lopez, O. Safety assessment by in vitro digestibility and allergenicity of genetically modified maize with an amaranth 11S globulin. *J. Agric. Food Chem.* 2004, 52, 2709–2714.

Siruguri, V., Bharatraj, D. K., Vankudavath, R. N., Rao Mendu, V. V., Gupta, V., Goodman, R. E. Evaluation of Bar, Barnase and Barstar recombinant proteins expressed in genetically engineered *Brassica juncea* (Indian mustard) for potential risks of food allergy using bioinformatics and literature searches. *Food Chem. Toxicol.* 2015, 83, 93–102.

Sollid L. M., Qiao, S.-W., Anderson, R. P., Gianfrani, C., Koning, F. Nomenclature and listing of celiac disease relevant gluten T-cell epitopes restricted by HLA-DQ molecules. *Immunogenetics,* 2012. 64, 455–460.

Sowka, S., Hafner, C., Radauer, C., Focke, M., Brehler, R., Astood, J. D., Arif, S. A., Kanani, A., Sussman, G. L. Scheiner, O., Beezhold, D. H., Breitender, H. Molecular and immunological characterization of new isoforms of the *Hevea brasiliensis* latex allergen Hev b 7, evidence of no cross-reactivity between Hev b 7 isoforms and potato patatin and proteins from avocado and banana. *J. Allergy Clin. Immunol.* 1999, 104(6), 1302–1310.

Springer, N. M., Stupar, R. M., Allelic variation and heterosis in maize. How do two halves make more than a whole? Genom. Res., 2007, 17, 264–275.

Stadler, M. B., Stadler, B. M. Allergenicity prediction by protein sequence. *FASEB J., 2003,* 17, 1141–1143.

Stupar, R. M. Into the Wild. The soybean genome meets its undomesticated relative. *Proc. Natl. Acad. Sci (USA),* 2010, 107, 21947–21948.

Taylor, S. L., Baumert, J. L. Worldwide food allergy labeling and detection of allergens in processed foods. *Chem. Immunol. Allergy* 2015, 101, 227–234.

Taylor, S. L., Baumert, J. L., Kruizinga, A. G., Remington, B. C., Crevel, R. W., Brooke-Taylor, S., Allen, K. J., Allergen Bureau of Australia and New Zealand, Houben, G. Establishment of reference doses for residues of allergenic foods, report of the VITAL expert panel. *Food and Chemical Toxicology*, 2014, 63, 9–17.

Taylor, S. L., Houben, G. F., Baumert, J. L., Crevel, R. R., Allen, K. J., Dubois, A. E., Knulst, A. C., Remington, B. C., Kruizinga, A. G., Blom, W. M., Brooke-Taylor, S. Understanding food allergen thresholds requires careful analysis of the available clinical data. *J. Allergy Clin. Immunol.* 2015, 135(2), 583–584.

Thomas, K., Aalbers, M., Bannon, G. A., Bartels, M., Dearman, R. J., Esdaile, D. J., Fu, T. J., Glatt, C. M., Hadfield, N., Hatzos, C., Hefle, S. L., Heylings, J. R., Goodman, R. E., Henry, B., Herouet, C., Holsapple, M., Ladics, G. S., Landry, T. D., MacIntosh, S. C., Rice, E. A., Privalle, L. S., Steiner, H. Y., Teshima, R., van Ree, R., Woolhiser, M., Zawodny, J. A multi-laboratory evaluation of a common in vitro pepsin digestion assay protocol used in assessing the safety of novel proteins. Reg. Tox. Pharmacol. 2004, 39(2), 87–98.

Tjon, J. M.-L., van Bergen, J., Koning, F. Celiac disease, how complicated can it get? Immunogenet. 2010, 62, 6411–651.

Turner, P. J., Gowland, M. H., Sharma, V., Ierodiakonou, D., Harper, N., Garcez, T., Pumphrey, R., Boyle, R. J. Increase in anaphylaxis-related hospitalizations but no increase in fatalities, An analysis of United Kingdom national anaphylaxis data, 1992–2012. *J. Allerg. Clin. Immunol.*, 2014, Doi.org/10.1016/j.jaci.2014.10.021.

Van Do, T., Elsayed, S., Florvaag, E., Hordvik, I, Endresen, C., Allergy to fish parvalbumins, Studies on the cross-reactivity of allergens from 9 commonly consumed fish. J. Allergy Clin. Immunol. 2005, 116, 1314–1320.

van Ree, R., Cabanes-Macheteau, M., Akkerdaas, J., Milasso J.-P., Coutelier-Bourhis, C., Rayou, C., Villalaba, M., Koppelman, S., Aalberse, R., Rodriguez, R., Faye, L., Lerouge, P. β(1,2)-xylose and α(1,3)-fucose residues have a strong contribution to plant glycoallergns. *J. Biol. Chem.* 2000, 275(15), 11451–11458.

Vejvar, E., Himly, M., Briza, P., Eichhorn, S., Ebner, C., Hemmer, W., Ferreira, F., Gadermaier, G., Allergenic relevance of nonspecific lipid transfer protein 2, identification and characterization of Api g 6 from celery tuber as representative of a novel IgE-binding protein family. *Mol. Nutri. Food Res* 57(11), 2061–2070.

Wagner, S., Breiteneder, H. *Hevea brasiliensis* latex allergen, current panel and clinical relevance. *Int. Arch. Allergy Immunol* 2005, 136, 90–97.

Walker, K. A., Hellmich, R. L., Lewis, L. C., 2000. Late-instar European corn borer (Lepidoptera, Crambidae) tunneling and survival in transgenic corn hybrids. *J. Eco. Ent* 93(4), 1276–1285.

Wong, G. W., Mahesh, P. A., Ogorodova, L., Leung, T. F., Fedorova, O., Holla, A. D., Fernandez-Rivas, M., Mills, E. N. C., Kummeling, I., van Ree, R., Yazdanbakhsh, M., Burney, P. The EuroPrevall-INCO surveys on the prevalence of food allergies in children from China, India and Russia, the study methodology. *Allergy*, 2005, 65(3), 385–390.

Wu, J.-L., Wu, C., Lei, C., Baraoidan, M., Bordeos, A., Madamba, M. R., Ramos-Pamplona, M., Mauleon, R., Portugal, A., Ulat, V. J., Bruskiewich, R., Wang, G., Leach, J., Khush, G., Leung, H. Chemical- and irradiation-induced mutants of indica rice IR64 for forward and reverse genetics. *Plant Molec Biology,* 2015, 59(1), 85–97.

Xu, Y. S., Kashner, M., Harada, L., Xu, A., Satter, J., Waseman, S. Anaphylaxis-related deaths in Ontario, a retrospective review of cases from 1986 to 2011. *Allergy Asthma Clin. Immunol.* 2014, 10(1), 38. Doi: 10.1186/1710-1492-10-38.

Zhuang, Y., Dreskin, S. C. Redefining the major peanut allergens. *Immunol. Res.* 2013, 55(1–3), 125–134.

PART VI

ALLERGEN IMMUNOTHERAPY AND ANTI IgE

CHAPTER 16

SPECIFIC IMMUNOTHERAPY: PRINCIPLES AND PRACTICE

WIQAR SHAIKH[1] and SHIFA WIQAR SHAIKH[2]

[1]*Professor of Medicine, Grant Medical College and Sir J.J. Group of Hospitals, Bombay Hon. Visiting Allergist, Bombay Hospital and Medical Research Centre, Hon. Physician and Allergist, Prince Aly Khan Hospital, Hon. Physician, Police Hospital and Byculla Jail, Mumbai, India, E-mail: drwiqar@gmail.com*

[2]*Allergy and Asthma Clinic, Shakti Sadan Co-op Housing Society Ground Floor, B-Block, Opp. Navjeevan Society Lamington Road, Mumbai–400007, India*

CONTENTS

16.1 INTRODUCTION

"Allergic diseases" represent the commonest of diseases of mankind. In the 20th century, a series of treatment options were discovered, which have helped ameliorate the symptoms of allergy sufferers. However, a large number of patients continued to suffer despite optimum avoidance measures and pharmacotherapy. In this quest for another treatment option, which could perhaps be a cure for "allergies," up came one of the most novel, yet effective of treatment modalities available to the allergist – "immunotherapy" for allergic diseases (also termed "specific immunotherapy" or SIT). Other synonyms for this treatment are desensitization, hyposensitization, allergy shots, allergy vaccines and allergen injection therapy. Discovered in 1911 by Leonard Noon (1911) at the St. Mary's Hospital in London, SIT has stood the test of time for the past 104 years and has now come to be accepted as the cornerstone of treatment for allergic diseases.

Leonard Noon provided the following guidelines, which hold true even today. They are as follows: (1) a negative phase of decreased resistance develops after injection treatment; (2) increased resistance to allergen challenge, measured by quantitative ophthalmic tests is dose dependent; (3) optimal interval between two injections should be 1 to 2 weeks; (4) sensitivity may increase if injections are too frequent; (5) overdoses may induce systemic reactions.

SIT involves the introduction of allergen extracts either subcutaneous (SCIT) or sublingual (SLIT) in increasing concentrations and decreasing frequency. The aim of SIT is to induce a state of "hyposensitization" with a diminished clinical response on natural re-exposure to the allergen.

16.2 IS THE EXISTENCE OF SPECIFIC IMMUNOTHERAPY JUSTIFIED?

Few medical treatments have been shrouded in as much controversy as the practice of SIT. The only compelling argument in favor of establishing a specific diagnosis in allergic disease is that when the offending allergen is identified, a specific treatment can be instituted. Only two specific treatments are available to the allergic patient; allergen avoidance and SIT. Medication, though useful, will only suppress symptoms but do little to modify the long-term disease process. SIT is at present the only specific, disease modifying, cost-effective treatment option. Indeed, SIT constitutes a true aetiological treatment that possibly prevents the emergence of new sensitizations. Undoubtedly, SIT would not have survived for the past 104 years, if it did not work!

16.3 SPECIFIC IMMUNOTHERAPY VACCINES: PREPARATION AND STANDARDIZATION

Safety, efficacy and reproducibility of specific allergy disease management are dependent on high quality allergen extracts for both in vivo diagnosis and for SIT. However, the term "allergic extract" is no longer used; the WHO changed it in 1988 to "allergen vaccine" (Bousquet et al., 1998).

Allergen vaccines (after being checked for potency, composition and stability) should be distributed as any one of the following:

1. Vaccines from a single source material;
2. Cross-reacting allergen mixtures;
3. Mixtures of non-cross-reacting allergens (with proven stability data).

Allergen products are manufactured by aqueous extraction of natural source materials inherently complex and variable in nature. The standardization procedure (Larsen et al., 1999) includes all aspects of extract preparation and handling including selection and collection of raw materials, extraction and production process as well as storage and distribution of manufactured goods. An important aspect of allergen standardization is batch-to-batch standardization, which in its optimal performance is a combination of scientific laboratory analyses and in vivo testing centered on the key reagent, the in-house reference preparation (IHRP). The IHRP is company specific, which explains why extracts differ from manufacturer to manufacturer. The IHRP is thoroughly and completely characterized to ensure the presence of all relevant allergens, and its biological activity is confirmed by the skin prick test as well as by clinical efficacy in trials of IT. Having established the IHRP, batch-to-batch standardization is performed by demonstrating that each new batch matches the IHRP in all respects. There is a 3-step laboratory procedure, which achieves this:

1. Complexity analysis using crossed immuno-electrophoresis, establishing a semi-quantitative relation between all antigenic components.
2. Determination of major allergen content.
3. Determination of overall IgE binding potency.

In the United States, standardization is done with a national reference ID50 EAL (intradermal dilution for 50-mm sum of erythema, determines the bioequivalent allergy unit) that is calculated using the intradermal skin test. The dilution is chosen when 50 mm of erythema is observed to the tested extract. The test is performed on a population known to be allergic to the allergen being tested. Once the process is complete, the allergen extracts are labeled with the same unit, the bioequivalent allergy unit (BAU), which is possibly, the unit most commonly used today. Other units used for labeling allergen extracts are weight/volume (w/v) and PNU (protein nitrogen units), both of which indicate a non-standardized extract.

It must be remembered that the allergen vaccine when sent across to the patient requires to be stabilized and needs to be stored at 4°C. It is therefore important to maintain a cold chain. Lyophilization and addition of a stabilizing agent such as 50% glycerol are other methods of stabilizing allergen preparations.

It is possible to attempt enhancement of an allergen vaccine using physical modification. Thus adsorbing the allergen vaccine with alum or cross-linking with formaldehyde or polyethylene glycol (PEG) are some of the methods used for enhancement. Such modified allergens are termed "allergoids."

16.4 CRITERIA FOR SELECTION OF PATIENTS FOR SPECIFIC IMMUNOTHERAPY

1. SIT is considered in selected patients with symptoms of allergic rhinitis or allergic asthma uncontrolled by avoidance measures and pharmacotherapy. Skin prick tests (SPT) should confirm which allergens are to be used.
2. Venom SIT is recommended for individuals with systemic reactions following insect stings such as bees and wasps (Reisman, 1994). Venom SIT has been shown to be superior to SIT with whole body stinging insects.
3. The remote evaluation and diagnosis of allergic disease and/or formulation of plans should not be done (Nelson et al., 1993) and has indeed been condemned and is not recommended by the American Academy of Allergy, Asthma and Immunology (Position Statement, 1986). In remote allergy practice, a laboratory simply asks for the blood of the patient by mail and runs a blood test to measure specific IgE levels to different allergens. The report of the blood test is then mailed back to the patient along with an SIT prescription, based on the results of the test. In remote allergy practice, a trained allergist never sees the patient; no history is taken nor is any physical examination conducted. Of great concern therefore is that remote practice promotes provision of clinical care by non-physician health providers. Besides, it is known that the SPT is a more reliable and reproducible test.

16.5 INDICATIONS FOR SPECIFIC IMMUNOTHERAPY

The efficacy of SIT has been confirmed in a large number of carefully controlled, clinical studies. As mentioned earlier, SIT represents a specific treatment for allergic diseases and unlike conventional pharmacological treatment, has the potential to alter the course of the disease with prevention of progression (Durham, 1994).

1. *Rhinitis:* SIT is advised to patients who are not symptom free despite receiving adequate pharmacotherapy. A Cochrane review

showed that SIT in patients with rhinitis showed considerable improvement with reduction in the symptom scores (Calderon et al., 2007). A meta-analysis done from various databases from 1966 to 2006, shows that sublingual immunotherapy with standardized extracts when compared with a placebo is more effective in patients with allergic rhinitis (Rush Immunotherapy Information).

2. *Allergic Asthma:* Long term use of SIT in house dust mite allergic children with asthma caused a reduction in the use of inhaled corticosteroids and improvement in lung functions. However, before starting SIT in a patient, one must evaluate the role of the allergen in the severity of the asthma exacerbation. Along with SIT one must make sure avoidance measures are followed strictly (Skripak and Wood, 2008).
3. *Insect Sting Allergy:* A recent study shows that children, who receive 3 to 5 years of Venom immunotherapy (VIT), have lasting benefits for up to 2 decades. VIT is the treatment of choice in insect sting allergies and is considered life saving in all patients (Golden, 2006).
4. *Drug Allergy:* The commonest drug allergy is seen to penicillin, NSAIDs and aspirin. Avoidance of the offending drug is the most effective form of treatment. However, in a few cases, where the drug may be essential for the patient, desensitization should be done. During desensitization standardized protocols should be implemented with a very high standard of care (Castells, 2006).
5. *Skin Allergy and Food Allergy:* Double blind placebo controlled studies involving SIT with respect to skin and food allergies are needed to establish clinical effectiveness (Niebuhr et al., 2008).

16.6 MECHANISM OF SPECIFIC IMMUNOTHERAPY

The following is the sequence of events in allergen specific immunotherapy (Akdis and Akdis, 2014; Fujita et al., 2012):

1. *Very Early Events:* The very early effects of SIT are related to mast cell and basophil desensitization. The intermediate effects are attributed to allergen specific T cells and the late effects are due

to the B-cells, IgE, mast cells, basophils and eosinophils. For a definitive decrease in the levels of IgE antibody, years of SIT may be needed. Right from the first dose in SIT, there is a considerable decrease in the mast cell and basophil activity, and degranulation. There is a reduction in the chances of anaphylaxis as SIT is continued. All this is followed by the bringing forth of a class of T regulatory (Treg) cells which are allergen specific and suppression of Th2 cells.

2. *Generation of Treg Cells and Peripheral T-cell Tolerance:* In this stage there is generation of allergen specific Treg cells. There is also a peripheral T-cell tolerance, which is marked by suppressed cytokine and proliferative responses against the offending allergen. Treg cells may be of two types, the naturally occurring thymic selected CD4+ and CD25+ Treg cells, and the inducible type 1 Treg cells (Tr1). The process initiation of T-cell tolerance starts with the autocrine action of IL-10 and TGF-beta (produced by antigen specific T-cells). It has been noted in various studies that CD4+ CD25+ Treg cells from atopic donors have a reduced capacity to suppress the CD4+CD25– T-cells. Thus, the conclusion that upregulation of Treg cells has a major role in SIT. All individuals have Th1, Th2 and Tr1 allergen specific subsets. These are present in varying amounts. The shift of balance between Th2 and TR1 could lead to the person either developing an allergy or recovering from it. Also, Treg cells are characterized by the expression of FOXp3 (transcriptional regulator). It is said to be the "MASTER SWITCH" gene for Treg development and function. Apart from suppressing Th2 cells, Treg cells use other mechanisms to suppress allergic inflammation. The sequence is: suppression of the antigen presenting cells (APCs), which in turn control the Th2 and Th1 cells; suppression of Th2 cells; suppression of IgG, IgA, IgE; mast cell, basophil and eosinophil suppression; remodeling of the target tissue after interaction with the resident tissue cells (Figures 16.1 and 16.2).

3. *Breg Cells:* Similar to Th cells, B cells can be classified into subsets according to the cytokines which they produce. One functional B-cell subset, the Breg cells (van de Veen et al., 2013), has

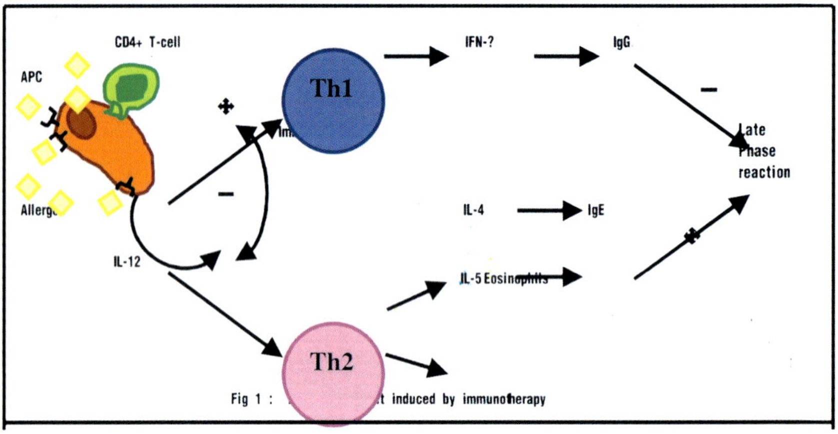

FIGURE 16.1 Th2 to Th1 shift induced by immunotherapy.

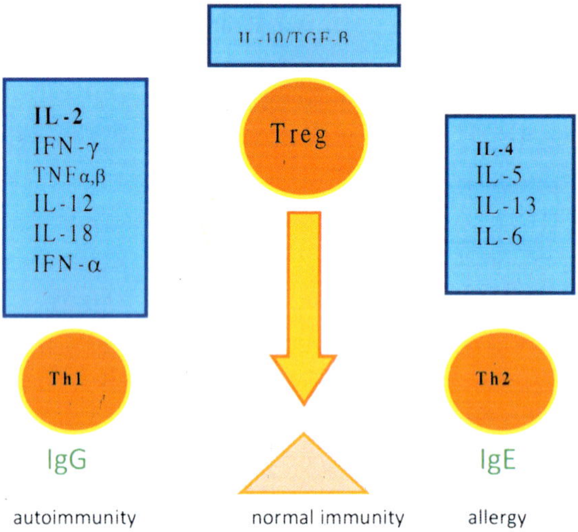

FIGURE 16.2 Role of T regulatory cells, TGF-Beta and IL-10 in Specific Immunotherapy.

recently been shown to contribute to the maintenance of the fine equilibrium required for developing tolerance. Breg cells control excessive inflammatory responses through IL-10, which inhibits proinflammatory cytokines and supports Treg cell differentiation.

As observed in TR1 cells, recently, highly purified IL-10-secreting Breg cells (BR1) cells were phenotypically and functionally characterized.

4. *Runt-Related Transcription Factor:* RUNX 1 impairs the expression of IL-2 and IFN-gamma and exerts suppressive activity (Klunker et al., 2009). Induction of RUNX1 and RUNX3 by TGF-beta plays an essential role in the generation and suppressive function of induced Treg cells. RUNX1 and RUNX3 bind to the FOXP3 promoter and activate the induction of FOXP3-expressing functional Treg cells.
5. *Modulation of Allergen-Specific IgE and IgG Subtype Responses During Allergen-SIT:* FcåRI bound IgE, which is found on mast cells and basophils is characteristic of atopic diseases. B-cell tolerance does not develop early, unlike T-cell tolerance. When the body is exposed to an allergen, the levels of specific IgE increase. This is also seen in the initial phase of SIT. In the later stages, specific IgE levels drop, which could be over a period of months to years. In patients suffering from seasonal rhino-conjunctivitis, the levels of pollen specific IgE remains low due to desensitization as a result of SIT. The clinical response in patients does not always correlate to the levels of specific IgE (the level of IgE falls late during the course of SIT), thus bringing in the role of IgG. The role of IgG is controversial in the response of SIT, as there are studies both proving and disproving its role in the clinical improvement of patients. The blocking effect of IgG is responsible, as it binds for the same sites as IgE and thus halts the allergic cascade. A detailed analysis of IgG reveals that SIT causes an increase in the levels of IgG, especially IgG4. The IgG4 levels have been shown to increase to almost 100 fold. Recent assays using flow-cytometry show that the blocking ability of IgG in SIT is not just dependant on the amount of the IgG antibody; it also depends on the subset of the antibody. IgG1 and IgG4 have been found to be responsible for a considerable amount of blocking activity. However, the role of IgG needs to be studied further. Another molecule that is important is the IL-10. IL-10 is responsible for inducing T-cell tolerance and also for shifting the balance from an IgE response to an IgG4

response. The shift from Th2 to Treg cells occurs with a few days of starting SIT, whereas, the reduction in IgE occurs after years. It must be emphasized that only high allergen doses generate specific Treg cells resulting in a normal immune response, whereas sub-optimal allergen doses generate a Th2 mediated allergen immune response (Figures 16.3 and 16.4).

6. *Suppression of Effector Cells and Inflammatory Responses During SIT:* The peripheral tolerance which develops as a result of SIT causes decrease in both acute and chronic allergic reactions. It decreases the release of histamine and causes a modulation in the threshold for basophil and mast cell activation. IL-10 is known to decrease the eosinophil function, reduces cytokine release from mast cells; it also reduces IL-5 production. IL-10 is also known to

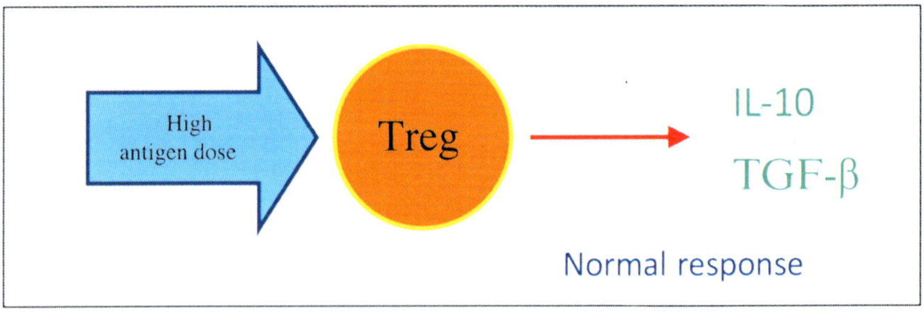

FIGURE 16.3 High allergen doses generate specific Treg cells and normal immune response.

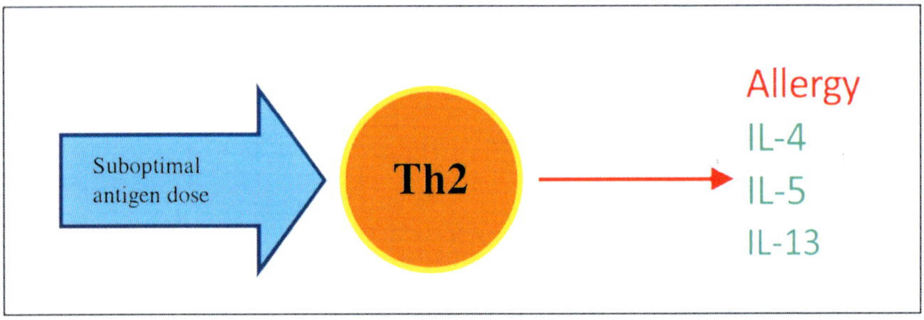

FIGURE 16.4 Suboptimal allergen doses generate a Th2 mediated allergen immune response.

cause prevention of mast cell degranulation. Reduction of the late phase reaction (LPR) forms an important part of SIT. Eosinophils play a major role in the LPR, unlike mast cells in the early phase. SIT is known to cause decrease in the levels of eosinophils and mast cells in the nasal and bronchial tissues.

Current theory postulates a shift from Th2 to Th1, along with increase in IgG4 and a decrease in IgE. Apart from FOXp3+ and Treg cells, there is also a role of transforming growth factor (TGF-α) and interleukin10 (IL-10). The role of Breg cells RUNX has also been recently discovered. Studies also show that there could be a major role played by antigen presenting cells (APC) like dendritic cells (DC) in the initiation and modulation of the allergic response.

16.7 WHAT WE ALREADY KNOW ABOUT IMMUNOTHERAPY IS?

1. SIT causes increase in Tr1 cells that secrete IL-10.
2. SIT increases the suppressive capacity of Tr1 and CD4+CD25+cells.
3. SIT decreases allergen specific T-cell proliferation, along with decreased Th1 and Th2.
4. IgG, especially IgG4 and IgG1 levels are increased by SIT.
5. Induction of both early and late phase reactions are reduced due to administration of SIT.
6. SIT causes increase in IL-10, CD4+CD25+FOXp3+ Treg cells and Breg cells, and a decrease in mast cells and eosinophils and their mediators.
7. Treatment with pharmacotherapy (beta2 agonists and glucocorticoids) helps in enhancement of the effects of SIT.
8. SIT is safe in all age groups above 6 years of age, and even in pregnancy.

16.8 WHAT WE STILL DO NOT KNOW ABOUT IMMUNOTHERAPY IS?

1. The exact molecular mechanism of the generation of the Treg and Breg cells in vivo.

2. Whether Treg cells are harmful because of the immune tolerance they develop, and their role in case of tumor antigens and chronic infectious agents?
3. Which adjuvants promote Treg and Breg cells?
4. What is the lifespan of SIT induced Treg and Breg cells?
5. What are the biomarkers and predictors for the success of SIT?
6. What are the mechanisms for the long-term maintenance of allergen tolerance following SIT?
7. What exactly is the contribution of the target tissue cells in the development of immune tolerance?
8. What is the optimal dose of SIT, particularly of SLIT?

16.9 ROLE OF HISTAMINE RECEPTOR IN MECHANISM OF SIT

Histamine enhances Th1 responses by triggering the H1 receptors, whereas, H2 receptors have a negative effect on both Th1 and Th2. In a double blind placebo controlled trial it was seen that use of levocetrizine along with SIT did not decrease in the H1:H2 receptor ratio as seen is the group treated with placebo and SIT. A high level of IL-10 was also observed in the group being treated by antihistamines suggesting an immunomodulatory effect of antihistamines (Akdis and Akdis, 2007, 2009a,b, 2014; Fujita et al., 2012; Francis et al., 2003; Klunker et al., 2009; Nouri-Aria et al., 2004; Palomares et al., 2010; van de Veen et al., 2013).

16.10 ADVENT OF SUBLINGUAL IMMUNOTHERAPY

Scadding and Brostoff (1986) first used sublingual immunotherapy (Scadding and Brostoff, 2004) and concluded that it is safe, and avoids side effects of injection immunotherapy. Since then, SLIT has been found to be the most effective non-injective route of administering SIT. However, oral immunotherapy (OIT), local nasal immunotherapy (LNIT) and local bronchial immunotherapy (LBIT) are too expensive, unsafe or ineffective. SLIT can be safely used at home. It is an essential adjuvant to pharmacotherapy in allergic diseases. SLIT is "CHEAP, SAFE and EFFECTIVE therapy."

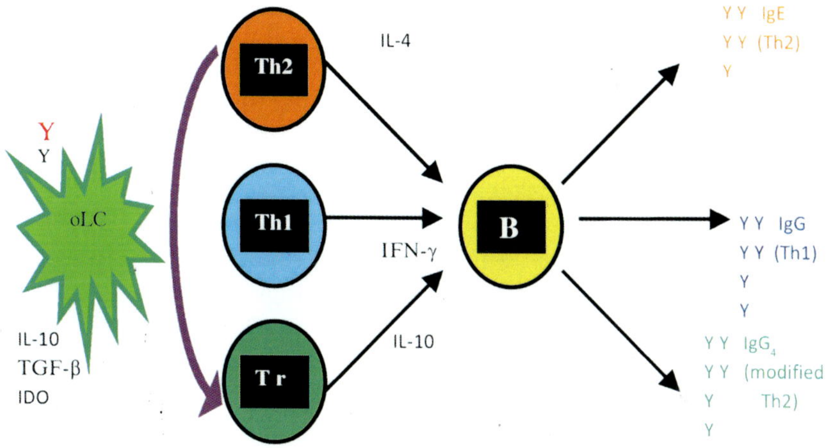

FIGURE 16.5 Role of oral Langerhans cells in SLIT.

16.11 MECHANISM OF SUBLINGUAL IMMUNOTHERAPY

SLIT has been shown to be well tolerated in all reported, double-blinded, placebo-controlled, randomized trials. Owing to its excellent safety and good compliance, SLIT has become an integral part of the ideal treatment in treating allergic diseases in the pediatric population. It is postulated that in SLIT, oral Langerhans cells engulf the allergen, and then pass it on to the draining lymph node. These lymph nodes produce IgG antibody and induce T lymphocytes (Figure 16.5) (Akdis and Akdis, 2014; Fujita et al., 2012).

16.12 MONTELUKAST AND IMMUNOTHERAPY

A recent study failed to show any benefits of montelukast when used along with SIT. On the contrary it showed that as compared with placebo, when montelukast was used, it led to a decrease in effectiveness in SIT (Majak et al., 2010).

16.13 LONG-TERM BENEFITS OF SIT

It has been shown that in patients suffering from rhinitis and asthma, SIT helps in reducing symptom scores (Jacobsen et al., 2007). It was also seen that, the benefits of the treatment were maintained for almost 6 years after stopping the SIT. SIT is also known to stop the progression from rhinitis to asthma.

Another study done in India showed that the beneficial effect of SIT (house dust mite immunotherapy) continued even a decade after stopping immunotherapy and the benefit could continue for approximately 28 years (Shaikh, 2005). This was proven by comparing the symptom scores and FEV1 of patients who received immunotherapy, to those who were in the control group (who did not receive immunotherapy).

16.14 SIT VERSUS INHALED CORTICOSTEROIDS

An open, parallel, comparative trial showed that, even though relief with inhaled corticosteroids (ICS), in this case Budesonide, in bronchial asthma patients was more instant as compared to SIT; the decline in the benefits after stopping the ICS was very rapid. This rapid decline was not seen on stopping the SIT. This study made a case for a combination of SIT and inhaled corticosteroids, wherein the relief is likely to be rapid as well as sustained (Shaikh, 1997).

16.15 SPECIFIC IMMUNOTHERAPY DURING PREGNANCY

SIT has been found to be safe during pregnancy. Two different studies from our clinic have shown that both SCIT and SLIT are safe during pregnancy (Shaikh, 1993; Shaikh and Shaikh, 2012) and should not only be continued in a pregnant patient but could also be initiated for the first time during pregnancy.

16.16 PRACTICE PARAMETERS IN SPECIFIC IMMUNOTHERAPY

It is imperative that practice parameters be set up and complied with when administering SIT.

1. As mentioned earlier, SIT can be safely administered during pregnancy (Shaikh, 1993; Shaikh and Shaikh, 2012). The incidence

of complications is much higher in pregnant patients who are not given SIT as compared to those who receive IT.

2. SIT is recommended only for inhalant allergens viz. pollen, fungi, insects, dusts and dust mites. SIT has no place as yet in the treatment of food allergies and allergies to animals.
3. Do not administer SIT to patients on beta-blockers. An alternative medication should be substituted for a beta-blocking agent (Executive Committee, 1989). It may be very difficult to reverse anaphylaxis in patients on beta-blockers.
4. Patients with underlying cardiac disease should be considered very carefully for SIT because of the risk of morbidity and mortality after anaphylaxis on the myocardium in these patients.
5. Malignancy, autoimmune diseases and immunodeficiency are contraindications to administration of SIT since the effects on the immune system are not well understood (Li et al., 2003).
6. Children below the age of 6 years should not be administered SIT in view of greater chances of anaphylaxis in young children as well as the reduced chances of response to anaphylaxis treatment (Shaikh, 1996). Similarly, results of SIT beyond the age of 50 years are not satisfactory.
7. An SIT prescription should not contain more than 6 allergens; in fact the lesser the number of allergens the better are the results (Bousquet et al., 1998).
8. SIT vaccines need to be stored in a refrigerator at a temperature between 2°C and 8°C. Also, the vial needs to be shaken but not warmed before use.
9. The patient should receive verbal and written information about SIT including a description of efficacy, possible complications, practical details of the duration of treatment, cost of the vaccines and who is to administer SCIT. SLIT of course, can be self-administered by the patient, but adequate instruction and training is essential.
10. The benefits of SIT are seen to begin around 6 months to 1 year after initiation. Following this aggressive, initiating phase, the patient must be placed on regular maintenance SIT for another 4 to 5 years. SIT has been shown to provide long-term benefits (Shaikh,

2005). The success of SIT is dependent on the patient receiving regular injections of the highest tolerated dose of the biologically standardized vaccine. It has been estimated that an optimal maintenance dose of 5–20 micrograms of major allergen per injection correlates with clinical efficacy (Durham et al., 1999).

11. Conventional SIT should be administered subcutaneously only and not intramuscularly or intravenously. Other forms of IT, such as oral (OIT) and local nasal (LNIT) have all been studied with inconsistent and varying results. SLIT is the only other form of SIT, which has been evaluated and found to be effective and safe (Canonica and Pasalacqua, 2003).
12. Do not be lackadaisical when administering SCIT. Following administration of the vaccine, the patient must be observed in the clinic for at least 30 minutes for development of any reactions.
13. SIT can cause local and systemic reactions. Local reactions are seen at the site of administration, viz. itching and/or swelling with erythema. Local reactions should be treated with oral anti-histamines, taken an hour before the vaccine is administered. Systemic reactions may occur as urticaria, acute attack of asthma or anaphylaxis. All these must be immediately and vigorously treated with adrenaline (epinephrine), parenteral anti-histamines and large doses of hydrocortisone. It has been shown that epinephrine is more effective in anaphylaxis when given intramuscularly as compared to subcutaneously (Simons, 2001). If there has been a reaction to the last SCIT injection, the next dose may need to be modified, decreased or even omitted. This is important in order to prevent systemic reactions to subsequent doses.
14. It is important to combine various other modes of treatment with SIT. Specific allergen avoidance measures and inhaled corticosteroids when combined with SIT, give superior results as compared to any of them used alone (Shaikh, 1997).
15. SIT should not be administered if the patient has fever or has an acute episode of bronchial asthma.
16. All forms of sport, exercise, alcohol and hot baths should be avoided for six to eight hours after an SIT injection since the increased blood circulation could precipitate an anaphylactic reaction.

17. SIT should be prescribed and administered by a qualified medical practitioner only and not by a technician.
18. Sublingual IT (SLIT) is a mode of delivery, which is not associated with a high risk of systemic reactions even with high dosage of allergens. The optimal dose of allergen for SLIT is not yet well established. In literature, the effective dose for SLIT varies between 3 to 500 times the dose used in SCIT. However, some guidelines recommend a dose between 50 to 100 times the one used for SCIT. In SLIT, high doses are more regularly effective than low doses. However, the precise dose for each allergen needs to be carefully assessed especially the content of major allergen. The sublingual-swallow method is generally used; the other method, sublingual-spit is not so commonly used (Canonica and Pasalacqua, 2003).

16.16.1 IS SPECIFIC IMMUNOTHERAPY REALLY EFFECTIVE?

Currently SIT remains the only effective, immunomodulatory treatment available for allergic rhinitis, allergic asthma, insect sting hypersensitivity and certain forms of drug allergy. Although a lot of controversy has been generated as regards SIT, the bulk of evidence in inhalant and insect sting allergy suggests that SIT is beneficial. Indeed, regardless of the mechanism of action or the associated immunologic changes, this cumbersome and prolonged therapy would have no place in medical treatment if it did not result in substantial benefit. Undoubtedly SIT has survived the trial of time (Ohman, 1991) and more importantly, a large body of clinical and immunologic information has accumulated through the years regarding its efficiency. It must be emphasized that classical allergen SIT, either rush or conventional, is a most appropriate and successful treatment maneuver for the reduction of an atopic patients' inflammatory bronchial burden. Several studies have shown that the success rate of SIT is from 80% to 90% (Badhwar and Druce, 1992; Bernstein, 1991; Brostoff and Scadding, 1991; Pichler and Stadler, 1989). It is possible that the benefits of SIT could be overestimated because of unpublished negative studies; however, an additional 33 such studies would be necessary to overturn the positive results of SIT (Abramson et al., 1995, 2000).

Unwarranted and untoward reactions do occur with currently available SIT and cannot be denied. The late Louis Tuft, an accomplished and devoted American allergist once said, "For God's sake, you're doing allergists and their sick patients a great disservice to emphasize deaths and other adverse effects associated with immunodiagnosis and therapy" (Bukantz and Lockey, 1991). Indeed, the WHO position paper on SIT concluded that allergen immunotherapy properly used, was both effective and relatively safe and is a necessary part of the management of allergic disease (Larsen et al., 1999). Successful SIT will reduce the severity of an allergic disorder, improve the quality of life of the allergy sufferer and diminish the risk and cost of pharmacotherapy. SIT thus remains the cornerstone of treatment in allergic diseases in contemporary medical therapeutics. This cornerstone treatment is of particular importance to India since approximately 29% of the Indian population is atopic. Thus, more than 250 million Indians suffer from one or more allergic diseases making this one of the largest allergy suffering population in any country on earth. Of greater concern is that more than 80% of allergy sufferers in India are below the age of 40 years, thus affecting the most productive years of a person's life (Shaikh and Shaikh, 2008).

SIT has been compared to pharmacotherapy (inhaled budesonide) in just one study so far (Shaikh and Shaikh, 2008). The results of this study clearly showed that budesonide acts faster than SIT in relieving the symptoms of asthma but the effects of the drug wane off the moment it is withdrawn. The beneficial effects of SIT on the other hand are slower to be seen clinically, but persist long after it has been withdrawn. It has also been shown that in patients having allergic rhinitis, SIT prevents the development of asthma, and this beneficial effect certainly cannot be achieved by any other mode of therapy (Linneberg et al., 2002; Moller et al., 2002). Yet another finding that puts SIT on a high pedestal is that several studies have now proved that SIT results in long-term benefits; the longest follow-up study continued for 15 years and also concluded that the beneficial effects of SIT could last for up to 23 years after it's cessation (Shaikh, 2005).

16.16.2 IMMUNOTHERAPY OF THE FUTURE!

Newer concepts are emerging in SIT. Research is being carried out to develop safe and efficient means of SIT.

IL-4 is known to play an important role along with Th2 cells in producing IgE antibodies in an atopic individual. IL-4 binds to IL-4 receptor (IL-4R) on the surface of certain cells triggering a cascade of events leading to clinical symptoms. "Altrakincept," is a soluble IL-4 receptor to which IL-4 binds instead of to cell surface IL-4R. Thus the effects of IL-4 are blocked by altrakincept. The advantage of IL-4R is that it needs to be administered once a week through an inhaler. Unfortunately, it has not been efficacious in clinical trials. Similarly, Mepolizumab (Anti-IL-5 monoclonal antibody) has undergone clinical trials, but like IL-4R has not been found to be significantly effective.

In view of work on the analysis of the "epitopes" the use of " allergen peptides" which are the active components of an individual allergen has been studied for sometime now. Respiratory allergies have usually been considered as immediate IgE antibody mediated responses, but attention is now turning to inflammatory responses that appear to be initiated by T cells. These cells respond to peptide fragments from allergens presented in combination with HLA class II molecules. Although classic SIT with allergen extracts down regulates these T cell responses, more efficient and safe methods are being sought. Peptides of relatively short chain length that contain epitopes for protein allergy molecules can, if prevented without co stimulatory signals, down regulate T cell, responses. Studies are underway with peptides from several common allergens (Exley et al., 1997).

An exciting new development in SIT is the possible advent of DNA based vaccines. CpG – ODN motifs (cytosine-phosphate-guanosine – oligodeoxynucleotides). These motifs mimic bacterial DNA and the vaccines are GpG-ODN coupled to an allergen. In one approach, the active immunostimulatory oligo dinucleotide moiety (ISS-ODN) is linked to the major allergenic component. This product is termed the "immunostimulatory conjugate." The importance of these DNA based vaccines is increased immunogenicity, decreased allergenicity and increased safety.

Possibly, an exciting target could be the CCR3 receptor on the eosinophil, which is responsible for accepting cytokine signals leading to eosinophil migration and blockage of which could result in significant clinical benefits.

Administration of allergen extracts can often cause life-threatening anaphylactic reactions. These are seen with SCIT and therefore other routes of mucosal administration are being researched. The problem of anaphylactic reactions can also be overcome by the use of recombinant allergen extracts.

The following is a list of the newer novel immunomodulatory approaches for allergen specific immunotherapy:

1. Fusion of major allergens expressed as a single recombinant protein with attenuated IgE binding and preservation of T-cell reactivity.
2. Chimeric allergens expressed as a single recombinant protein with attenuated IgE binding and preservation of T-cell reactivity.
3. Fragments of major allergens.
4. Peptides of major allergens.
5. Polymers of major allergens (trimerised allergens).
6. Unrefolded native or recombinant allergens.
7. Mixture of several major recombinant allergens.
8. CpG oligonucleotide-conjugated allergens Monophosphoryl lipid A combined with allergens, given in pre-seasonal treatment.
9. Allergens coupled to virus like particles.
10. Intra-lymphatic vaccination administered directly into the lymph node.
11. Targeting FcεRII fusion of allergens with human FcεRII.
12. Modular antigen translocation vaccines.

16.17 IMMUNOTHERAPY IN INDIA

It is unfortunate that in India, the lack of adequate and proper training in SIT reflects in its improper use. Either SIT is used for an inadequate length of time or the prescription itself is improper. It is commonly seen that SIT was discontinued within a few months after initiation. In several cases, the prescription itself contains more than 6 allergens, sometimes even 12 or more allergens. It is also usual to see allergens such as foods and animal danders used in SIT prescriptions. Finally, not surprisingly, SIT has been prescribed for conditions such as contact dermatitis, psoriasis and even migraine. With such indiscriminate usage, added to the poor availability of quality, standardized allergens, SIT itself and the specialty of "allergy" is a condemned area of medicine for patients, general practitioners and general physicians.

Interestingly, there have however been studies on SIT published from India (Shaikh, 1993, 1997, 2005; Shaikh and Shaikh, 2012), which also reflect on the practice of SIT in the country. However, much more is needed. An important step forward has been the constitution of a "National Expert Committee on the Standardization of Allergens in India" under the Ministry for Health and Family Welfare. It is hoped that this Committee would become the watchdog for Allergy practices in India.

In conclusion, SIT is the RAISON D'ETRE for the specialty of allergy. You remove immunotherapy and the very existence of the allergist is threatened. SIT is an important part of our treatment of allergic diseases. Its importance in our treatment plans will increase as we recognize the potential for subtle complications from pharmacotherapy.

KEYWORDS

- **asthma**
- **immunotherapy**
- **pregnancy**
- **rhinitis**
- **subcutaneous**
- **sublingual**

REFERENCES

Abramson, M. J., Puy, R. M., Weiner, J. M. Is allergen immunotherapy effective in asthma? A meta-analysis of randomized controlled trials. *Am. J. Respir. Crit. Care Med.* 1995, 151, 969–974.

Abramson, Puy, R. M., Weiner, J. M., Allergen immunotherapy for asthma. *Cochrane Database Syst Rev.* 2000.

Akdis, C. A., Akdis, M., Mechanisms and treatment of allergic disease in the big picture regulatory T cells. *J Allergy Clin Immunol* 2009, 123, 735–746.

Akdis, M., Akdis, C. A., Mechanisms of allergen-specific immunotherapy: Multiple suppressor factors at work in immune tolerance to allergens. *J Allergy Clin Immunol* 2014, 133, 621–631.

Akdis, M., Akdis, C. A., Mechanisms of allergen-specific immunotherapy. *J Allergy and Clin Immunol* 2007, 119, 780–789.

Akdis, M., Akdis, C. A., Therapeutic manipulation of immune tolerance in allergic disease. *Nat Rev Drug Discov* 2009, 8, 645–660.

Badhwar, A. K., Druce, H. M. Allergic Rhinitis. In: Bush, R.K. (ed). *Med. Clin. North America: Clinical Allergy*. 1992, 789–803.

Bernstein, L., Preventive therapy in the, U. S. A, In Morley, J., (ed). *Preventive Therapy in Asthma*. London: Academic Press, 1991, 219–230.

Bousquet, J., Lockey, R., Malling, H. J. Allergen immunotherapy: therapeutic vaccines for allergic diseases. A WHO position paper. *J Allergy Clin Immunol* 1998, 102, 558–562.

Brostoff, J., Scadding, G. K. In: Brostoff, J., Scadding, G. K., Male, D., Roitt, I., (eds.). *Clinical Immunology*. London: Gower Medical Publishing, 1991, 17.

Bukantz, S. C., Lockey, R. F. Adverse effects and fatalities associated with immunotherapy. In: Lockey, R. F., Bukantz, S. C. (eds.). *Allergen Immunotherapy*. New York: Marcel Dekker Inc., 1991, 233.

Calderon, M. A., Alves, B., Jacobson, M., Hurwitz, B., Sheikh, A., Durham, S. (2007). Allergen injection immunotherapy for seasonal allergic rhinitis. *Cochrane Database of Systematic Reviews 2007*, Issue 1. Art. No.: CD001936.

Canonica, G. W., Pasalacqua, G., Non-injection routes of immunotherapy. *J Allergy Clin Immunol* 2003, 111, 437–448.

Castells, M. (2006). Desensitization for drug allergy. Curr Opin Allergy Clin Immunol. 2006, 6, 476–81.

Durham, S. R. Immunotherapy. Current Medical Literature: *Allergy* 1994, 2(4), 91–96.

Durham, S. R., Walker, S. M., Varga, E.-M., et al. Long term clinical efficacy of grass-pollen immunotherapy. *N. Engl. J. Med* 1999, 341, 468–75.

Executive committee. Position statement—beta adrenergic blockers, immunotherapy and skin testing. *J Allergy Clin Immunol.* 1989, 84, 129–30.

Exley, M. A., Rogers, B. L., Irwin, J., Peptides for allergy immunotherapy. In: Roberts A.M., Walker M.R. (eds). *Allergic Mechanisms and Immunotherapeutic Strategies*. Chichester: John Wiley and Sons, 1997, 151–76.

Francis, J. N., Till, S. J., Durham, S. R., Induction of IL-10+CD4+CD25+ T cells by grass pollen immunotherapy. *J Allergy Clin Immunol* 2003, 111, 1255–1261.

Fujita, H., Soyka MB, Akdis, M., Akdis, C. A., Mechanisms of Allergen – Specific Immunotherapy. *Clin & Transl Allergy* 2012, 2, 2.

Golden, D. B. K. Insect sting allergy and venom immunotherapy. *Ann. Allergy, Asthma and Immunology* 2006, 96, S16–S21.

Jacobsen, L., Petersen, B. N., Wihl, J. Å., Løwenstein, H., Ipsen, H., Imunotherapy with partially purified and standardized tree pollen extracts. IV. Results from long-term (6-year) follow-up. *Allergy* 2007, 52, 914–920.

Klunker, S., Chong, M. M. W., Mantel, P. Y., Palomares, O., Bassin, C., Ziegler, M., et al. Transcription factors RUNX1 and RUNX3 in the induction and suppressive function of Foxp31 inducible regulatory T cells. *J Exp Med* 2009, 206, 2701–2715.

Larsen, J. N., Wikborg, T., Vega, M. L., Lowenstein H. Manufacturing and standardizing allergen vaccines. In: Lockey, R. F., Bukantz, S. C. (eds.). *Allergens and Allergen Immunotherapy*, 2nd edition. New York: Marcel Dekker, Inc. 1999, 207–320.

Li, J. T., Lockey, R., Bernstein, I. L., et al. (eds.). Allergen immunotherapy: A Practice parameter. *Ann Allergy Asthma Immunol* 2003, 90 (suppl): 1–40.

Linneberg, A., Henrik, N., Frolund, L., et al. Copenhagen Allergy Study. *Allergy* 2002, 57, 1048–1052.

Majak, P., Rychlik, B., Puaski, L., Bauz, A., Agnieszka, B., Bobrowska-Korzeniowska, M., Kuna P., Stelmach, I., Montelukast treatment may alter the early efficacy of immunotherapy in children with asthma. *J Allergy Clin Immunol* 2010, Jun; 125, 1220–1227.

Moller, C., Dreborg, S., Ferdousi, H. A., et al. Pollen immunotherapy reduces the development of asthma in children with seasonal rhinoconjunctivitis (the PAT study). *J Allergy Clin Immunol* 2002, 109, 251–256.

Nelson, H. S., Areson, J., Reisman, R. A prospective assessment of the remote practice of allergy. *J Allergy Clin Immunol.* 1993, 92, 380–386.

Niebuhr, M., Kapp, A., Werfel, T., Specific immunotherapy (SIT) in atopic dermatitis and food allergy. *Hautarzt* 2008, 59, 44–50.

Noon, L. Prophylactic inoculation against hay fever. *Lancet* 1911, 1, 1572–1573.

Nouri-Aria, K. T., Wachholz, P. A., Francis, J. N., Jacobson, M. R., Walker, S. M., Wilcock, L. K., Staple, S. Q., Aalberse, R. C., Till, S. J., Durham, S. R., Grass pollen immunotherapy induces mucosal and peripheral IL-10 responses and blocking IgG activity. *J Immunol.* 2004, 172, 3252–3259.

Ohman, J. L. Clinical and immunologic responses to immunotherapy. In: Lockey, R. F., Bukantz, S. C. (eds.). *Allergen Immunotherapy*. New York: Marcel Dekker Inc., 1991, 209–232.

Palomares, O., Yaman, G., Azkur AK, Akkoc, T., Akdis, M., Akdis, C. A., Role of Treg in immune regulation of allergic diseases. *Eur J Immunol* 2010, 40, 1232–1240.

Pichler, W. J., Stadler, B. M. (eds.). *Progress in Allergy and Clinical Immunology*. Toronto: Hogrefe and Huber Publishers, 1989, 387–390.

Position Statement: American Academy of Allergy and Clinical Immunology. The remote practice of allergy. *J. Allergy Clin. Immunol.* 1986, 77, 651.

Reisman, R. E. Insect stings. *New Eng. J. Med.* 1994, 331, 523–527.

Rush immunotherapy information. Rush/Rapid immunotherapy vs. Conventional Immunotherapy. *TRAAC* website. [Online].

Scadding, G. K., Brostoff, J., Low dose sublingual therapy in patients with allergic rhinitis due to house dust mite. *Clin Allergy* 1986, 16, 483–491.

Shaikh, W. A., Immunotherapy in Children. *Pediatric Pulmonology Update* 1996, vol. 8, 6–7.

Shaikh, W. A., A retrospective study on the safety of immunotherapy in pregnancy. *Clin Exp Allergy* 1993, 23, 857–860.

Shaikh, W. A., Immunotherapy vs. inhaled budesonide in bronchial asthma: an open, parallel, comparative trial. *Clin Exp Allergy.* 1997, 27, 1279–1284.

Shaikh, W. A., Long-term Efficacy of House Dust Mite Immunotherapy in Bronchial Asthma: A 15-year Follow-Up Study. *Allergol International* 2005, 54, 443–449.

Shaikh, W. A., Shaikh, S. W., A prospective study on the safety of sublingual immunotherapy in pregnancy. *Allergy* 2012, 67, 741–743.

Shaikh, W. A., Shaikh, S. W., Allergies in India: an analysis of 3389 patients attending an allergy clinic in Mumbai, India. *J Indian Med Assoc* 2008, 106, 220–224.

Simons, K. J., Epinephrine absorption in adults: intramuscular versus subcutaneous injection. *J Allergy Clin Immunol* 2001, 108, 871–873.

Skripak, J. M, Wood, R. A. Efficacy of Long-term Sublingual Immunotherapy as an Adjunct to Pharmacotherapy in House Dust Mite-Allergic Children with Asthma. *Pediatrics* 2008, 122, S222.

van de Veen, W., Stanic, B., Yaman, G., Wawrzyniak, M., Sollner, S., Akdis, D. G., et al. IgG4 production is confined to human IL-10-producing regulatory B cells that suppress antigen-specific immune responses. *J Allergy Clin Immunol* 2013, 131, 1204–1212.

CHAPTER 17

ALLERGEN IMMUNOTHERAPY

S. NARMADA ASHOK[1] and P. K. VEDANTHAN[2]

[1]*Consultant Pediatrician and Director, Nalam Medical Centre and Hospital, Tamilnadu, India*

[2]*University of Colorado, Denver, Colorado, USA; Christian Medical College, Vellore, Tamilnadu, India*

CONTENTS

17.1 INTRODUCTION

With the increasing costs of newer medications and increasing number of sufferers, continuous dependence on just pharmacotherapy is unsustainable. Both patients and physicians are seeking more specific and long term control of allergic disorders (Calderon et al., 2012).

Allergen specific immunotherapy has confirmed effectiveness and tolerability for many years now (Calderon et al., 2012). The benefits of allergen specific immunotherapy continue several years after discontinuation of the treatment. Moreover, specific products for allergen specific immunotherapy have shown to have disease-modifying capacities of allergic diseases and also to reduce the risk of new sensitizations (Calderon et al., 2012). Recent initial studies have shown that allergen specific immunotherapy probably has a role in the treatment of food allergy (Frew, 2010). Allergen immunotherapy, much as it is practiced today, was introduced in 1911 by Leonard Noon and John Freeman (Nelson, 2014).

17.2 DEFINITION

Specific allergen immunotherapy is the administration of increasing amounts of specific allergens to which the patient has type I immediate hypersensitivity.

It is used for the treatment of allergic rhinitis, allergic asthma and hymenoptera sensitivity in the following scenarios:

1. Inadequate symptom control despite pharmacotherapy and avoidance measures.
2. Desire to reduce the morbidity from allergic rhinitis and/or asthma or reduce the risk of anaphylaxis from a future insect sting.
3. When the patient experiences undesirable side effects from pharmacotherapy.
4. When avoidance of implicated allergens is not possible.
5. When economic benefit from allergen immunotherapy is sought (George MS et al., 2012).

The use of immunotherapy by injection for inhalants (Pollens, HD mite, animal danders) for treatment of allergic rhinitis and allergic asthma is supported by randomized, controlled clinical studies. Injection immunotherapy with hymenoptera venom is well established. There are a few studies, which suggest that patients with atopic dermatitis who are sensitive to inhalant allergens may benefit, although this indication requires more investigation. Immunotherapy for food allergy, on the other hand, is still being investigated.

The methodology of practicing immunotherapy varies between countries. American allergists tend to treat polysensitization using mixtures of antigens, in contrast to European colleagues who prefer monotherapy. Another difference in clinical practice is that the allergen extracts used in the United States are prepared in the allergist's office, where as those used in Europe are usually supplied by the manufacturer in their final form.

17.3 MECHANISM OF ACTION OF IMMUNOTHERAPY

The physiopathology of allergic diseases is complex and influenced by many factors, including genetic susceptibility, route of exposure, antigen/allergen dose, and time of exposure, structural characteristics of the allergen/antigen and co exposure with stimulators of innate immune response, such as infections or commensal bacteria. Allergens enter the body through the respiratory tract, gut, conjunctiva, skin or insect stings.

To understand the mechanism of SIT, it is important to first review aspects of allergic reactions, including 'early' and 'late phase' responses. The initial component of the allergic reaction is sensitization, which involves the differentiation and clonal expansion of allergic specific Th2 cells, which in turn, stimulate production of IL-4 and IL-13 to induce an antibody class switch production of allergen specific IgE antibodies. Allergen specific IgE molecules attach to cells, such as mast cells and basophilic leukocytes, to complete the sensitization process. When an allergen is re-encountered, cross linking of allergen-specific IgE bound to FcεR1 on mast cell surface occurs to trigger the release of vasoactive amines mainly histamine, tryptase, chymase, kininogenase (which generates bradykinin), or heparin immediately and leukotrienes, prostaglandins and other chemokines four to six hours later. Late-phase reaction may occur as a consequence of ongoing generation of mast cell mediators and the activation of allergen-specific Th2 cells to generate a variety of cytokines (IL4, 5, 9 and 13) which have a wide range of effects, including smooth muscle cell activation, increased endothelial cell adhesion and basophil transmigration and recruitment of eosinophils to further the development of an inflammatory milieu. Additionally, a Th2 cell activation induced apoptosis of interferon-α producing Th1 cells further shifts the balance towards a Th2 profile. This exaggerated and dysregulated Th2 cell pattern of response underlies the pathophysiology of many atopic diseases (Viswanathan et al., 2012).

SIT attempts to attenuate this immune dysregulation in allergic reactions by inducing immunologic and clinical tolerance. It has been shown to suppress both early and late phase allergic responses in the skin, nose and lungs.

Cellular and molecular events that take place during the course of AIT can be classified into four stages:

1. Decrease in mast cell and basophil activity and degranulation (local desensitization) start to take place within hours.
2. Generation of allergen-specific T reg and regulatory B reg cells and suppression of allergen-specific effector T-cell subsets. They produce IL10 and transforming growth factor (TGF-α) to suppress activity of allergen-specific Th2 cells with the subsequent recruitment of other inflammatory effector cells (Figure 17.1) (Viswanathan and Busse, 2012).

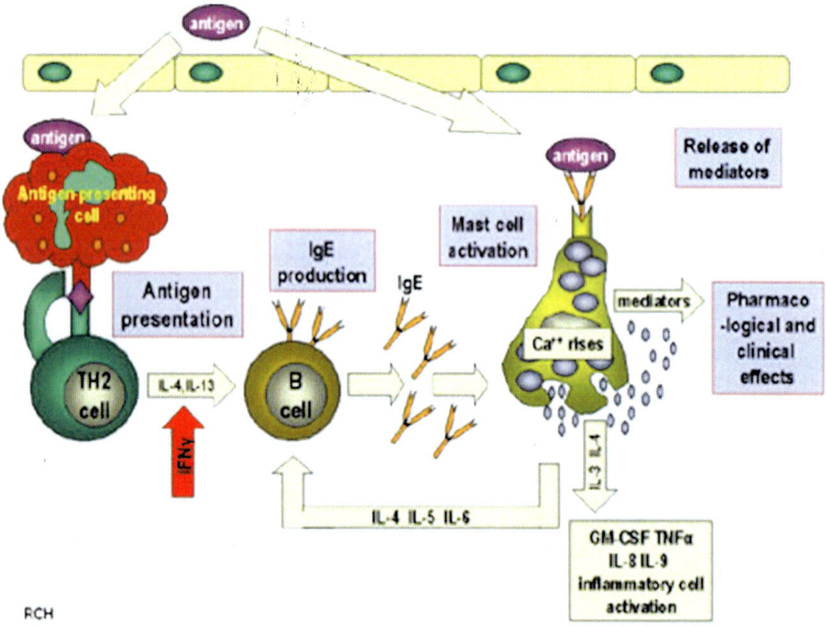

FIGURE 17.1 Aspects of allergic reaction—early and late phase responses. (Courtesy of Microbiology and Immunology On-line and the University of South Carolina School of Medicine.)

3. Regulation of antibody isotypes demonstrating an early increase in specific IgE levels, which later decrease and an early and continuous increase in specific IgG4. The production of allergen specific IgG antibodies disrupts the interaction between the allergen and mast cell-bound IgE by directly competing for the same epitope.
4. The fourth group of events takes place after several months, with decrease in tissue mast cells and eosinophils and release of their mediators. It is accompanied by a decrease in Type I skin test reactivity. Multiple cell types in the blood and affected organs show changes and contribute to allergen-specific immune tolerance development (Akdis and Akdis, 2014; Viswanathan and Busse, 2012).

Overall these events results in an immune deviation from a Th2 cell pattern (allergic) of response to more of a Th1 (non-allergic) and T reg cell pattern and induce peripheral T-cell tolerance to allergens which correlates with clinical improvement in allergic inflammation (Akdis and Akdis, 2014; Viswanathan and Busse, 2012).

17.3.1 MECHANISM OF ACTION – SUBLINGUAL IMMUNOTHERAPY

Similar to what is observed in SCIT, SLIT affects both humoral and cell-mediated immune responses. Thus, SLIT results in a dose dependent increase of allergen-specific IgG4, even if this effect is less intensive than that induced by SCIT and mostly evident for seasonal aeroallergen. SLIT also reduces mucosa infiltration by effector cells (neutrophils and eosinophils), increases allergen-specific IL-10 production and modulates Th1 and Treg activity in the oral mucosa. The peculiar characteristic of antigen presenting cells in the oral mucosa was suggested to be responsible for the modulation of IL-10 and TGF-α secreting Treg observed following sublingual immunotherapy. However, the immunologic effects of sublingual immunotherapy are nevertheless partially unclear (Piconi et al., 2014) (Figure 17.2).

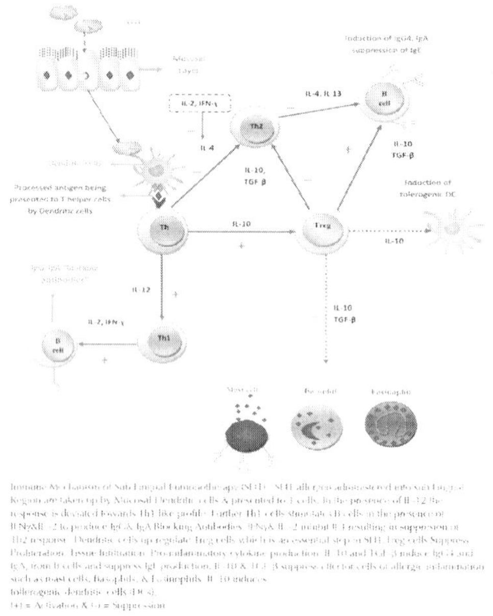

FIGURE 17.2 Mechanism of action of immunotherapy (Authors wish to acknowledge Mr. Prashanth, Dr. B. V. Balachandra, Dr. P. K. Vedanthan for lending the diagram on "Mechanism of Action: Sublingual Immunotherapy").

17.4 TYPES OF IMMUNOTHERAPY

Immunotherapy can be classified depending on the route of administration and the duration of administration.

17.4.1 ROUTE OF ADMINISTRATION

17.4.1.1 Subcutaneous Route (SCIT)

It is the established form of treatment and involves administering gradually increasing doses of injections at fixed intervals.

17.4.1.2 Sublingual Route (SLIT)

It is the emerging alternate route of administration of immunotherapy and involves taking gradually increased doses of allergen extract under the tongue and then spit or swallowed. It works through allergen interaction with pro-tolerogenic Langerhan's cells in the oral mucosa, which leads to the down-regulation of the allergic response (Stacey Jones, Wesely Burks, Christophe Duphont).

17.4.1.3 Epicutaneous Route (EPIT)

It uses a novel delivery of allergen to the skin surface through application of an allergen-containing patch to activate skin Langerhan's cells, with migration to lymph nodes and down regulation of effector cell responses. Only limited studies are available with regard to this mode of immunotherapy (Stacey Jones, Wesely Burks, Christophe Duphont).

17.4.1.4 Oral Immunotherapy (OIT)

It has been studied more than a decade in clinical trials and has the largest body of evidence among emerging therapies for food allergy. OIT acts by activation of gut mucosal dendritic cells, which affects the allergic response through immunomodulation of tissue and circulating effector cells (Stacey Jones, Wesely Burks, Christophe Duphont).

17.4.1.5 Intranasal Route

Local nasal immunotherapy consists of spraying allergen extracts into the nasal cavity. It was first investigated at the end of 1970s, with encouraging clinical data. It is performed by the administration of natural biological or chemically-modified allergen extracts in a soluble form. It demonstrates significant reduction in the treatment of ragweed and grass pollen induced allergic rhinitis. Further studies are required to document the safety and efficacy prior to wide use (Moinegon and Mascarell, 2012).

17.4.1.6 Intra-Lymphatic Route

It involves administering the allergen doses directly into the lymph nodes thereby reducing the dose and duration of immunotherapy. However, it is not well studied and the developments are necessary including the need to assess efficacy and to optimize treatment dose in large phase three studies. It also requires complex equipments and associated with training of skilled personnel, which may hinder its broad use in humans (Moinegon and Mascarell, 2012).

17.5 DURATION OF IMMUNOTHERAPY

17.5.1 CONVENTIONAL IMMUNOTHERAPY

It involves administering the doses in incremental dosages over 12 weeks. It is performed as an outpatient procedure. The rate of systemic reactions is around 15 (6–34) %. The main disadvantage is prolonged duration of the up dosing phase (Nelson, 2014).

17.5.2 CLUSTER IMMUNOTHERAPY

The buildup takes about 7 weeks. The rate of systemic reactions is 9 (5–12)%. Studies have shown it is comparable to conventional immunotherapy (Taber et al., 2005.) It can also be done as an outpatient procedure. It reduces the time to maintenance schedule by 46% (Harold S. Nelson, 2014; Taber et al., 2005).

17.5.3 RUSH IMMUNOTHERAPY

The build up takes only about 3–4 days. It can be done as an outpatient/inpatient procedure. But the main problem is with systemic side effects and is about 22%.

17.5.4 ULTRA RUSH IMMUNOTHERAPY

The build up is about 1–2 days. It is done as an inpatient procedure only with strict monitoring. The systemic side effects rates may be intolerable (Nelson, 2014). Used when protection is urgently required after a serious anaphylactic reaction.

17.6 IMMUNOTHERAPY IN INDIVIDUAL CONDITIONS IMMUNOTHERAPY FOR ASTHMA

Immunotherapy has been widely used for allergic asthma, although, the introduction of effective inhaled therapies has changed the general pattern of asthma care. Current drug therapies for asthma aim to suppress airways inflammation and relieve the bronchospasm. None of these are curative and asthma recurs on cessation of treatment. Allergen avoidance helps in some patients but although extreme forms of allergen avoidance can improve asthma control, there is only limited evidence for benefit with the degree of allergen avoidance. Specific allergen immunotherapy offers the important opportunity of deviating the immune response away from the 'allergic' pattern and towards 'non allergic' or protective response. However, immunotherapy remains controversial as a treatment for asthma because of the potential side effects (Frew, 2010). GINA guidelines updated in 2015 categorically states that compared to pharmacological and avoidance options, potential benefits of allergen immunotherapy (SCIT or SLIT) must be weighed against the risk of adverse effects and the inconvenience and cost of the prolonged course of therapy, including for SCIT the minimum half-hour wait required after each injection (GINA Guidelines, 2015). Although the incidence of severe systemic reactions with subcutaneous allergen immunotherapy is low, asthmatics are particularly susceptible to severe bronchospasm during such reactions. This risk factor needs to be given a serious thought before starting the patient on immunotherapy (Walker S. Metal). In conclusion, immunotherapy is a valid but controversial treatment for asthma. Patient selection and antigen selection are crucial factors to determine the course of response to AIT in asthma.

17.6.1 IMMUNOTHERAPY FOR ALLERGIC RHINITIS

It is a useful treatment for allergic rhinitis, especially when the range of allergens responsible is narrow. The allergic basis of rhinitis should be carefully assessed based on both history and skin or blood tests and other causes of nasal symptoms should be excluded. This difficulty in determining clinical relevance contributes to the reported lower degree of efficacy in SIT trials with perennial allergens compared with SIT for seasonal allergies (Frew, 2010). However, number of studies has concluded that there is significant advantage of using immunotherapy for allergic rhinitis patients and it improves the quality of life (Zeldin, et al., 2008; Johansen et al., 2005; Malling, 2003; Nelson, 2009). In summary, there is level Ia evidence for its efficacy in adults and children to support both subcutaneous and sublingual immunotherapy for allergic rhinitis. Patients report improvements in symptom control and quality of life although many continue to require concomitant pharmacotherapy. The patient choice is important in the decision whether to use the subcutaneous or sublingual route.

17.6.2 IMMUNOTHERAPY FOR VENOM HYPERSENSITIVITY

Anaphylaxis to Hymenoptera venom is relatively rare but can be fatal. Venom-specific IgE antibodies may be found in certain individuals in high concentration, which can lead to fatal anaphylaxis even years after exposure to stings. The purpose of venom immunotherapy is twofold: to reduce the risk of fatality and to improve the patient's quality of life by allowing him/her to go out and work or play without worrying about the possibility of a serious allergic reaction. Venom immunotherapy has been able to reduce the risk of systemic reactions to 10% and the reactions which occur are also mild. Venom immunotherapy is the only specific treatment currently available for reducing the systemic reactions and has been proven to be extremely effective (Anthony J. Frew, 2010; Nelson, 2014).

17.6.3 IMMUNOTHERAPY FOR FOOD ALLERGY

Food allergy is common with more than 170 foods reported to cause food – induced allergic reactions. Some progress has been accomplished over the past 5 years, with the focus on allergen-specific immunotherapy and prevention of anaphylaxis. None of these therapies are ready for clinical use because of the uncontrolled nature of the clinical trials, small number of subjects studied in aggregate and uncertain safety profiles (Jones et al., 2014).

17.6.4 IMMUNOTHERAPY FOR ATOPIC DERMATITIS

There is initial data indicating that SCIT is effective for atopic dermatitis when it is associated with aeroallergen sensitivity, especially for patients with dust mite sensitivity who have mild to moderate disease (Bussmann et al., 2006; George and Saltoun, 2012).

17.6.5 IMMUNOTHERAPY FOR ALLERGIC CONJUNCTIVITIS

A Cochrane systemic review done with analyzing 811 studies involving 3958 participants found that SLIT is effective in reducing total and individual ocular symptom scores in subjects with allergic rhinoconjunctivitis or conjunctivitis where as ocular drops did not have any benefit. Hence sublingual immunotherapy may be indicated for allergic conjunctivitis (Calderon et al., 2011).

In summary, the main indications for immunotherapy are:

(a) High dose-subcutaneous immunotherapy is indicated in the following cases:
   1. Patients presenting with symptoms induced by exposure to allergens.
   2. Patients exposed to a prolonged season presenting with symptoms induced by successive pollen seasons.
   3. Patients with allergic rhinitis and lower respiratory disease during peak exposure to the allergen.
   4. Patients in whom H_1–antihistamines and moderate doses of topical glucocorticoids do not control symptoms sufficiently.
   5. Patients who do not wish to undertake constant or prolonged pharmacotherapy.
   6. Patients in whom pharmacotherapy causes side effects (Viswanathan and Busse, 2012).

(b) High dose-sublingual immunotherapy may be indicated in the following cases:
   1. Clearly selected patients with rhinitis, conjunctivitis, and/or asthma caused by allergy to pollen/house dust mites

2. Patients whose symptoms are inadequately controlled with conventional pharmacotherapy.
3. Patients who have had systemic reactions during specific immunotherapy by injections.
4. Patients who have compliance problems with or refuse immunotherapy by injections (Viswanathan and Busse, 2012).

(c) Indications for allergen immunotherapy in patients with reactions to hymenoptera stings:

1. Patients with a history of a systemic reaction to a hymenoptera sting (especially if such a reaction is associated with respiratory symptoms cardiovascular symptoms or both) and demonstrable evidence of clinically relevant specific IgE antibodies.
2. Patients older than 16 years with a history of systemic reaction limited to the skin and demonstrable evidence of clinically relevant specific IgE antibodies.
3. Adults and children with a history of a systemic reaction to imported fire and demonstrable evidence of clinically relevant specific IgE antibodies.
4. Potential indication: for large local reactions in patients who have frequent and disabling large local reactions (Cox et al., 2011).
5. Immunotherapy is currently investigational for food hypersensitivity and not indicated in urticaria. Cox et al(2011).

17.7 SAFETY OF IMMUNOTHERAPY

17.7.1 SAFETY OF SUBCUTANEOUS IMMUNOTHERAPY

SCIT is safe when undertaken in selected individuals in a specialist clinic with adequate facilities and trained health professionals. Patients treated with SCIT are at risk of both local and systemic adverse reactions but in the vast majority of cases, symptoms are readily reversible if they are recognized early and treated promptly.

The incidence of systemic reactions in patients receiving subcutaneous immunotherapy varies between 5% and 35% (Frew, 2010). The incidence of systemic reaction is more severe with patients with uncontrolled asthma or exacerbation (Frew, 2010). Co-existing cardiac disease might be exacerbated by diverse reactions to SIT (Frew, 2010).

Incidence of local reactions associated with allergen immunotherapy is fairly common with a frequency ranging from 26% to 82% of patients and 0.7% to 4% injections (Cox et al., 2011). Large local reactions do not appear to be predictive of subsequent systemic reactions (Frew, 2010). However, some patients with a greater frequency of large local reactions might be at an increased risk of future systemic reactions (Nelson, 2014; Frew, 2010).

The majority of serious systemic reactions from allergen immunotherapy occur within 30 minutes after an injection and hence patient should remain in the physician's office/clinic for at least 30 minutes (Cox et al., 2011).

World Allergy Organization Subcutaneous Immunotherapy systemic reaction grading system (Table 17.1) has been used extensively to grade the systemic reactions associated with subcutaneous immunotherapy (Canonica & Cox et al., 2013).

TABLE 17.1 Systemic Reaction Grading System*

Grade 1	Grade 2	Grade 3	Grade 4	Grade 5
Symptoms/signs of one organ system present Cutaneous – pruritus, urticaira, flushing or sensation of heat or warmth	Symptoms/signs of more than one organ system present or asthma responding to bronchodilator	Asthma not responding to bronchodilator	Lower or upper respiratory failure with or without loss of consciousness	Death
Angioedema (not Laryngeal, tongue, uvular) Rhinitis – sneezing, rhinorrhea, nasal pruritus and/or nasal congestion, itchy throat	Abdominal cramps, vomiting or diarrhea	Laryngeal, uvula or tongue edema with or without stridor	Hypotension with or without loss of consciousness	
Conjunctival erythema, pruritus or tearing	Uterine cramps			
Nausea, metallic taste or headache				

(Adapted from Canonica & Cox et al. (2013); https://waojournal.biomedcentral.com/articles/10.1186/1939-4551-7-6.)

Adequate equipment and medications should be immediately available to treat anaphylaxis.

The following are suggested equipments and medications for the management of immunotherapy systemic reactions:

1. Stethoscope and sphygmomanometer;
2. Tourniquet, syringes, hypodermic needles and catheters;
3. Aqueous epinephrine HCl 1:1,000 wt/vol;
4. Equipment to administer oxygen by mask;
5. Intravenous fluid set up;
6. Short acting H1 antihistamine (diphenhydramine) for injection and oral use (preferably liquid) Corticosteroids (Solucortef) for IM/IV injection;
7. Appropriate equipment to maintain airway;
8. Glucagon kit for patients receiving beta-blockers (Nelson, 2014).

17.7.2 SAFETY OF SUBLINGUAL IMMUNOTHERAPY

Sublingual immunotherapy appears to be better tolerated than subcutaneous immunotherapy. The majority of SLIT adverse events are local reactions (e.g., oromucosal pruritus) that occur during beginning of treatment and resolve within a few days or weeks without any medical intervention. A few cases of SLIT related anaphylaxis have been reported but there have been no fatalities. Risk factors for the occurrence of SLIT related severe adverse events have not yet been established, although there is some suggestion that patients who have had prior systemic reactions to SCIT may be at increased risk.

World allergy organization grading system has been used for local adverse events.

The grading is done as Grade 1 – mild, Grade 2 – moderate and Grade 3 – severe. The symptom/signs that are taken into account are pruritus, swelling of mouth, tongue, lip, throat irritation, nausea, abdominal pain, vomiting, diarrhea, heart burn and uvular oedema. Grades 1 and 2 does not require discontinuation of immunotherapy but Grade 3 is a severe reaction and requires discontinuation. SLIT related serious adverse events are graded using the same grading system used for subcutaneous immunotherapy (Cox et al., 2011).

17.8 IMMUNOTHERAPY IN SPECIAL SITUATIONS IN CHILDREN

Immunotherapy for children is effective and well tolerated. It has been shown to prevent the new onset of allergen sensitivities in mono-sensitized patients, as well as progression of allergic rhinitis to asthma (Nelson, 2014). Therefore immunotherapy should be considered along with pharmacotherapy and allergen avoidance in the management of children with allergic rhinitis/rhino conjunctivitis, allergic asthma and stinging insect hypersensitivity.

Studies of children receiving allergen immunotherapy have demonstrated significant improvement in symptom control with less pharmacotherapy, and hence reduced total health care costs (Cox et al., 2011).

The lower most age for starting immunotherapy in children is generally 5 years. There has been report of effectiveness in children as young as 3 years. A randomized double blind, placebo controlled study assessing the efficacy of grass pollen – specific allergen immunotherapy over 2 pollen seasons showed that immunotherapy was effective for childhood seasonal allergic asthma in children aged 3 to 16 years (Roberts et al., 1999).

The preventive allergy treatment study (PAT) which is an European multicenter study involving 210 children has showed effectiveness not only in immediate clinical effects but also preventing development of asthma in children with allergic rhinoconjunctivitis upto 7 years after treatment (Jacobsen et al., 2007; Valovrita, 1999)

Hence, immunotherapy can be safely used in children after careful selection of the patient and has long-term benefits. Sublingual immunotherapy is preferred as it negates the need for repeated injections but cost is a major factor for non-compliance (Daigle and Rekkerth, 2015)

17.8.1 IN PREGNANCY

Immunotherapy can be continued but is usually not initiated nor built up in the pregnant patient. There have been no reports of increased incidence of prematurity, toxaemia, abortion, neonatal death and congenital malformation compared to general population. The incidence of adverse events is not increased during pregnancy. Studies suggest that allergen immunotherapy might prevent allergic sensitization in the child (Cox et al., 2011).

17.8.2 IN AUTOIMMUNE DISEASE

There is some concern about the use of immunomodulatory treatments in patients with autoimmune disorders, immunodeficiency treatment or malignant disease. Although there is no hard evidence that SIT is actually harmful to these patients some clinicians feel uncomfortable. The risk and benefits of the treatment has to be discussed with the patient.

17.9 IMMUNOTHERAPY SCHEDULES AND DOSES PATIENT SELECTION

1. Suitable candidates for immunotherapy should be carefully selected.
2. They should have demonstrated sensitivity (prick skin testing or ImmunoCap) to the allergens under consideration.
3. There need to be clinical correlation of patients' symptoms with allergen reactivity.
4. Finally the degree of symptoms must be of sufficient severity and duration to warrant the risk, expense and inconvenience of immunotherapy (Nelson, 2014).
5. The physician and patient would discuss the benefits, risks and costs of the appropriate management options and agree to the management plan (Cox et al., 2011).

17.9.1 SELECTION OF ALLERGENS

Immunotherapy is effective for pollen, animal allergens, dust mite, mould/fungi and hymenoptera hypersensitivity. There are limited data on the efficacy of cockroach immunotherapy. In choosing the components for a clinically relevant allergen immunotherapy extract, the physician should be familiar with local and regional aerobiology and indoor and outdoor allergens, considering the potential allergens in the patient's environment. Multi allergen immunotherapy has not been well studied and has produced conflicting results, with some demonstrating significant clinical improvement where as others showing no benefit over pharmacotherapy and environmental control measures (Cox et al., 2011).

17.9.2 ALLERGEN EXTRACT SELECTION

Extracts used for SCIT are complex mixtures. The extracts used for mixing can differ in concentrations depending on the allergen used. Extracts are available in two forms: (a) standardized and (b) non-standardized. Currently, US FDA has approved 19 standardized allergen extracts, including grass pollens, dust mites, cat, ragweed and hymenoptera. Non-standardized extracts have been used for decades and analysis of the literature has found it to be safe and effective (Daigle and Rekkerth, 2015). However, when possible standardized extracts should be used to prepare the allergen immunotherapy extract sets (Cox et al., 2011).

To retain a clinically relevant concentration of treatment, it is recommended that the volume of each allergen added reflects the recommended dose, and that after the first allergen subsequent additions only replace diluents. Examples of the doses recommended for representative extracts are listed in Table 17.2.

17.9.3 MAJOR ALLERGEN

The extracts are standardized based on the amount of major allergen in the constituent and the major allergen is the highly purified protein that

TABLE 17.2 Recommended Doses of Extracts for Subcutaneous Immunotherapy

Allergen extract	Effective doses
Short ragweed	6–12.4 mcg
Cat dander	15 mcg
Dust mite Der p1	7 mcg
Dust mite Der f1	10 mcg
Fungi	Highest tolerated dose
Insects	Highest tolerated dose
Animals	Highest tolerated dose

Adapted and modified from tables from "Harold S. Nelson. Allergen immunotherapy. (Textbook of allergy for the clinician. Editors, P. K. Vedanthan, Harold S. Nelson, Shripad N. Agashe, P. A. Mahesh, Rohit Katial, 2014. pp. 203–216;" and "Barbara Daigle, Donna J. Rekkerth. Practical recommendations for mixing allergy immunotherapy extracts. Allergy Rhinol 2015, Spring 6(1), e1–e7.")

induces immediate skin responses in >80% in a large panel of allergic patients and significant proportion of total IgE (>10%) can be allergen specific. Absorption of the allergen from the source material reduces specific IgE to the extract. It also accounts for a significant proportion of the extractable protein in the source material (Chapman, 2008)

These extracts should be performed by persons experienced and trained in handling allergenic products. A customized allergen immunotherapy extract should be prepared from a manufacturer's extract or extracts in accordance to the patient's clinical history and skin tests and might consist of single or multiple allergen (Cox et al., 2011). The guidelines as to how the extracts has to be prepared and the responsibility of the physician varies between countries but should be strictly adhered to in all countries both for legal and medical purposes.

17.9.4 PRINCIPLES OF MIXING OF ALLERGENS

Consideration of the following principles is necessary when mixing allergen extracts:

Cross Reactivity of Allergen Extract – The selection of allergens should be based on the cross-reactivity of clinically relevant allergens. When pollens are cross reactive, selection of a single pollen within the cross reactive genus will suffice (Eguideline, 2014). However, treatment with the specific allergens causing the clinical problem may be the most effective approach in inducing tolerance. If partially reactive binding sites are contributed by multiple allergens in the treatment vials, the concentration of cross reacting segments of the allergen may be greater than the target dose and could induce as side effect that might be uncomfortable for the patient. A common approach to addressing the reactive allergens is to use mixes. For prescriptions that include dust mites, either an extract containing two most common species, *Dermatophagoides pteronyssinus* and *Dermatophagoides farinae*, or the individual extracts is recommended because although the two species are similar, they are sufficiently different that both are necessary for effective treatment. The use of mixes can both help to reduce the safety risk of cross-reactive allergens and address the limitations of cross-reactivity when treating to achieve tolerance (Cox et al., 2011; Daigle and Rekkereth, 2015).

Relationship of pollen allergens is more challenging as cross reactivity among the major allergen affects formulation. Protein family content (molecular classification) rather than botanical taxonomy is a superior way to address cross reactivity issues (Weber, 2007). A knowledge about the common allergenic plants and their cross reactivity in the area from where the patient comes will aid us to select the major allergens for immunotherapy. In India the common allergic plants (Table 17.3) vary with season and place (Singh, 2014).

The commonest family these grasses, weeds and trees belong to are given below and also their cross reactivity potential (Table 17.4).

The other families do not have high cross allergenicity and hence when mixing allergen extract individual allergens have to be included. However, where related plants appear to have adequate cross-reactivity and extracts

TABLE 17.3 Common Allergic Plants in India

Spring (Feb–April)	Autumn (Sep–Oct)	Winter (Nov–Jan)
Grasses		
Cynodon dactylon	Bothriochloa pertusa	Cynodon dactylon
Dicanthium annualtum	Cenchrus ciliaris	Eragrostis tenella
Imperata cylindrical	Hetropogon contortus	Phalaris minor
Paspalum distichum	Pennisetum typhoides	Poa annua
Poa annua	Sorghum vulgare	
Polypogon monspeliensis		
Weeds		
Canabis sativa	Amaranthus spinosus	Ageratum conyzoides
Chenopodium murale	Artemisia scoparia	Argemone Mexicana
Parthenium hysterophorus	Cassia occidentalis	Chenopodium album
Suaedafruticosa	Ricinus communis	Asphedelous tenuifolius
Plantago major	Xanthium strumarium	Ricinus communis
Trees		
Ailanthus excels	Anogeissus pendula	Cassis siamea
Holoptelea integrifolia	Eucalyptus sp.	Salvadaro persica
Prosopis juliflora	Prosopis juliflora	Mallotus phillipensis
Putranjiva roxburghii	Cedrus deodara	Cedrus deodara

Source: Singh (2014).

have similar potency, it appears wise to use the most prevalent member (Weber, 2007). Hence knowledge about the common allergenic pollens, trees and weeds is important to prepare the allergenic extract.

17.9.5 OPTIMIZATION OF THE DOSE OF EACH CONSTITUENT

The maintenance concentrate should be formulated to deliver a dose considered to be therapeutically effective for each of its constituent components. The maintenance concentrate vial is the highest concentration allergy immunotherapy vial. (e.g., 1:1 weight/vol vial). The projected effective dose is the maintenance goal and the maintenance dose is the dose that provides therapeutic efficacy without significant

TABLE 17.4 Cross Reactivity Potential*

Family of the genus and species	Cross-reactivity
Grass family	**Grass allergen interrelationship**
Pooideae	Strong cross allergenicity noted between members
Chloridoideae	Cross reactivity noticed among members with Bermuda strongest inhibitor
Panicoideae	More cross reactivity with Pooideae than Chloridoideae
Juncaceae	Cross-allergenicity within families noticed
Cyperaceae	No cross reactivity noted
Typhaceae	No cross reactivity noted
Areceae	No cross reactivity noted
Trees–Rosidae Family	
Sapindaceae	Disparity present
Salicaceae	Strong skin test correlation
Elaeagnaceae	Questionable cross reactivity with Oleaceae
Betulaceae	Strong cross allergenicity
Flowering trees and weeds	**Asteridae family**
Amaranthaceae	Strong cross allergenicity noted
Oleaceae members	Strong cross allergenicity
Artemisia species	Strong cross allergenicity among short, giant, western and false ragweeds.

*Adapted from Weber (2007).

TABLE 17.5 Protease Content of Allergens – Trypsin Equivalent

Pollens	<1 mg
Cat and Dog dander	<1 mg
House dust mites (US)	<5 mg
Alternaria alternata	29 mg
American cockroach	168 mg
A. fumigates	212 mg
Penicillium notatum	242 mg

adverse local or systemic reactions and may not always be the projected effective dose (Cox et al., 2011; Eguideline, 2014).

Proteolytic Enzymes and Mixing – Some allergenic products used for immunotherapy naturally include proteases. Proteases are enzymes that degrade other proteins and are the reason for allergy incompatibility. The allergenic products with the highest protease activity are insect and fungal (mold) extracts. Certain mixtures of fungi and insects are also incompatible (Table 17.5) (Cox et al., 2011; Daigle and Rekkereth, 2015).

17.9.6 ALLERGEN IMMUNOTHERAPY EXTRACTS HANDLING

1. The extract should be stored at 2–8°C to reduce the rate of potency loss.
2. Extract manufacturers conduct stability studies with standardized extracts and it is their responsibility to ship extracts under validated conditions
3. In determining the extract expiration date, consideration must be given to the fact that the rate of potency loss over time is influenced by several factors like the storage temperature, stabilizers and bactericidal agents, concentration and the volume of the storage vials
4. It is necessary to maintain a customized individual maintenance concentrate of the allergen immunotherapy and serial dilutions labeled with the patient's name and birth.
5. Mixing of antigens in a syringe is not recommended.
6. Color coding for the dilutions should be followed (*see*, Figure 17.3) (Cox et al., 2011)

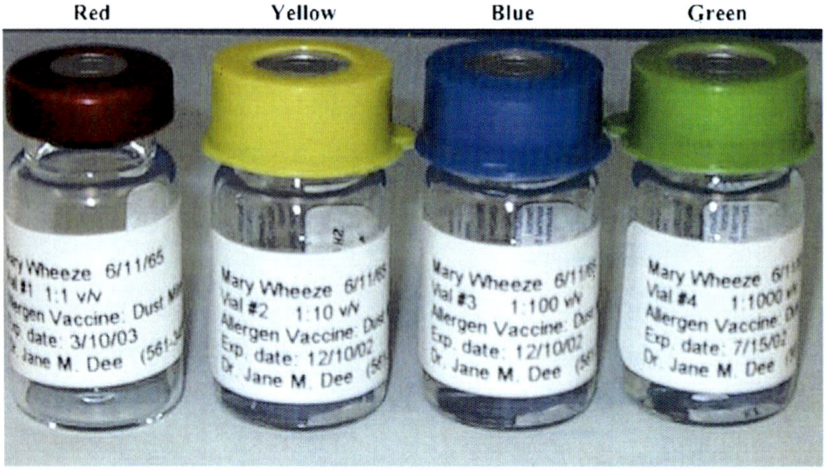

FIGURE 17.3 Extracts in various dilutions and color coded. (Source: https://www.aaaai.org/Aaaai/media/MediaLibrary/PDF%20Documents/Practice%20and%20Parameters/Allergen-immunotherapy-Jan-2011.pdf)

17.9.7 SCHEDULES AND DOSES: STARTING DOSES

There are two phases of allergen immunotherapy administration: the initial build up phase, when the dose and concentration of allergen immunotherapy extract are increased and the maintenance phase, when the patient receives an effective therapeutic dose over a period of time. If the starting dose is too dilute, an unnecessarily large number of injections will be needed, resulting in a delay in achieving a therapeutically effective dose. On the other hand, if the starting dose is too concentrated, the patient might be at increased risk of having systemic reaction. Usual starting dilutions from the maintenance concentrate are 1:10,000 (weight/vol) or 1:1000 (weight/vol) (Cox et al., 2011).

17.9.8 METHOD OF SELECTION OF ADEQUATE DOSE

What constitutes an ideal dose can only be determined by double blind placebo controlled trial however such a dose response study is very rarely conducted and also there is the problem with measuring of dosing and potency and its variability even among standardized extracts. With all these limitations, the dose of the major allergen remains the only effective way to determine the maintenance dose for allergen immunotherapy. In children the strength of the extract remains the same but the volume used is about half the adult dose used for maintenance therapy (Nelson, 2014).

17.9.9 FREQUENCY OF BUILD UP INJECTIONS

A number of schedules are used for the build up phase of immunotherapy. The most commonly used schedule is for increasing doses of allergen immunotherapy extract to be administered 1 to 3 times per week. This weekly schedule is recommended in most of the allergen extract package inserts. With this schedule, a typical patient can expect to reach a maintenance dose in 3–6 months, depending on the starting dilution and the occurrence of reactions. It is acceptable for patients to receive injections more frequently. The interval between injections is usually empiric but may be as short as 1 day without occurrence of systemic reactions if there is a need to approach the maintenance dose as quickly as possible due to personal schedule or seasonal (Cox et al., 2011).

17.9.9.1 Use of Premedication

Premedication might reduce the frequency of systemic reactions and increases the proportion of patients who achieve target maintenance dose in conventional schedule. However, when antihistamines are used there is a concern around the fact that antihistamines might mask a minor reaction that would otherwise alert a physician to an impending systemic reaction.

Other attempts to reduce the occurrence of systemic reactions, such as addition of epinephrine to the allergen immunotherapy extract or use of concomitant steroids are not justified and might delay the onset of systemic reaction beyond the waiting time when the patient is in the physician's office.

However in cluster and rush immunotherapy schedules premedication with either oral antihistamine alone or with combination of ketotifen, methylprednisolone and theophylline while using an inhalant allergen have shown to reduce the risk of systemic reaction from 72% to 27% (Cox et al., 2011; Nelson, 2014).

Omalizumab pretreatment has shown to improve the safety and tolerability of cluster and rush immunotherapy schedules in patients with moderate persistent asthma and allergic rhinitis. Also it has been shown to be effective when given in combination with immunotherapy (Cox et al., 2011).

17.9.10 MAINTENANCE SCHEDULES

Once a patient reaches a maintenance dose the interval between injections often can be progressively increased, as tolerated up to an interval of 4 weeks for inhalant allergens and up to 8 weeks for venom. In case of sublingual immunotherapy involving placing the vaccine either as a tablet or in solution under the tongue for 1–2 min without swallowing, the optimum dosage, duration of treatment and frequency of administration of SLIT have not yet been established. Much higher dosages of allergen are used than for subcutaneous immunotherapy, which is typically 30–50 times greater than conventional subcutaneous immunotherapy. Several regimens have been employed including daily dosing with or without an initial up dosing phase, three times per week and weekly thereafter (Nelson and Cox, 2012).

17.10 PREDICTING THE RESPONSE TO IMMUNOTHERAPY

It is the clinical response that determines the efficacy of the immunotherapy program. There are a few biomarkers to monitor the efficacy; they are mostly of research interest at this time.

17.11 NOVEL APPROACHES TO ALLERGEN IMMUNOTHERAPY

1. Strategies by altering the shape of intact allergens – fusion of major allergens, chimeric allergen, polymeric allergen, unrefolded allergens – allergoids (Cox et al., 2012; Walker et al., 2014).

2. Strategies by fragmenting allergens – allergen fragments and peptides.
3. Conjugation of allergens immune response modifiers – immunostimulatory oligonucleotide sequence of DNA containing a CpG motif and 3-deacylate monophospholipid A.
4. Using mixtures of recombinant allergens.
5. Combination of immunotherapy with anti-IgE.
6. Intra lymphatic vaccination.

KEYWORDS

- **allergen immunotherapy**
- **allergen selection**
- **subcutaneous immunotherapy**
- **sublingual**
- **venom hypersensitivity**

REFERENCES

Akdis, M., Akdis, C. Mechanisms of allergen-specific immunotherapy: multiple suppressor factors at work in immune tolerance to allergens. *J Allergy Clin Immunol* 2014, 133(3), 621–623.

Allergy immunotherapy. http://www.allergy.org.au/patients/allergy-treatment/immunotherapy.

Allergy shots (Immunotherapy). http://www.aaaai.org/conditions-and-treatments/treatments/allergy-shots-(immunotherapy).aspx.

Bussmann, C., Bockenhoff, A., Henke, H., Novak, N. Does allergen – specific immunotherapy represent a therapeutic option for patients with atopic dermatitis? *J Clin Allergy Immunol* 2006, 118, 1292–1298.

Calderon et al. EAACI: A European declaration on Immunotherapy. Designing the future of allergen specific immunotherapy. *Clinical and Translational Allergy* 2012, 2, 20. http://www.ctajournal.com/content/2/1/20.

Canonica et al. Sublingual immunotherapy: World Allergy Organization position paper 2013 update. *World Allergy Organ J.*, 2014, 7(1), 6. http://eguideline.guidelinecentral.com/I/57869-immunotherapy/20.

Chapman, M. D. *Allergen Nomenclature IUIS Allergen Nomenclature*. 2008, http://www.allergen.org/7_BRP_65_MDC_Allergen_Nomenclature_08.pdf

Cox, L., Nelson, H., Lockey, R. Allergen immunotherapy: A practice parameter third update. Task force report. *J Allergy Clin Immunol*. January 2011, S1–55.

Daigle, B., Rekkerth, D. J. Practical recommendations for mixing allergy immunotherapy extracts. *Allergy Rhinol* 2015, 6(1), e1–e7.

Frew, A. J. Allergen Immunotherapy. *J Allergy Clin Immunol* 2010, 125(2), S306–313.

Gaur, S. N., Singh, B. P., Singh, A. B., Vijayan, V. K., Agarwal, M. K. Guidelines for practice of allergen immunotherapy in India. *Indian J Allergy Asthma Immunol* 2009, 23(1), 1–21.

George, M. S., Saltoun, C. A. Allergen Immunotherapy: definition, indications and reactions. *Allergy, Asthma Proc* 2012 May–June, 33(Suppl 1), S9–11.

Jacobsen et al. Specific immunotherapy has long term preventive effect of seasonal and perennial asthma: 10 year follow up on the PAT study. *Allergy* 2007, 62(8), 943–948.

Jones, S., Burks, W., Duphont, C. State of the art on food allergen immunotherapy: oral, sublingual and epicutaneous. *J Allergy Clin Immunol*. 2014, 133(2), 318–324.

Malling, H. J. Immunotherapy for rhinitis. *Curr Allergy Asthma Rep*. 2003, 3, 204–209.

Marseglia, G. L., Incorvaia, C., Rosa, M. L., Fraiti, F., Marcucci, F. Sublingual immunotherapy in children facts and needs. *Italian Journal of Pediatrics* 2009, 35, 31.

Moingeon, P., Mascarell, L. Novel routes for allergen Immunotherapy. *Immunotherapy*. 2012, 4(2), 201–212.

Nelson, H. S. Allergen immunotherapy. *Textbook of Allergy for the Clinician*. Editors P. K. Vedanthan, H. S. Nelson, S. N. Agashe, P. A. Mahesh, R. Katial. 2014, pp. 203–216.

Nelson, H. S. Multi allergen immunotherapy for allergic rhinitis and asthma. *J Allergy Clin Immunol* 2009, 123(4), 763–769. doi: 1016/j.jaci.2008.12.013. ePub Feb 13.

Nelson, M. R., Cox, L. Allergen immunotherapy extract preparation manual. *AAAAI Practice Management Resource Guide*, 2012 edition.

Piconi et al. Immunological effects of sublingual immunotherapy: Clinical efficacy is associated with modulation of programmed cell death ligand 1, IL 10 and IgG4. http://www.jimmunol.org/cgi/doi/10.4049/jiimmunol 1002465.

Roberts, G., Hurley, C., Lack, G. Grass pollen immunotherapy as an effective therapy for childhood seasonal allergic asthma. *J Allergy Clin Immunol* 2006, 117, 263–268.

Senti, G., Johansen, P., Gomez, M. J., Varica, P. B. M., Kundig, T. M. Efficacy and safety of allergen-specific immunotherapy in rhinitis, rhino conjunctivitis and bee/wasp venom allergies. *Int Rev Immunol* 2005, 24(5/6), 519–513.

Singh, A. B. Pollen and fungal aeroallergen associated with allergy and asthma in India. *Global Journal of Immunology and Allergic Diseases*, 2014, 2, 19–28.

Tabar, A. I., Echechipía, S., García, B. E., et al. Double blind comparative study of cluster and conventional immunotherapy schedules with Dermatophagoides pteronyssinus. *J Allergy Clin Immunol* 2005, 116(1), 109–118.

Valovirta, E. PAT – the preventive allergy treatment study design and preliminary results. *Wien Med Wochenschr*. 1999, 149(14/15), 442–443.

Viswanthan, R. K., Busse, W. W. Allergen Immunotherapy in allergic respiratory diseases: From mechanism to meta-analyses. *Chest* 2012, 141(5), 1303–1314.

Walker, S. M., et al. Immunotherapy for allergic rhinitis. BSACI guidelines. *Clinical and Experimental Allergy*, 2011, 41, 1177–1200.

Weber, R. W. Cross reactivity of pollen allergens: impact on allergen immunotherapy. *Ann Allergy Asthma Immunol.* 2007, 99, 203–212.

Werfel, T., Breuer, K., Rueff, F., et al. Usefulness of specific immunotherapy in patients with atopic dermatitis and allergic sensitization to house dust mites: a multi center, randomized, dose response study. Allergy 2006, 61, 202–205. http://www.ginaasthma.org/local/uploads/files/GINApocket04clean2_1.pdf.

Zeldin, Y., Weiler, Z., Magen, E., et al. Safety and efficacy of allergen immunotherapy in the treatment of Allergic rhinitis and Asthma in real life. *IMAJ Bol 10.* December 2008, 869–873.

CHAPTER 18

SUBLINGUAL IMMUNOTHERAPY

PARANJOTHY KANNI, NAGENDRA PRASAD KOMARLA, and A. B. SINGH

Bengaluru Allergy Centr, Bengaluru, India

CONTENTS

18.1 INTRODUCTION

Allergy is on the increase worldwide. Today people are becoming more and more aware about the allergens and the Sublingual Immunotherapy (SLIT). Allergens are molecules with capacity to elicit IgE responses in human (reactive antibodies induce allergy symptoms). Identifying causative allergens and feeding allergy subjects in small quantities through Sublingual route (SLIT) on daily basis over a period of time induce tolerance in the body by producing blocking antibodies (IgG), which reduces the allergy symptoms. Sublingual immunotherapy emerged in the year 1980 in the midst of safety issues of traditional century old subcutaneous immunotherapy (SCIT). Study by Scadding and Brostoff introducing Sublingual immunotherapy (SLIT) with very low doses and followed by another controlled trial after a gap of four years. A major turn on first meta-analysis evaluating the data from the first 22 controlled studies, demonstrated the efficacy and safety of SLIT in seasonal allergic rhinitis. Now, the studies of dose-response clearly demonstrate that the clinical efficacy of SLIT depends upon the administrated dosage, as already proved since long time for SCIT. Systematic revision of the literature showed that SLIT has no dose dependence of safety, which allowed the development of new formulations of SLIT without up dosing phase. SLIT is considered a suitable alternative to injections.

18.2 DEVELOPMENT OF SLIT

Allergen-specific immunotherapy has been shown to be highly effective (Bosquet et al., 1998), reduces allergy symptoms and use of relief medications, modify the natural history of allergic disease such as development of asthma in allergic rhinitis patients (Moller et al., 2002) and as well development of new sensitization (Des-Roches et al., 1997) and markedly improves "quality of life." Immunotherapy is the only available therapy that treats the underlying cause of the allergic disease with proven long-term benefits. Recent past, the subcutaneous immunotherapy was the main approach to immunotherapy and because of its occasional risk of severe side effects, which confines to use by specialist centers. Sublingual immunotherapy (SLIT) initiated as an alternative routes of administration of specific immunotherapy. Now SLIT is widely used in several European countries and in USA, the safety profile and convenience of this route of administration have been recognized as attractive. SLIT is particularly interesting treatment option for the pediatric population where safety is paramount, home based therapy.

The mechanisms of action of SLIT are similar but probably not identical to SCIT. Oral mucosa has a specific organization of APC (antigen presenting cells) and DC (dendritic cells) along with expression of adhesion molecules as ICAM 1. Treg cells which regulate IL-10 and TGF-*Beta* is the major response of the immune system to specific immunotherapy by mucosal route, in production of IgA, IgG and IgG4 instead of IgE (Jutel et al., 2006; Nouri-Aria et al., 2004). The local reduction of expression of ICAM 1, involved in inflammation (Passalacqua et al., 1999). This is confirmed by the decrease of nasal eosinophils and mediators during SLIT (Bagnasco et al., 2005; Marogna et al., 2005). The contact with oral mucosa is a critical step in the mechanisms of action of SLIT. When allergen immediately swallowed, the treatment fails to respond and responds only with high doses of allergen when compare to SCIT dose. The bio distribution studies performed with radio labeled allergens have shown that allergen persist for couple of hours in the mouth after administration (Bagnasco et al., 2005). Uptake of allergen in the mouth is by dendritic cells (Macatonia et al., 1995). SLIT is more than symptomatic treatment and modifies natural history of the disease. Immunotherapy is not the last choice to be used when drugs do not work (Bousquet et al., 1998), but is complimentary to pharmacotherapy and must be used together. Immunotherapy should be initiated in the early phases of disease and SLIT represents a good friendly choice compare to SCIT.

Specific immunotherapy is a very powerful tool, which is currently underutilized in the treatment of allergies. SLIT has many advantages over SCIT and has been well proven to work for pollens and dust mites. SLIT improves symptoms and reduces the reliance on conventional medications. SLIT is endorsed by World Health Organization committee on SLIT as a viable alternative to SCIT.

To prove the effectiveness of SLIT Double Blind Placebo Controlled studies are vital. Double-dummy, double-blind study by Quirino et al. (1996) compared SLIT versus SCIT in grass pollen (n=20), therapy for 12 months with 2.4 fold higher cumulative dose compared to SCIT. The SCIT and SLIT were equally effective according to subjective clinical parameters. The decrease symptom score (p=0.002) as well as medication score (p=0.0039 in SLIT and p=0.002 in SCIT) were observed.

Khinchi et al. (2000) with birch pollen with cumulative dose of Bet v 1 was about 210 times (1470 mcg) higher than SCIT dose (70 mcg). Both therapies showed significantly reduced total score of rhino-conjunctivitis,

conjunctivitis, and rhinitis and medication intake during pollen season of first year.

Open study by Bernardis et al. (1996) compared SLIT with SCIT in *Alternaria tenuis* allergic patients (n=23), showed improvement in clinical symptoms in both and specific nasal provocation had statistically significant difference in favor of SLIT.

Swiss study (Andre et al., 2000) investigated efficacy of SLIT versus SCIT to pollen allergy. A yearly post-seasonal evaluation of symptom and drug consumption was done. After three years there was neither statistical difference in the efficacy between the two treatment groups nor in the number of adverse reactions.

WHO and EAACI reviewed literature on SLIT on DBPC trials published in peer-reviewed journals and with adequate methods and statistical trials published analysis are considered, seven of these studies performed in pediatric patients. Most frequently reported side effect is local (sublingual itch and sometime gastrointestinal complaints such as stomach ache or nausea), which were of short period and self-resolving.

Andre et al. (2000) reviewed safety aspects of controlled trails performed with vaccines of a single manufacturer. About 690 subjects were enrolled (347 active + 343 placebo), 218 of them children (103 active + 115 placebo). The large majority of event was mild and had similar incidence in active and placebo, with the exception of the oral and gastrointestinal side effects, which were more frequent in SLIT, which were very mild. The occurrence of side effects and dropouts was similar in adults and children.

No near fatal or severe systemic event has been reported with SLIT. The adverse events observed in SCIT are 0.5–6% (Ostergaard et al., 1986). Comprehensive review by Stewart and Lockey (1992) on SCIT reported 0.8–46.7% with conventional schedules, 0–16% with modified allergens and 0–21% with accelerated or rush schedules. These are on average higher than report in SLIT. No fatality has ever been reported with SLIT, which is at variance with SCIT, where more than 50 cases are well documented (Lockey et al., 2001).

The use of SLIT in children is safe, efficacious and good adherence to treatment. Published position paper is not recommended to start SCIT immunotherapy before 5 years of age, reason behind is difficulty to recognize the early symptoms of systemic reaction, the reduced response to emergency treatment for reactions and possibly child develop new sensitizations during treatment (Malling and Weeke, 1993). In 2001 Allergic Rhinitis and its Impact of Asthma (ARIA) document by WHO established that immunotherapy, comprising SLIT route administration be started in early life, but minimal age of starting treatment was not specified (Bosquet et al., 2001).

Di Rienzo's first study on children recruiting 268 children aged 2–15 years followed a period of 3 months to 7 years, adverse reactions reported 3%, 7 events with abdominal pain, rhinitis, conjunctival itching did not require treatment and one case of urticaria treated with antihistamines and no other serious adverse reactions were reported (Rienzo et al., 1999).

18.3 THE ECONOMIC EVALUATION SLIT VS. SCIT

SLIT offered clinical benefits comparable to SCIT. The total cost spend by SLIT of three year treatment is of 416 Euro and for SCIT is about 482 Euro. For SLIT cost 255 Euro and for SCIT costs about 176 Euro. Both direct and indirect cost (injection administration, traveling and potential waiting time-loss of income for injection at doctor's office), SLIT represents less expensive relative to subcutaneous administration from all perspectives (Pakladnikova et al., 2008). However, from a patient's perspective, SCIT offers less expensive alternative to patients who do not experience loss of income and travel costs associated with treatment.

Economic advantages offered by immunotherapy for allergic rhinitis and asthma review shows that studies aimed at determining cost of illness and studies focused on either on a simpler cost comparison amongst available therapeutic alternatives or directly comparing alternatives using full economic evaluations (cost-effectiveness, cost-utility measures, etc.) in comparison with standard pharmaceutical treatment have shown that immunotherapy is beneficial to health care systems which can bring more clinical outcome at a reduced cost versus standard therapy (Berto and Frati, 2008).

Many double-blind placebo controlled studies confirm the efficacy of subcutaneous injection immunotherapy (SCIT) for treatment of allergic rhinitis (Calderon et al., Cochrane sys rev AIT in allergic rhinitis, 2007) and for asthma (Abramson et al., Cochrane sys rev AIT for asthma, 2003). SCIT is currently the standard immunotherapy with well-ascertained clinical efficacy.

Despite SCIT clinical and disease modifying efficacy, SCIT has some disadvantages such as patient non friendly due to regular injections, which are sometime painful locally, fear among children and few adults, increased indirect cost due to frequent visit to doctor's office and lost working or school hours. SCIT prolonged time for build-up phase to reach maintenance level of treatment and by adverse reactions.

SCIT undoubtedly has clinical efficacy, but it displays several inconveniences, such as the need to visit doctor for injection, its invasiveness, which many patients, especially children do not tolerate psychologically and possible side effects. SLIT with DBPC studies demonstrate clinical and immunological efficacy, but direct comparisons between SCIT and SLIT have thus far been very poor. SLIT is friendlier with patients and accepted easily.

Sublingual Immunotherapy (SLIT) was born although in the year 1980 in the middle of the debate about safety issues of traditional effective Subcutaneous Immunotherapy (SCIT), it has gained momentum and patient's acceptance is more than SCIT. Drop out cases are rarely seen as the patients can easily administer at home itself and need not go to a doctor for the SCIT shot! Study by Scadding and Brostoff introducing SLIT used very low doses. Tari et al. (1990) used much higher dose than previous trial and generated positive results. Passalacqua and Canonica reviewed in 2005 with three year study of Marcucci et al (2005) and 5 year study by Marogna et al. demonstrated clinical efficacy together anti-inflammatory effect of SLIT. Concerning the safety, reviewed by Giadro conclude that anaphylactic reaction never occurred. The frequency of reactions, most of which local and short-lived, occurred after SLIT, is higher in frequency ($p < 0.0001$) with low dosages compared to higher dosages. Kleine-Tebbe in 2006, tested safety of SLIT with dosage of up to 1,000,000 SQ Units with confirmatory results. Fiocchi et al. in the year 2006 showed no contraindications to SLIT in children aged less than 5 years. And subsequently several clinical trials showed promising results and on the basis of 22 trials on SLIT WAO published a position paper on SLIT and similarly

EAACI released position paper in favor of its efficacy. ARIA guidelines on SLIT recommend SLIT for children beyond three years old. SLIT long-term efficacy is recorded, first published 7 years and recently beyond 15 years showing the sustained efficacy of SLIT (Maurizio Marogna et al.).European Medical Agency (EMA) approved SLIT under guidelines on the clinical development of products for specific immunotherapy for treatment of allergic diseases effective from 2009 and United States (US) FDA approved in the year 2014. Now it is globally well recognized and it is on its way for FOOD sensitivity showing promising results.

18.4 MANAGEMENT OF ALLERGY WITH SLIT

Patients are given questionnaire to fill up the details to get information to know the cause of the allergy. Blood samples are taken for testing with ELISA or Phadia. The allergen sensitivity is conformed with SPT and the personalized prescription are generated. SLIT drops with unique diluent formulations can be given for better absorption of allergens through mucous membrane. The limitation of drops is storing in a stipulated temperature in refrigerator. The dose generated by the dropper is variable and few patients consume two weeks, which was meant for four weeks. In some cases, it is used to stretch for two months, which was dispensed for one month. The generation of proper dose maintenance is difficult and storing SLIT bottles in refrigerators found unavailable in certain living conditions.

SLIT tablets and SLIT Stripes are solid forms of SLIT, patients adherence is good. Patients are taking the medication for 5-year period and they have witnessed the effectiveness of SLIT in the management of their allergy problems (Jones and Lympany, 2008). SLIT tablets are preferred over the SLIT drops.

18.5 PREPARATION OF ALLERGENIC EXTRACTS

Sourcing of the materials like House Dust mites, pollen, cockroaches should be done with utmost care. Sorting, purification from other debris and selection of the proper particle size of the materials are also important for efficient extraction. Defatting is done by cold extraction process. The extraction is then done with aqueous solvents like physiological Saline or phosphate buffer solution cocoa's solution or some suitable solvents at 4–5°C. Organic solvents are to be avoided. The extraction medium contains preservatives such as phenol or parabens or any other suitable preservatives. It may also contain, if necessary, stabilizers such as Human Serum Albumin, Glycerol or Sucrose, or epsilon amino caproic acid (EACA) or other suitable stabilizers. The extraction is carried out for a minimum time (about 2 hours) duration to avoid degradation or denaturation. Low molecular weight (5000 Da) non-allergenic material should be removed, by stirred cells or gel filtration. The extract should be sterilized by sterile filtration using 0.22 micron membranes at 4°C. The extracts are then assayed for the protein content using Modified Lowry's or Bicinchoninic Acid (BCA) or any other suitable protein estimation methods. The extracts can then be lyophilised and stored at –20°C to –40°C. These allergenic extracts are then used to prepare diagnostic and therapeutic formulations (Jones and Lympany, 2008; Manda et al., 2011).

18.6 PREPARATION OF SLIT FORMULATIONS

SLIT drops, SLIT tablets, SLIT stripes are available today for the efficient management of different kinds of allergy.

Diagnostic Solutions for Skin Prick Test (SPT): Purified sterile allergenic extracts are diluted with sterile glycerinated buffer saline and adjusted to the potency required for SPT. The preparation is done in clean room under Laminar Air Flow cabinet. The solution is filled into the sterile vials, sealed and labeled with all relevant particulars.

SLIT Drops: This is more popular and dispensed by the allergists to patients as a personalized medicine for their allergy symptoms. SLIT drops can be prepared in a pharmacy attached to the allergy clinic/nursing home/hospital itself. Allergens are dissolved in the SLIT diluent and dispensed at their appropriate potency requirements of the patients. SLIT diluent contains excipients like Mannitol, Sorbitol, pH buffer components preservatives, flavors and purified water. They are prepared in Clean rooms under Laminar Air Flow cabinets.

SLIT Tablets (compressed): Allergens are mixed with excipients like mannitol, crospovidone, hydroxy propyl methylcellulose, croscarmellose sodium, lubricants such as talc and magnesium stearate, sweeteners like sucralose, flavors and preservatives. They are blended well and compressed into Tablet dosage forms (Gaur et al., 2010; Prasad et al., 2010).

SLIT Tablets (non-compressed): Active allergenic extracts are dissolved in a SLIT Suspension diluent, mixed by effective stirring. Correct quantities are metered using micro pipets and casted into preformed blister wells. The filled blisters are then lyophilized. The blisters are then closed and sealed with the lidding material. The molded tablets are analyzed for their potency and dispensed to the patients (Kanni and Komarla, 2015).

SLIT Films: Active allergenic extracts are dissolved into viscous SLIT diluent solutions by effective mixing and stirring and casted into glass plate troughs and dried at low temperatures (European Medicines Agency, 2009; Mondoulet et al., 2009). The films are then cut into required size, analyzed, approved by Quality control and dispensed to the patients. The dosage is comparable to SCIT and there is no need to start the Build-up phase. One can initiate the calculated Maintenance dose from day one with no systemic side effects and noticed 4–5% local side effects at the sublingual mucous membrane, which disappears in few days. The maintenance duration overtake build up phase, which amounts months without any adverse event.

18.7 EVALUATION OF THE ALLERGENIC EXTRACTS AND DOSAGE FORMS

Allergen extracts are complex mixtures derived from natural sources and as such prone to natural variation. Standardization is very much necessary to control variation and ensure consistency and reproducibility for Quality Safety and Efficacy of allergy management. Based on the ICH guidelines emphasizing on for the Quality, Safety and efficacy, European Medicine Agency have brought out guidelines for the manufacture and Quality of Allergen products. India also brought out guidelines in the year 2009 and being reviewed currently with the experts in the field (Kanni and Komarla, 2015; Paranjothy and Nagendra, 2013; Paranjothy et al., 2013).

Allergen Extracts: In-House reference Standards (IHR) is prepared in the laboratory and kept as the primary standard. When extraction procedure has been established, three batches are selected to verify the reproducibility and one of the best among them is selected to represent as IHR. All batches prepared subsequently are standardized and controlled in comparison with this IHR. It is preferable to prepare a fresh IHR once in a year for effective controlling and monitoring of manufacturing batches. US-FDA authorizes general standards of some allergens and if they are available these Standard allergens can be procured and used as primary standards.

IHR should be carefully defined including assessment of dry weight, protein content and composition, major allergen content and total allergenic activity by in-vivo and in-vitro methods. Protein content can be found out by Microkjeldhal or Modified Lowry's or BCA or by automated amino acid analysis.

Dosage Forms/Formulations: The Assay method has to be developed specifically for each formulation considering the excipients they possess taking principles of the methods adopted for the extracts. Pharmaceutical factors such description of the dosage form, disintegration time, dissolution, pH, and hardness, weight variation, also to be tested and evaluated.

Stability Testing: Criteria, methods and limits should be established. In Europe, allergenic activity between 30 and 300% is accepted. In US, limits between 50 and 200% of the labelled activity is accepted. Storing samples at –20°C, refrigerated temperature (5°C), room temperature (25°C) are recommended. The frequency of withdrawal for testing could be of every 3 months for a period of 12 months or 24 months whichever is appropriate for the product.

18.8 CONCLUSION

The search for *Gold Standard* treatment for Allergy continues to be an important matter of debate in the management of allergic disease. SLIT has proven to be better than SCIT. Another area Epicutaneous Immuno Therapy (EPIT) (Aktar, 2014; Manda et al., 2011; Mondoulet et al., 2009) is also catching up as an intermediate between SLIT and SCIT. Allergen incorporated soluble polymeric micro needles can be administered by transdermal route and is emerging as a viable alternative to both SLIT and SCIT. Allergens will be picked up by Langerhans cells in the Epicutaneous layer and they are involved in cellular responses. The needles can be fabricated to be long enough to penetrate the stratum corneum, but short enough to not come into contact with nerve endings and hence EPIT is a painless treatment. Nevertheless, SLIT is getting established in most cases of allergy management and the future and the road ahead seems to be for SLIT formulations.

KEYWORDS

- **allergenic extracts**
- **allergy**
- **excipients**
- **Epicutaneous**
- **immunotherapy**
- **Langerhans cells**
- **SCIT**
- **SLIT**
- **sublingual**

REFERENCES

Abramson, M. J., Puy, M. R., Weiner, J. M., Allergen immunotherapy for asthma, Cochrane database Sys rev 2003, CD001186.

Aktar, N., Microneedles an alternative approach to transdermal drug delivery. *Int. J. Pharm. Pharmaceut. Sci.*, 2014, 6, 18–25.

Andre, C., Vatrinet, C., Galvain, S., Carat, F., Sicard, H. Safety of sublingual swallow immunotherapy in children and adults. *Int. Arch. Allergy Immunol.* 2000, 121, 229–234.

Bagnasco, M., Altrinetti, V., Pesce, G. Pharmacokinetics of Der f p 2 allergen and derived monomeric allergoid in allergic volunteers. *Int. Arch. Allergy Immunol.* 2005, 138, 197–202.

Bernardis, P., Agnoletto, M., Puccinelli, P., Parmiani, S., Pozzan, M. Injective versus sublingual immunotherapy in *Alternaria tenuis* allergic patients. *J. Investig. Allergol. Clin. Immunol.* 1996, 6, 55–62.

Berto, P., Frati, F. Economic studies of Immunotherapy a reviews. *Curr. Opinion Allergy Clin. Immunol.* 2008, 8, 585–589.

Bosquet, J., Lockey, R., Malling, H. J. World Health Organization Position paper. Allergen Immunotherapy: therapeutical vaccines for allergic diseases. *Allergy* 1998, 53(suppl. 50), 13–15.

Bosquet, J., Van Cauwenberge, P., Khaltaev, N. ARIA workshop group, World health Organization. Allergic Rhinitis and its impact on asthma. *J. Allergy Clin. Immunol.* 2001, 108(suppl. 5), S147–S334.

Bousquet, J., Lockey, R. F., Malling, H. J. Allergen immunotherapy: therapeutic vaccines for allergic diseases. World Health Organization. American Academy of Allergy, Asthma and Immunology. *Ann. Allergy Asthma Immunol.* 1998, 81, 401–405.

Calderon, M. A., Alves, B., Jacobson, M., Hurwitz, B., Sheikh, A., Dhuram, S., Allergen injection immunotherapy for seasonal allergic rhinitis. Cochrane database of Systematic reviews 2007, issue 1. Art. No: CD 001936. doi: 10.1002/14651858.CD-001936pub2.

Des-Roches, A., Paradis, L., Menardo, J. L., Bouges, S., Daures, J. P., Bousquet, J. Immunotherapy with a standardized *Dermatophagoides pteronysinus* extract. VI. Specific immunotherapy prevents the onset of new sensitization in children. *J. Allergy Clin. Immunol.* 1997, 99, 450–453.

Di Rienzo, V., Pagani, A., Parmiani, S. Post-marketing surveillance study on the safety of sublingual immunotherapy in children. *Allergy* 1999, 54, 1110–1113.

European Medicines Agency, Guidelines on Allergenic Products, Production, Quality Aspects, 20, May 2009.

Fiocchi, A., Assad, A., Bahna, S., Food allergy and the introduction of solid foods to infants and children below 5 years. *Annals of Allergy, Asthma and Immunology* 2006, 97, 10–21.

Gaur, S. N., Singh, B. P., Singh, A., Vijayan, V. K., Agarval, M. K. Guideline for practice of Allergen immuno therapy. *Indian J. Allergy Asthma Immunoblot.* 2009, 23, 1–21.

Giadro, G. B., Marcucci, F., Sensi, L., Incorvaia, C., Frati, F., Ciprandi, G. The safety of sublingual-swallow immunotherapy: an analysis of published studies. *Clin. Exp. Allergy* 2005, 35, 1407–1408.

Jones, M. G., Lympany, P. *Allergy Method and Protocols,* 1st edition, 2008, pp. 133–145.

Jutel, M., Akdis, M., Blaser, K. Mechanisms of allergen specific immunotherapy: T-cell tolerance and more. *Allergy* 2006, 61, 796–807.

Khinchi, M. S., Poulsen, L. K., Carat, F., Andre, C., Malling, H. J. Clinical efficacy of sublingual-swallow and subcutaneous immunotherapy in patients with allergic rhinoconjunctivitis due to birch pollen. A double-blind, double-dummy placebo-controlled study. *Allergy* 2000, 54(suppl. 63), 24.

Kleine-Tebbe, Ribel, M., Herald, D. A., Safety of a SQ standardized grass pollen tablet for sublingual immunotherapy, a randomized placebo-controlled trial. Allergy, European Journal of allergy and immunology , 2006, 61(2), 181–184.

Lockey, R. F., Nicoara-Kasti, G. L., Theodoropoulos, D. S., Bukantz, S. C. Systematic reactions and fatalities associated with allergen immunotherapy. *Ann. Allergy. Asthma Immunol.* 2001, 87(suppl. 1), 47–55.

Macatonia, S. E., Hosken, N. A., Litton, M. Dendritic cells produce IL-12 and direct the development of Th1 cells from naïve CD4+ T cells. *J. Immunol.* 1995, 154, 5071–5079.

Malling, H. J., Weeke, B. Immunotherapy: Position paper. *Allergy* 1993, 48(suppl. 14), 9–35.

Manda, P., Modepalli, N., Juluri, A., Pranjothy, K. L. K., Nagendra Prasad, K. Sublingual Immunotherapy using Allergens from house Dust Mites. AAPS (American Association of Pharmaceutical Scientists), 25th October 2011.

Marcucci. The safety of sublingual-swallow immunotherapy: Clinical and Experimental Allergy 2005, vol. 35, 565–571.

Marogna, M., Spadolini, I., Massolo, A. Clinical, functional and immunologic effects of sublingual immunotherapy in birch pollinosis: 13-year randomizes controlled study. *J. Allergy Clin. Immunol.* 2005, 115, 1184–1188.

Maurizio Marogna, Igino Spladolini, Alessandro Massolo, Giogio Walter Canonica, Giovanni Passsalacua, Long lasting effects of Sublingual Immunotherapy according to it's duration of 15 year prospective studies, Allergy and Clinical immunology, 2010, 126, 969–975.

Moller, C., Dreborg, S., Ferdousi, H. A. Pollen immunotherapy reduces the development of asthma in children with seasonal rhinoconjunctivitis (the PAT study). *J. Allergy Clin. Immunol.* 2002, 109, 251–256.

Mondoulet, L., Dioszeghy, V., Ligouis, M., Dupont, C., Benhamou, P. H. Clinical and Experimental Allergy, 2009, 40, 659–667.

Nagendra Prasad, K. V., Paranjothy, K. L. K., Surendran B. R., Prathima, J., Srivastava, D., Hima Sravanthi, G. Preparation and standardization of STRIPE for SLIT. XXIX EAACI Congress, London June 2010. Abstract No. 65.

Nanjundaiah, Paranjothy Kanni, Nagendra Prasad Komarla, 67th Indian Pharmaceutical Congress, at Mysore India December 2015, Poster presentation on "Formulation and evaluation of (non-compressed) Lyophilized tablets of House dust mite extract for sublingual immune therapy."

Nouri-Aria, K. T., Wachholz, P. A., Francis, J. N. Grass pollen immunotherapy induces mucosal and peripheral IL-10 responses and blocking IgG activity. *J. Immunol.* 2004, 172, 3252–3259.

Ostergaard, P. A., Kaad. P. H., Kristensen, T. A prospective study on the safety of immunotherapy in children with severe asthma. *Allergy* 1986, 41, 588–593.

Pakladnikova, J., Krcmova, I., Vlcek. Economic evaluation of sublingual vs. subcutaneous allergen immunotherapy.*J. Ann. Allergy Asthma Immunol.* 2008, 100, 482–489.

Paranjothy, K., Dhruva, Nagendra, P. Isolation of House Dust Mite and formulation of its purified extract into Sublingual tablets for Immunotherapy, ISMA conference at Vienna Austria, 2013.

Paranjothy, K., Nagendra P. Custom made SLIT Tablets for Allergy Disorders. EAACI-WAO 2013 congress, Milan June 2013. Abstract No. 158.

Paranjothy, K., Nagendra, P. Formulation and Evaluation of custom made Sublingual films of House Dust mite extract for immunotherapy. EAACI 2014 Congress June 2014, Copenhagen.

Passalacqua, G., Albano, M., Riccio, A. Clinical and immunologic effects of a rush sublingual immunotherapy to Parietaria species: A double-blind, placebo-controlled trial. *J. Allergy Clin. Immunol.* 1999, 104, 964–968.

Quirino, T., Lemoli, E., Siciliani, E., Parmiani, S., Milazzo, F. Sublingual versus injection immunotherapy in grass pollen allergic patients. A double blind (double dummy) study. *Clin. Expe Allergy* 1996, 26, 1253–1261.

Scadding and Brostoff. Low dose sublingual low therapy in patients with allergic rhinitis due to house dust mite. *Clinic Allergy*, 1986, 16(5), 483–491.

Stewart, G. E., Lockey, R. F. Systemic reactions from allergen immunotherapy. *J. Allergy Clin. Immunol.* 1992, 90, 567–578.

Tari, M. G., Mancino, M., Monti, G. Efficacy of sublingual immunotherapy in patients with rhinitis and asthma due to house dust mites. A double-blind study, *J. Allergy Clin. Immunol.* 1990, 86, 521–531.

CHAPTER 19

ANTI IGE THERAPY IN ALLERGIC ASTHMA AND ALLERGIC RHINITIS

AGAM VORA

Vora Clinic, Soni Shopping Center,Borivali West, Mumbai-400092

CONTENTS

ABSTRACT

Immunoglobulin E (IgE) has long been regarded as the major trigger of hypersensitivity and acute allergic reactions. Allergic Asthma and rhinitis are chronic inflammatory diseases of the airways and the prevalence of these allergic conditions is steeply rising around the world. Targeting IgE in these conditions has significantly improved the medical management of allergic asthma and rhinitis. Many asthmatic patients with moderate-to-severe persistent asthma continue to experience symptoms, even with currently available varied therapeutic options. Similarly, patients with moderate-to-severe allergic rhinitis who are inadequately controlled with current treatment protocols have a significant unmet medical need. Such patients have a heavy negative impact on daily functioning and are at greater risk of developing serious comorbidities, like asthma and chronic rhinosinusitis. Omalizumab is a humanized monoclonal antibody that binds serum IgE. Anti-IgE therapy using omalizumab reduces circulating free IgE levels and blocks both early and late-phase reactions to allergen challenge. It has been proven to be effective for allergic asthma and is currently being evaluated for use in a number of other atopic conditions, one of the most promising being allergic rhinitis. Omalizumab is relatively well tolerated and has a favorable safety profile.

19.1 INTRODUCTION

Clinical studies with omalizumab have shed new light on the multifaceted roles of IgE in immune homeostasis and in allergic disease. In recent times, a significant rise in the prevalence of two common allergic conditions, asthma and allergic rhinitis is seen. According to recent estimations 300 million people worldwide suffer from asthma and by the end of next decade the figure is estimated to reach 400 million. According to the Centers for Disease Control (CDC), 1 in 14 people have asthma (World Health Organization, 2007). Roughly 20% to 50% of the population is found to suffer from allergic rhinitis (AR) (Bousquet et al., 1991). Symptomatic allergic rhinitis has a strong negative impact on productivity and performance of an individual. New-generation oral H1 antihistamines and intranasal glucocorticosteroids are the first-line treatment for AR. However, there is a significant proportion of patients with AR who do not respond to standard therapy and pose a significant challenge in patient management.

Asthma poses a significant healthcare burden in India. Although there is a paucity of accurate epidemiological data to estimate prevalence of asthma or the allergic asthma, a multicenter study conducted in India to understand prevalence of bronchial asthma in adults by the Asthma Epidemiology Study Group of the Indian Council of Medical Research (ICMR) found the prevalence to be 2.38% (Aggarwal et al., 2006). In India up to 26% people suffer from allergic rhinitis and alarmingly 80% of asthmatic adults and 75% of asthmatic children suffer from symptoms of rhinitis (Pitts et al., 2008). Considering Indian population of 1 billion plus, the burden of rhinitis and asthma in the country is substantial. Unfortunately, in India both diseases still remain under-recognized, under-estimated and under-treated.

Currently, bronchodilators and anti-inflammatory agents, concurrent with other drugs such as anti-leucotrienes, are used in management of majority of asthma patients, but these therapies do not provide symptomatic relief to all the patients. Hence significant proportion of asthmatic patients fall under the category of difficult-to-treat patient population (Pitts et al., 2008). Although difficult-to-treat patient population is less than 20% of the asthma patients, utilization of healthcare resources is significantly higher, as these patients require frequent emergency department visits and seek care in other urgent care facilities. The Global Asthma Physician and Patient Survey concluded that asthma management has substantial unmet medical need. Severe persistent asthma patients who are poorly controlled in spite of treatment according to Global Initiative for Asthma (GINA) guidelines step IV, represent a challenging population with significant unmet medical need (CDC, 2005). Some of the reasons quoted for this non-maintenance of therapeutic effects are; patient non-adherence, lack of response to pharmacotherapy, poor inhalation, presence of co-morbid diseases, triggers such as respiratory infections, indoor and outdoor allergens. These patients who experience frequent exacerbations requiring emergency department visits or hospitalizations, will derive significant benefit from novel anti immunoglobulin-E (IgE) antibodies which are specifically designed to target airway inflammatory mechanism (Storms, 2003).

19.2 ROLE OF IGE

Human immunoglobulin E (IgE) plays a pivotal role in the inflammatory response to allergens in atopic patients and plays a critical role in the pathogenesis of atopic-allergic conditions like rhinitis and bronchial asthma (Spector, 1999). IgE antibodies function through activation of several receptors. The two primary receptors are the "high-affinity receptor," FcεRI, and the "low-affinity receptor," CD23. IgE plays an important role in the regulation and expression of both high and low affinity receptors.

Levels of IgE are highly correlated with the development of asthma and bronchial hyper-responsiveness. Higher serum level of allergen-specific IgE is the characteristic of allergic diseases, such as rhinitis and asthma. In such conditions IgE is directed towards environmental or aeroallergens. On the other hand, IgE against foods are associated with food allergy and eosinophilic disorders of the gastrointestinal tract (Erwin, 2011).

The primary role is played by IgE in type I hypersensitivity reactions, where it binds to high-affinity IgE receptors (FcεRI) on mast cells and basophils. Binding to the receptor occurs via the Cε3 domain on the Fc fragment. Direct relationship of levels of FcεRI expression and serum levels of IgE exists. Any reduction in serum levels of IgE can result in significant decreases in expression of FcεRI receptors (Malveaux et al., 1978). In addition to mast cells and basophils, high-affinity FcεRI are also expressed on dendritic cells (DCs), especially type II DCs that promote Th2 responses.

Attachment of IgE to the FcεRI on DCs is associated with increased allergen uptake and initiation of allergic response. Moreover, IgE also binds low-affinity receptors (FcεRII, CD23) on DC and other antigen presenting cells. Attachment of IgE to this receptors result in attenuation of the immune response. Considering the central role of IgE in the pathogenesis of allergic diseases including asthma and allergic rhinitis, IgE-mediated immunologic pathways have become lucrative target for therapeutic agents. The anti-IgE antibody inhibits IgE functions via blocking free serum IgE and inhibiting their binding to cellular receptors. As serum IgE level drops, IgE receptor expression on inflammatory cells in the context of allergic cascade also drops (D'Amato et al., 2010). It represents a very interesting therapeutic option for asthmatic patients.

Multiple studies concluded that IgE-mediated positive reactions to skin prick tests for common aeroallergens are detectable in severe asthmatics, ranging from about 50%–80% (ENFUMOSA, 2003). This lead to inclusion of anti-IgE therapy in 2006 within step 5 of the Global Initiative for Asthma guidelines (GOLD) as add-on therapy to inhaled and eventually oral corticosteroids, long-acting β2-agonists (LABA), and other controller medications, such as leukotriene-modifiers and theophylline. GINA guidelines of 2014 recommends use of anti-IgE therapy before oral corticosteroids within step 5 (GINA, 2014).

19.3 OMALIZUMAB

Omalizumab is a recombinant anti-IgE monoclonal antibody developed for the treatment of allergic diseases associated with high circulating IgE levels. Currently omalizumab is the only IgE-targeted therapy approved by EMEA (European Agency for the Evaluation of Medicinal Products) and FDA (Food and Drug Administration) for allergic asthma. It is indicated in the treatment of moderate-to-severe and severe persistent allergic asthma poorly controlled with regular treatment (D'Amato et al., 2010; Pelaia et al., 2011).

Upon allergen cross-linking of mast cell-bound IgE, spontaneous release of a granule-associated substance, such as histamine is released. Within short time, de novo synthesis of key lipid mediators such as cysteinyl/leukotrienes is initiated from membrane phospholipids. Subsequently within few hours, the activated mast cells are also capable of the synthesis and release of a large number of cytokines, such as interleukin (IL)-4, IL-6, IL-9, IL-13, and tumor necrosis factor (TNF)-alpha. This sequential and programmed cascade of events results in the initiation of early and late-phase allergic reactions (D'Amato et al., 2010; Erwin, 2011; Pelaia et al., 2011). Omalizumab blocks initiation of inflammatory process by reducing serum IgE levels, as well as FcεRI and FcεRII receptor expression on inflammatory cells. Omalizumab attaches to the binding site of IgE (Cε3 domain) for the high-affinity receptor, and results in prevention of free-serum IgE from attaching to mast cells and other IgE receptor-expressing cells, thereby preventing IgE-mediated immune responses.

19.4 CLINICAL EXPERIENCE

Omalizumab attaches with free circulating IgE regardless of antigen specificity, which indicates that reducing free IgE may limit more chronic aspects of allergic inflammation involving T-cell antigen presentation and further activation. Thus, omalizumab is potential therapeutic agent for atopic disorders caused by either perennial or seasonal allergens, as well as by multiple other sensitizations (Erwin, 2011).

Multiple controlled clinical trials have proven therapeutic advantage of omalizumab. Efficacy results of omalizumab as anti-asthmatic therapeutic agent were demonstrated by the investigator in late 1990s. Investigator demonstrated that intravenous administration of the agent (initially called anti-IgE antibody E25) inhibited early and late-phase allergic asthmatic responses which were induced by allergens (Fahy et al., 1997). In subsequent pivotal clinical trials confirming efficacy of omalizumab, omalizumab has been administered subcutaneously. Subcutaneous administration of omalizumab to patients diagnosed with moderate-to-severe asthma at intervals of 2 or 4 weeks significantly reduces the incidence and frequency of asthma exacerbations. Additionally, it also lead to steroid-sparing effect as indicated by reduced use of inhaled corticosteroid (ICS). Immediately after the first Omalizumab injection, level of free serum IgE drops down. It is clinically evident that after a standard course of therapy, both early- and late-phase asthmatic reactions to inhaled allergens gets alleviated (Fahy et al., 1997). Additionally, these studies have also established a relation between reduction in circulating and sputum eosinophilia and nonspecific bronchial hyper responsiveness.

A number of clinical trials have concluded superior efficacy and safety of omalizumab in adolescents and adults with moderate-to-severe asthma (Pelaia et al., 2011). Omalizumab has been administered as add-on to treatment with ICS and other anti-asthma drugs. Omalizumab reduced asthma exacerbations and corticosteroid requirement compared with placebo in patients with moderate-severe allergic asthma, further reducing emergency room visits and hospitalizations (D'Amato et al., 2010). The patients which benefited the most with omalizumab treatment are the patients on highest ICS doses and having poorest lung function.

The pivotal trial INNOVATE (Investigation of Omalizumab in severe Asthma Treatment), showed substantial advantage of omalizumab in patients given high-dose ICS combined with LABA and other controller medications. Omalizumab reduced the rate of clinically significant asthma exacerbations as compared to the control group (0.68 versus 0.91, p = 0.042). There were also improvements in FEV1 percent predicted values (p = 0.043), and total asthma symptom scores (p = 0.039). Rate of severe exacerbations [defined as a peak expiratory flow or FEV1 < 60% of personal best] was halved (0.24 versus 0.48, p = 0.002), and the rate of emergency room visits was reduced (0.24 versus 0.43, $p = 0.038$). The safety profile was similar throughout the study arms. Bousquet and colleagues further confirmed the advantages of omalizumab which were seen in INNOVATE trial (Humbert et al., 2005).

A double-blind, randomized, placebo-controlled trial studied patients with severe IgE-mediated asthma who required fluticasone 1000 µg/day or more to control symptoms. Of those roughly half of the patients were concomitantly taking LABA. Patients were randomized to take either omalizumab or placebo. The dose of fluticasone was maintained for 16 weeks and then tapered for 16 weeks. Doses of fluticasone were reduced more in patients who received omalizumab compared to those who received placebo (reductions of 57.2% versus 43.3%, $p = 0.003$). In patients treated with omalizumab, the doses of fluticasone were reduced by at least 50% compared to placebo-treated patients (74% versus 51%, $p = 0.001$). Patients who were taking LABA and omalizumab were able to maintain or achieve improvement in asthma. Moreover, these patients needed fewer rescue drugs despite the substantial reductions in fluticasone doses (Holgate et al., 2004).

In a meta-analysis of eight trials covering 2037 mild-to-severe allergic asthmatics, omalizumab therapy lead to either reduction or withdrawal of ICS use by over 50% (OR 2.50, 95% CI 2.02 to 3.10) Omalizumab lead to complete withdrawal of their daily steroid intake: (OR 2.50, 95% CI 2.00 to 3.13) (four trials) and was also effective in reducing asthma exacerbations as an adjunctive therapy to ICS (OR 0.49, 95%CI 0.38 to 0.64, four trials) Omalizumab was also proved to be an effective agent which will help taper the steroid dose (OR 0.47, 95% CI 0.37 to 0.60, four trials) (Walker et al., 2006). Reductions of steroid use and of asthma exacerbations were the primary outcomes in this systematic review while secondary outcome measures included lung function, use of rescue medication, asthma symptoms, and health-related quality of life.

A study conducted by Busse et al. (2011) had 419 children, adolescents, and young adults as patient population with persistent allergic, moderate-to-severe asthma, showed that treatment of omalizumab for 60 weeks significantly improved asthma control, nearly eliminated seasonal spikes in asthmatic exacerbations, and also decreased the need for inhaled corticosteroids. Recently, multiple Phase IV studies confirmed the efficacy of omalizumab in patients affected by severe persistent allergic asthma treated with omalizumab for 5–12 months.

The SOLAR (Study of Omalizumab in co-morbid Asthma and Rhinitis) study designed to evaluate efficacy of omalizumab in coexisting with moderate-to-severe asthma and moderate-to-severe persistent rhinitis in adolescents and adults. As evaluated by the Asthma Quality-of-Life Questionnaire and Rhinitis Quality-of-Life Questionnaire, omalizumab resulted in significant improvements in quality of life related to both asthma and rhinitis. The study interestingly showed reciprocal pathophysiologic correlation in allergic asthma and rhinitis. The large Phase III trials of omalizumab in allergic rhinitis have demonstrated its efficacy in ameliorating symptoms and improving quality of life for patients with intermittent and persistent allergic disease (Adelroth et al., 2000; Casale et al., 2001; Chervinsky et al, 2003). In patients with rhinitis, initial responses (e.g., ragweed-induced nasal volume) were seen on day 7 and peaked on day 42.

The PERSIST trial evaluated effectiveness of add on therapy with Omalizumab in real-life scenarios in a heterogeneous population of 158 patients. Evaluations were performed at week 16 and week 52. The study results have showed better physician-rated effectiveness (measured through GETE), greater improvements in quality of life, higher reductions in rates of severe exacerbations, and greater reductions in healthcare utilization than reported in any efficacy studies conducted until 2009, involving omalizumab in the treatment of severe persistent allergic asthma. At 52 weeks, >72% had a good/excellent GETE rating ($p < 0.001$), >84% had improvements in total AQLQ score of _0.5 points ($p < 0.001$), >56% had minimally important improvements in EQ-5D utility scores (PZ0.012), and >65% were severe exacerbation-free ($p < 0.001$) (Brusselle et al., 2009).

EASE study was a 52 week, post-marketing study in which 146 Indian patients were selected to assess the efficacy and safety of omalizumab. Interim analysis of the results of EASE study at week 16, were presented at different conferences. The results show that there was statistically significant reduction ($p = 0.046$) in the number of patients experiencing one or more asthma exacerbations. FEV1 levels improved significantly and there was a significant reduction in ICS dose. Significant improvement was seen in composite and mean ACQ scores. The number of days missed at college/work, number of patients requiring hospitalization, also reduced significantly ($p = 0.039$ and $p = 0.021$, respectively) (EASE, 2012).

In eXpeRience, a 2-year registry, which completed in 2013, Omalizumab was evaluated in 943 patients for its real-world effectiveness, use and safety. The results confirmed significant improvements in patient outcomes. The proportion of patients with clinically insignificant exacerbations increased from 6.8% during the 12-month pre-treatment period to 54.1% and 67.3% at Months 12 and 24, respectively. Symptoms and rescue medication use at Month 24 were reduced by >50% from baseline. Maintenance OCS use was lower at Month 24 (14.2%) compared with Month 12 (16.1%) and baseline (28.6%). Overall, Omalizumab demonstrated an acceptable safety profile (Braunstahl et al., 2013).

Center for Health Outcomes and Pharmaco-Economic Research, University of Arizona reviewed 24 'real-life' studies of omalizumab in the management of severe allergic asthma. The review included unique 4117 patients from 32 countries with significant heterogeneity in patient characteristics, physicians and healthcare settings. Benefits of omalizumab therapy may extend up to 2–4 years, and the majority of patients treated on omalizumab will continue benefiting for multiple years. Omalizumab has positive short- and long-term safety profiles which was very similar to already established in various randomized clinical trials. Significant improvement in lung function was evident in this review. In the first 16 weeks of treatment, FEV1 improved by up to 22%. Improvement rates over 1 year improved up to 25%, and an improvement over 4 years was up to 19%. At first 16 weeks of treatment, severe exacerbations declined by 82%. At 6 months, reductions in exacerbations were up to 84%, while at 1-year reduction rates were up to 80%. Reductions in severe exacerbations are likely to be sustained at 2 years by 73.2% and 4 years by 70%. Significant dose reductions in OCSs in association with omalizumab treatment were noted as well. In patients treated for more than 16 weeks, the mean dose reduction was 30%. Estimates of OCS dose reductions at 1 year were up to 50%, with a decline of 66% at 2 years. At first 16 weeks of treatment, one study reported a decline of 83% in hospitalizations. Beyond the initial 16 weeks, reductions in hospitalization rates were up to 96% at 1 year. Annual visits to the emergency department decreased by up to 53% in the first year and by 80% in the first 3 years of omalizumab therapy (Abraham et al., 2007).

19.5 SAFETY

Omalizumab is found to be well-tolerated with comparable incidence of adverse events with placebo. A recent and detailed analysis of the safety of omalizumab included 12 controlled, phase IIb–III clinical trials and more than 5243 patients. The most commonly reported adverse events with omalizumab therapy were reactions at injection site (45%), viral infections (23%), upper respiratory tract infections (20%), sinusitis (16%), headache (15%), and pharyngitis (11%). Injection site reactions of any severity occurred in 45% of omalizumab recipients and 43% of placebo recipients. Most of these injection site reactions occurred within 1 hour of injection, resolved within 8 days. The frequency of these injection site reactions decreased with subsequent dosing. This side effect profile has been confirmed by real-world studies, which made it feasible to perform long-term follow up to 3 years (Pelaia et al., 2011). Rarely events such as urticaria, dermatitis, and pruritus may occur with omalizumab. Multiple clinical trials and post marketing studies reported the frequency of anaphylactic reactions with omalizumab to be very low, ~0.1% and ~0.2%, respectively. Baring few incidences, majority of these reactions occur within 2 hours of the first and subsequent subcutaneous injections. Till date, no cases of anti-omalizumab monoclonal antibodies have been detected. Additionally, there is no evidence of any complications associated with the reduced levels of circulating IgE or antibodies against omalizumab (Deniz and Gupta, 2005).

The socioeconomic and health care burden imposed by asthma is substantial and is considerably skewed towards patients with severe asthma, especially when inadequately controlled. As discussed above omalizumab has proven to be effective as add-on therapy in patients with poorly controlled, moderate-to-severe allergic asthma and allergic rhinitis, considerably reducing asthma exacerbations and corticosteroid requirements.

Severe asthma, especially when poorly controlled, impose heavy burden on healthcare resources. As omalizumab is effective as an add-on therapy in patients with poorly controlled, moderate-to-severe allergic asthma and allergic rhinitis, it is poised to reduce the asthma exacerbations and corticosteroid requirement. Reduction in the exacerbation is likely to substantially reduce the mortality and morbidity of the asthmatic patients, thereby reducing the healthcare expenditure. Published cost-effectiveness analyses affirms the notion that omalizumab is cost-effective in patients with uncontrolled severe allergic (IgE-mediated) asthma despite other controller medications with a history of severe exacerbations and hospitalization. Even though incremental cost effect of omalizumab treatment was seen, cost could be justified by health benefits and overall improvement in quality of life achieved (Abraham et al., 2007; Sullivan and Turk, 2008).

There is real-world evidence as well, to suggest that treatment with Omalizumab has a significant influence on the direct and indirect costs in management of severe allergic asthma. It has been observed that, there are improvements in asthma control (ACT and ACQ) and asthma-related quality of life (AQLQ and mini-AQLQ), as well as reductions in OCS use along with noticeable reductions in numbers of days of missed work or school due to asthma (Braunstahl et al., 2013).

19.6 PATIENT'S SELECTION FOR OMALIZUMAB THERAPY

Omalizumab has been indicated as add-on therapy in patients aged 6 years or more with severe persistent allergic asthma and following characteristics (Holgate et al., 2009):

- multiple documented severe asthma exacerbations;
- symptomatic despite high dose ICS and LABA therapy;
- frequent daytime symptoms or night-time awakenings;
- reduced lung function (FEV1 < 80%);
- a positive skin test or in vitro reactivity (radio allergosorbent test [RAST]) to a perennial aeroallergen.

Omalizumab dose and dose frequency in India is based on baseline serum total IgE level (30–1500 IU/mL) and body weight (20–200 kg). As per the EU guidelines, it is mandated that omalizumab treatment should only be initiated in patients with confirmed IgE-mediated asthma. Physicians should therefore ensure that patients with IgE below 76 IU/mL have an unequivocal RAST to a perennial allergen before starting therapy.

19.7 CONCLUSION (PLACE IN THERAPY)

First of its kind, omalizumab is first anti-IgE antibody approved in more than 27 countries. The development of a humanized, selective anti-IgE monoclonal antibody is a paradigm changing clinical advance in blocking the allergic cascade, not only in allergic asthma but also in allergic rhinitis.

Omalzumab can be expected to fill the huge unmet medical need in the management of severe-persistent, allergic (IgE mediated) asthma patients; who remain symptomatic despite treatment with high dose ICS and LABA. Benefits of omalizumab have been confirmed by improvements in important clinical parameters as exacerbation rates, emergency visit rates, symptom scores, and quality of life scores. Anti-IgE therapy (omalizumab) is now included in GINA guidelines (Step 5), as add-on therapy with ICS and LABA plus other controller medications. With the availability of omalizumab as an effective therapeutic option to physicians, management of difficult to treat population has become easy. Multiple clinical trials have demonstrated the efficacy of omalizumab in reducing allergic airway inflammation and its clinical manifestations. Omalizumab has shown to have overall good safety profile and is generally well tolerated. Only rare event of anaphylaxis have been reported and no events of development of serum-sickness, serum-sickness like syndrome or thrombocytopenia are seen.

Omalizumab as therapeutic option in asthma care can be cost-effective if appropriate and thoughtful patient selection based on patient selection algorithm, described earlier in this article, is considered. It is recommended to evaluate treatment response to omalizumab after 16 weeks of therapy. Treatment should only be continued in responders. Overall, omalizumab offers a significant advancement in treatment of difficult-to-treat population and may fulfill an important need in patients with moderate-to-severe allergic asthma.

KEYWORDS

- **anti-IgE**
- **asthma**
- **immunoglobulin-E**
- **omalizumab**
- **rhinitis**

REFERENCES

Abraham, I., Alhossan, A., Lee, C. S., Kutbi, H., MacDonald, K., *Allergy*. 2016 May, 71(5), 593–610.

Adelroth, E., Rak, S., Haahtela, T., et al. Recombinant humanized mAb-E25, an anti-IgE mAb, in birch pollen induced seasonal allergic rhinitis. *J Allergy Clin Immunol.* 2000, 106, 253–259.

Aggarwal, A. N., Chaudhary, K., Chhabra, S. K., et al. Prevalence and risk factors for bronchial asthma in Indian adults: a multicenter study. *Indian J Chest Dis Allied Sci* 2006, 48, 13–22.

Bousquet, J., Heijaoui, A., Becker, W. M., Cour, P., Chanal, I., Lebel, B., et al. Clinical and immunologic reactivity of patients allergic to grass pollens and to multiple pollen species. Clinical and immunological characteristics. *J Allergy Clin Immunol* 1991, 87, 737–746.

Braunstahl, G. J. et al. The eXpeRience registry: The 'real-world' effectiveness of omalizumab in allergic asthma. *Respiratory Medicine* 2013, 107, 1141–1151.

Brown, R., Turk, F., Dale, P., Bousquet, J., Cost-effectiveness of omalizumab in patients with severe persistent allergic asthma. Allergy. 2007, 62(2), 149–153.

Brusselle, G., et al. "Real-life" effectiveness of omalizumab in patients with severe persistent allergic asthma: The PERSIST study. *Respiratory Medicine* 2009, 103, 1633–1642.

Busse, W. W., Morgan, W. J., Gergen, P. J., et al. Randomized trial of omalizumab (anti-IgE) for asthma in inner-city children. *N Engl J Med.* 2011, 364(11), 1005–1015.

Casale, T. B., Condemi, J., LaForce, C., et al. Effect of omalizumab on symptoms of seasonal allergic rhinitis. *JAMA*. 2001, 286, 2956–2967.

CDC. National Surveillance of Asthma: United States, 2001–2010. http://www.cdc.gov/nchs/data/series/sr_03/sr03_035.pdf. (Retrieved November 16 2015).

Chervinsky, P., Casale, T., Townley, R., et al. Omalizumab, an anti-IgE antibody, in the treatment of adults and adolescents with perennial allergic rhinitis. *Ann Allergy Asthma Immunol.* 2003, 91, 160–167.

D'Amato, G., Perticone, M., Bucchioni, E., Salzillo, A., D'Amato, M., Liccardi, G., Treating moderate-to-severe allergic asthma with anti-IgE monoclonal antibody (omalizumab): an update. *Eur Ann Allergy Clin Immunol.* 2010, 42(4), 135–140.

Deniz, Y. M., Gupta, N., Safety and tolerability of omalizumab (Xolair®), a recombinant humanized monoclonal anti-IgE antibody. *Clin Rev Allergy Immunol* 2005, 29(1), 31–48.

EASE Interim analysis poster presented at ERS 2012.

ENFUMOSA (European Network For Understanding Mechanisms Of Severe Asthma) Study Group. The ENFUMOSA cross-sectional European multicentre study of the clinical phenotype of chronic severe asthma. *Eur Respir, J.,* 2003, 22(3), 470–477.

Erwin, W. G., Anti-IgE Therapy in Asthma. Available from URL: http://www.medscape.org/viewarticle/530088, Accessed 19th September 2011.

Fahy, J. V., Fleming, H. E., Wong, H. H., et al. The effect of an anti-IgE monoclonal antibody on the early- and late-phase responses to allergen inhalation in asthmatic subjects. *Am J Respir Crit Care Med.* 1997, 155, 1828–1834.

Global Initiative for Asthma (GINA). Global strategy for asthma management and prevention 2014 (revision). Available at: www.ginasthma.org.

Holgate, S. T., Chuchalin, A. G., Hebert, J., et al. Efficacy and safety of a recombinant anti-immunoglobulin E antibody (omalizumab) in severe allergic asthma. *Clin Exp Allergy* 2004, 34(4), 632–638.

Holgate, S., Buhl, R., Bousquet, J., Smith, N., Panahloo, Z., Jimenez, P., The use of omalizumab in the treatment of severe allergic asthma: A clinical experience update. *Respir Med.* 2009 Aug, 103(8), 1098–1113.

Humbert, M., Beasley, R., Ayers, J., et al. Benefits of omalizumab as add-on therapy in patients with severe persistent asthma who are inadequately controlled despite best available therapy (GINA 2002 step 4 treatment), INNOVATE. *Allergy* 2005, 60, 309–316.

Malveaux, F. J., Conroy, M. C., Adkinson, N. F. Jr, Lichtensterin, L. M., IgE receptors on human basophils. Relationship to serum IgE concentration. *J Clin Invest.* 1978, 62, 176–181.

Pelaia, G., Gallelli, L., Renda, T., Romeo, P., Busceti, M. T., Grembiale, R. D., et al. Update on optimal use of omalizumab in management of asthma. *J Asthma Allergy*. 2011, 4, 49–59.

Pitts, S. R., Niska, R. W., Xu, J., Burt, C. W., National Hospital Ambulatory Medical Care Survey: 2006 emergency department summary. National Health Statistics Reports; No 7. Hyattsville, MD: National Center for Health Statistics. 2008.

Prescribing Information: Xolair® (Omalizumab powder and solvent for solution for injection), Novartis Healthcare Private Limited, India. Dated 22 Jan 14 based on IPL dated 16 Jul 13 Corr. 11 Dec 2013.

Spector, S. L., Allergic inflammation in upper and lower airways. *Ann Allergy Asthma Immunol* 1999, 83, 435–444.

Storms, W. W., Unmet needs in the treatment of allergic asthma: potential role of novel biologic therapies. *J Manag Care Pharm*. 2003 Nov–Dec, 9(6), 534–543.

Sullivan, S. D., Turk, F., An evaluation of the cost-effectiveness of omalizumab for the treatment of severe allergic asthma. *Allergy*. 2008 Jun, 63(6), 670–684.

Walker, S., Monteil, M., Phelan, K., Lasserson, T. J., Walter, E. H., Anti-IgE for chronic asthma in adults and children. *Cochrane Database Syst Rev* 2006, 2, CD003559.

World Health Organization. Global Surveillance, Prevention and Control of Chronic Respiratory Diseases: A Comprehensive Approach, 2007.

INDEX

H

I

P

T

U